Human Nutrition

Human Nutrition

Current Issues
and Controversies

EDITED BY

A. Neuberger

Lister Institute of Preventive
Medicine and Charing Cross
Hospital Medical School, London

T. H. Jukes

Department of Biophysics
and Medical Physics
Department of
Nutritional Sciences
University of California,
Berkeley

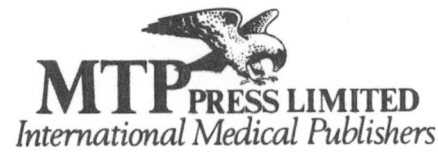

MTP PRESS LIMITED
International Medical Publishers

Published in UK by
MTP Press Limited
Falcon House
Lancaster, England

British Library Cataloguing in Publication Data

Human nutrition: current issues and controversies.
  1. Nutrition
  I. Neuberger, Albert II. Jukes, T. H.
  613.2   TX353

ISBN-13: 978-94-011-6260-9   e-ISBN-13: 978-94-011-6258-6
DOI: 10.1007/978-94-011-6258-6

Contents

List of Contributors

S BLAZA
Animal Studies Centre
Pedigree Petfoods
Freeby Lane, Walton-on-the-Wold
Melton Mobray
Leicestershire LE14 4RT
England

H F DELUCA
Department of Biochemistry
University of Wisconsin—Madison
420 Henry Mall
Madison, WI 53706, USA

G S GARROW
Clinical Research Centre
Division of Clinical Investigation
Watford Road
Harrow, Middlesex HA1 3UJ,
England

L GREEN
Department of Nutrition and Food
  Science
Massachusetts Institute of
  Technology
77 Massachusetts Avenue
Cambridge, MA 02139, USA

N JENKINS
Department of Oral Physiology
The Dental School
University of Newcastle-upon-Tyne
Newcastle-upon-Tyne NE1 8ST,
  England

T H JUKES
University of California
Berkeley
RSSF, 1414 Harbour Way So.
Richmond, CA 94804, USA

A NEUBERGER
The Lister Institute of Preventive
  Medicine
Charing Cross Hospital Medical
  School
The Reynolds' Building
St Dunstan's Road
London W6 8P, England

G M OWEN
Bristol-Myers Company, International
  Division
345 Park Avenue
New York, NY 10154, USA

A L OWEN
Owen Associates Inc.
251 Hilton Road
Westport, CT 06880, USA

D RALT
Department of Nutrition and Food
  Science
Massachusetts Institute of
  Technology
77 Massachusetts Avenue
Cambridge, MA 02139, USA

S R TANNENBAUM
Department of Nutrition and Food
  Science
Massachusetts Institute of
  Technology
77 Massachusetts Avenue
Cambridge, MA 02139, USA

S G SRIKANTIA
Postgraduate Department of Food
  and Nutrition
University of Mysore
Manasagangotri
Mysore 570012, India

J H YOUNG
Department of History
Emory University
Atlanta, GA 30322, USA

Preface

This new volume deals with a number of important and current topics in human nutrition that we hope will be of general interest to those concerned with this subject. We have first of all a chapter by J. S. Garrow and S. Blaza on energy requirements, which has a direct bearing on the problem of obesity, and which largely affects the populations of developed and affluent countries. This is followed by a chapter on fluoride and the fluoridation of water, under the authorship of G. N. Jenkins. The addition of fluoride to drinking water has given rise to a great deal of discussion both amongst scientists and the public at large, and the present account tries to give the scientific background and a critical evaluation of established facts. The chapter by G. Owen on the nutritional status of North Americans is also likely to be of interest to other countries, as the techniques used and the problems encountered are similar to those encountered in other parts of the world. A chapter on nitrates, nitrites and nitrosamines by S. R. Tannenbaum discusses a topic which again has engendered widespread interest amongst a large number of people, and where a balanced presentation of the relevant facts is particularly important. One of the fields in which biochemistry, physiology and nutrition have made enormous advances over the last few years is that of vitamin D and the new knowledge acquired on control of the metabolism of calcium and phosphorus. This information is critically discussed by H. DeLuca.

The developing world, which comprises the majority of mankind, has always had its special nutritional problems, and these vary from country to country. The problems chosen by S. G. Srikantia appear to be of special importance, and these are vitamin A deficiency, protein energy malnutrition, and pellagra. Whilst more knowledge is still required on many of these topics, the chief difficulty is in applying existing knowledge to the complex social, economic and political realities of the various countries concerned. We have a chapter by J. Harvey Young who deals with nutritional eccentricities, also choosing entirely American examples. This account emphasizes the different problems facing scientists and others who are concerned with putting sound nutritional advice to the population at large. These difficulties emphasize the fact that human beings are not entirely rational and irrational considerations play a large part in attitudes adopted by individuals and groups to many problems, but particularly with respect to the diet people wish (or are persuaded) to consume. In the last contribution one of us (T. H. Jukes) discusses the widespread use of laetrile, a substance which has received much publicity, especially in the USA. Several important topics in nutrition have not been covered, but we have tried to deal with the fields which are of particular importance at the present time.

Thomas H. Jukes
Albert Neuberger

1
Energy requirements in human beings

J. GARROW AND S. BLAZA

INTRODUCTION

A dietary source of energy must occupy a central place in any nutrition
scheme, since energy requirements must be met even at the expense of protein
requirements. However, dietary energy requirements are difficult to define in
any species, and particularly so in human beings. The nutritional objective of
livestock farmers is clear: they have to raise their animals as profitably as
possible. For a given strain of pig, for example, a certain ration can be shown to
be optimum to yield the most meat at least cost, but such criteria do not apply
in human nutrition. The human nutritionist cannot play safe and recommend
a minimum of energy in the diet. It is possible to define 'enough' vitamin C, and if
the requirement is exceeded not much harm is done, but the same latitude does
not apply to energy intake. Grossly excessive and grossly deficient energy
intakes are both damaging to health.

At least in the short term, there is no need for energy intake to match
expenditure, since a temporary excess or deficit can be met by adjustment of
the energy stores of the body, chiefly in the form of fat. In the long term, of
course, intake must match output, but alterations in the energy stores of the
body are themselves associated with alterations in metabolic rate, and hence in
energy requirements. Therefore, to discuss energy requirements it is necessary
to consider in turn energy expenditure, energy stores, and then the adaptive
responses which tend to stabilize energy balance.

Energy units

Until the change to SI (Système Internationale) units, human energy intake
and expenditure was usually expressed as kilogramme calories (kcal). The SI
unit is the joule (J), and the conversion:

$$1 \, kcal = 4.18 \, kJ$$

Since direct calorimeters are usually calibrated with respect to electrical
standards, the rate of heat output by direct calorimetry is expressed as watts:

$$1 \, watt = 1 \, J/s, \quad so \quad 1 \, kcal/min = 70 \, watts.$$

1

When energy expenditure is measured by indirect calorimetry, the heat equivalent of the respiratory exchange can be calculated using the Weir formula[1]. However, a fundamental limitation of the accuracy of indirect calorimetry is that the mixture of expired gases does not necessarily reflect the metabolic mixture being produced in the tissues. CO_2 may be stored in the tissues, so the apparent RQ may not equal the metabolic RQ. For this reason it is prudent to report the results obtained in indirect calorimetry in terms of oxygen uptake, rather than converting to heat production using an assumed value for the heat equivalent of oxygen which may not be correct. However, to provide the reader with an easy conversion of oxygen uptake to energy expenditure the following equation will suffice:

$$\text{Oxygen uptake (ml/min)} \times 7 = \text{kcal/day}.$$

ENERGY EXPENDITURE

Techniques for measurement of energy expenditure

(a) Direct calorimetry

The classical studies on human energy expenditure were performed by Atwater and Benedict[2] with a direct calorimeter. This was a copper box 2.15 m long, 1.22 m wide, and 1.93 m high. The subject entered through an aperture 49 cm wide and 79 cm high; the aperture was then sealed with a sheet of plate glass embedded in molten beeswax. Great care was taken to ensure that there was no heat gradient across the walls of the calorimeter, and the heat produced but the imprisoned subject was exactly removed by careful regulation of the flow of cold water through pipes inside the chamber. In the ensuing 70 years there have been considerable advances[3,4,5] making calorimetry less arduous for both the subject and the investigators, but the accuracy of the original apparatus has not been surpassed. The great advantage of direct calorimetry is its accuracy and ease of calibration. An electrical heat source, or a lamp burning ethyl alcohol or butane, can be used as a reference standard, and the observed heat production should agree with the theoretical value within 1 %[6]. The disadvantages of direct calorimetry are that it is expensive, laborious and slow. The design of a relatively simple direct calorimeter[7], which was constructed by the Division of Bioengineering at the Clinical Research Centre in 1976, is shown in Figure 1.

The calorimeter chamber (2 m wide by 1.7 m deep by 2 m high) is constructed of slabs of expanded polystyrene (P) 20 cm thick, faced on the inner and outer surfaces with sheet aluminium. Access to the chamber is by a door in which there is a pass-through hatch (H), with clear plastic panels hinged in the inner and outer faces; this also provides a window. The chamber is furnished with a bed, chair, table, small television set and radio–tape recorder. The great majority of patients admitted to our metabolic unit are quite willing to spend a period of 26 hours in this chamber on several occasions.

The air inside the chamber (volume approximately 6 m^3) is circulated by an axial fan (F) along a duct into a plenum chamber 10 cm deep covering the

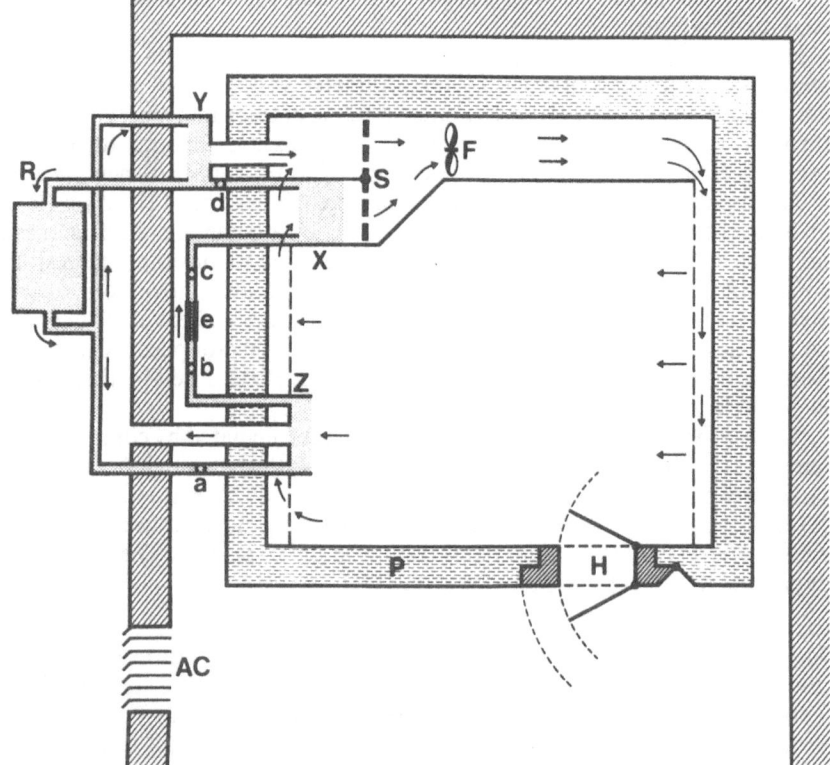

Figure 1 Diagram of the direct calorimeter at the Clinical Research Centre, Harrow. For description see text

whole area of the right-hand wall of the chamber. The inner wall of this chamber is made from perforated hardboard, so the air escapes into the chamber and flows in a laminar fashion from right to left across the chamber and enters a similar plenum chamber on the left-hand wall. From here it is sucked down to the duct, where part of the stream of air passes through a heat exchanger (X), and part bypasses the heat exchanger. The proportion of the circulating air which is cooled in the heat exchanger is determined by the position of the shutter (S), which is driven by a servo motor which is sensitive to the temperature gradient across the walls of the chamber. Thus, if the thermistors mounted on the inner and outer aluminium skins of the chamber detect a new outward flow of heat across the walls, the servo motor is instructed to move the shutter so a larger proportion of the circulating air is cooled, and if the net movement of heat through the walls is inward the shutter moves in the opposite direction to reduce the amount of heat extracted from the circulating air. In this way the heat flow across the walls is kept close to zero over any long period, so any heat produced by the subject in the calorimeter is quantitatively extracted in the heat exchanger. Heat loss by convection and evaporation is not separately measured, since evaporative heat loss is recovered by the heat exchanger as the water vapour is condensed on the cold metal surface.

In order to supply fresh air to the subject, without affecting the heat transfer, about 50 l/min of air is taken into the calorimeter from the shell space through a small heat exchanger (Y), and an equal volume of calorimeter air is extracted through a similar heat exchanger (Z). Air passing through these heat exchangers is cooled to 6°C, so the change of water vapour is negligible.

The supply of cold water for the cooling system is fed from a reservoir (R) in an adjacent room, which is maintained at 4°C by a commercial refrigeration unit. The main flow of water passes from this reservoir to the outgoing fresh-air cooler (Z), then through a reference heat (e) which introduces exactly 100 watts into the stream of water, then through the main heat exchanger (X), and so back to the reservoir. A second stream separately supplies the incoming fresh-air cooler (Y). The temperature of the water is measured by thermistors at points a, b, c and d.

The heat loss of the subject in the calorimeter is calculated by comparing the temperature rise across the reference heater (e) with that which occurs in the same stream of water across heat exchangers (X) and (Z). Since the rise across (e) is known to represent a heat uptake of 100 watts, the heat uptake from the calorimeter is easily calculated and displayed on a recorder. The cost of this apparatus at 1976 prices was about £15 000.

(b) Other methods

Alternative methods for measuring human energy expenditure have been discussed in some detail elsewhere[8]: the main conclusions are summarized in Table 1. The direct calorimeter is the most expensive and most accurate. All forms of indirect calorimetry share an error of 2–5 %, since this is the error in analysing respiratory gases and converting the results to equivalent heat production (see above). The one respect in which respiration chambers are better than direct calorimeters is that they are cheaper, and therefore it is

Table 1 Relative merits and limitations of apparatus designed to measure energy expenditure in man

Apparatus	Approx. cost (£1000s)	Feasible duration of measurement (h)	Range of activities measured	Detection of artefact	Approx. error in measurement (%)
Direct calorimeter	5–50	5–36	quite good	good	1
Respiration chamber	1–10	5–240	good	good	2–5
Ventilated hood	0.5–2	1–5	poor	good	2–5
Douglas bag	0.5–2	0.1–0.2	moderate	poor	2–5
Portable respirometer	0.5–2	0.2–1.0	quite good	poor	2–5
Heart rate	0.5–5	12–72	excellent	poor-good	5–10

practicable to make them larger and more luxurious, and hence to hope that subjects will tolerate a longer period of continuous measurement. However, large chambers carry a heavy penalty in having a slow response time, so it may not be possible to observe, for example, the increase in metabolic rate following a meal because the effect of one meal merges into that of the next.

Estimates of energy expenditure based on observations of heart rate are inaccurate[9], especially in relatively sedentary subjects in whom heart rate is determined more by posture[10] and emotional influences[11] than by metabolic requirements.

Components of energy expenditure

(a) Basal metabolism
When indirect calorimetry was introduced into clinical medicine it was mainly for the purpose of diagnosing thyroid disease. At the Mayo Clinic by 1929 some 60 000 individuals had their 'basal metabolic rate' measured[12]: that is energy output while physically and mentally at rest, at least 12 hours after taking food, and in a thermoneutral environment. These conditions were used to try to obtain a standardized test, in which a change in metabolic rate due to thyroid disease would be most likely to be detected. Basal metabolism is usually measured in the early morning, after an overnight fast.

In fact, conditions at this time of day are not very standard. Figure 2 shows the average hourly heat losses in six obese women who each spent two 26 hour periods in the direct calorimeter (Blaza, unpublished). The change from a sleeping rate of about 60 watts (0.9 kcal/min or 3.6 kJ/min) to the average daytime rate of about 90 watts (1.3 kcal/min or 5.4 kJ/min) takes place rather unsteadily between the hours of 0700 and 0900, which is the time at which 'BMR' is usually measured. The fall from daytime rate back to the sleeping

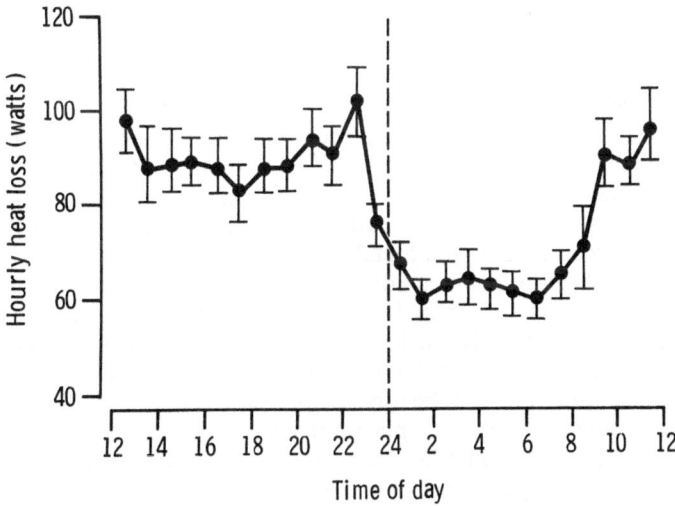

Figure 2 Hourly heat losses in six obese patients, each measured in the direct calorimeter on two occasions

level occurred in these women between 2300 and 0100. This diurnal rhythm is to some extent influenced by patterns of sleep and activity, but the changes cannot be abolished however rigorously the environmental factors are controlled[13].

However, it is obviously dangerous to attach too much significance to any measurement of BMR at one time of day, since a measurement on the same subject, under the same conditions but at a different time of day, would probably give an answer which differed by some 20%.

(b) Thermogenesis

It is implicit in the definition that 'basal' metabolism is a minimum value, so any change must be an increase. This is not necessarily true in special cases, e.g. during hypothermia, but for practical purposes the generalization is true. Metabolic rate will, of course, increase during physical activity, which is considered in the next section. The present heading, 'thermogenesis', is used to cover all those situations in which metabolic rate is raised above basal levels in the resting subject.

One of the commonest and most important stimuli for thermogenesis is food. After a meal resting metabolic rate increases, and reaches a maximum about 1 hour after the meal[14]. The effect then decreases, and is no longer detectable about 5 hours after a meal supplying 1000 kcal (4.2 MJ). The total extra energy expended as a result of dietary-induced thermogenesis is about 10% of the energy value of the meal. This is an approximate figure, because it is difficult to make an accurate measurement of the effect in man. Some workers[15] make the mistake of obtaining a 'baseline' measurement of metabolic rate before the meal, and then observing the increase above this baseline when the meal has been consumed. Reference to Figure 2 will show the error of this type of protocol: if the meal is given at 0900 the 'baseline' does not give a good indication of what the metabolic rate would have done without the meal, and indeed the rate would not fall to 'baseline' values for another 15 hours, regardless of any dietary-induced thermogenesis. Therefore, to make an accurate estimate of the thermogenesis caused by a meal, it is necessary to perform at least two studies on the same subject over the same period of the day, but to include the meal on one occasion and omit it on the other.

It was taught by Rubner and his pupils[16] that dietary protein had a 'specific dynamic action', not possessed by other dietary energy sources such as carbohydrate, fat or alcohol. This teaching was based on observations of dogs, and it was suggested that the metabolism of protein as an energy source necessarily involved loss of metabolic energy in the oxidation of amino acids and formation of urea[17]. In man dietary manoeuvres can greatly alter the rate of deamination and urea production: e.g. a meal containing a large amount of gelatine will increase urea production, since the amino acid composition of gelatine is such that it cannot be used for protein synthesis. If it were the case that urea production was an important determinant of 'specific dynamic action' then the effect should be much more marked after a meal of gelatine than after an isoenergetic meal of glucose, but this is not so[14].

An extreme case of dietary-induced thermogenesis would be the 'luxuskonsumption' postulated by Neumann[18]. He reported that he had

6

increased his energy intake by some 100 000 kcal (420 MJ) over a period of one year, but did not show the expected steady weight gain: it seemed, therefore, that the excess energy was being burned off by some thermogenic process. Twenty years later Gulick[19] repeated the experiment on himself with similar results. Over the ensuing half-century many attempts have been made to prove[20,21] or refute[22-24] the idea that a 'luxuskonsumption' mechanism exists, and there has been no clear victory for either side. At present, the best that can be said is that during long periods of overfeeding or underfeeding changes in energy expenditure occur which tend to minimize the extent of energy imbalance[25]. The nature of these adaptive mechanisms is discussed later in this review.

Other factors which may affect resting metabolic rate are the environmental temperature, emotional stress, certain drugs and hormones – notably thyroid hormones and the catecholamines. The effects of severe heat and cold stress are of more interest to those studying thermoregulation than those who are concerned with nutritional requirements. Severe cold stress can indeed increase metabolic rate[26-29], and hence energy requirements, but the changes in microclimate around the average person who has normal clothing and shelter are too small to make a significant contribution to energy expenditure. People living in extreme climates may incur extra energy costs if, for example, they have to move about in very heavy insulating clothing[30], but this is a special case of physical activity, not of resting thermogenesis.

Drugs such as salicylates, caffeine and dinitrophenol cause an increase in metabolic rate, but there is no circumstance in which the normal use of these drugs would affect energy requirements in the long term. Thyroid hormones will certainly increase resting metabolic rate by some 30%, and this increase can be sustained for many months if necessary. Noradrenalin infused intravenously at a rate sufficient to cause a five-fold increase in the basal level will cause an increase in metabolic rate of some 20% while the infusion continues, and it is likely that both catecholamines and thyroid hormones are involved in thermogenic reactions in general[31].

The effects of anxiety on metabolic rate are very difficult to investigate, since the effect, if any, is small. Therefore, it is necessary to study the subject in a relaxed and steady state, and then cause a high level of anxiety without otherwise affecting the experimental conditions. Apart from any ethical considerations, this is a very difficult task. Landis[32] made a heroic study of his own, and his colleagues', reactions to severe sleep deprivation, gastric intubation and electric shocks, and there was little to show for all this bravery in terms of metabolic response.

(c) Physical activity

There is considerable confusion about the magnitude of the contribution made by physical activity to total energy expenditure, and hence to energy requirements. The National Academy of Sciences and National Research Council (1964) Report on Dietary Allowances says 'Although physical activity is the major variable affecting calorie requirements, no simple procedure has been derived for estimating calorie allowances in relation to expenditure of physical energy'. Table 2 is based on the 'arbitrary example' given in the above

Report, which indicates the energy expenditure of the 'reference' man and woman, who are deemed to spend 8 hours per day lying, 6 hours sitting, 6 hours standing, 2 hours walking, and 2 hours in other activities requiring an expenditure at 4.5 kcal/min for men or 3.0 kcal/min for women. If, for comparison, we postulate a 'very inactive' and a 'very active' man and woman similar estimates of energy expenditure can be made, and it can be seen from Table 2 that a very inactive lifestyle would be expected to yield a saving of about 682 kcal/day for the reference man, and 336 kcal/day for the reference woman. On the other hand if they were employed in a heavy manual occupation, so 8 hours a day was spent at the highest rate, the extra energy expended would be about 840 and 588 kcal for the reference man and woman respectively. These differences agree fairly well with the observed difference in energy expenditure between people in very sedentary, or very strenuous, occupations[33-35].

However, as the quotation above indicates, there is no simple procedure for relating energy allowances to physical activity. The calculations in Table 2 are plausible, but they depend on the assumption that a person who was in the habit of spending 20 hours of the day either lying or sitting would have the same resting metabolic rate as someone who habitually undertook strenuous work for 8 hours per day. This is an improbable assumption. The very sedentary person would almost certainly lack the physique to perform very

Table 2 Postulated energy expenditure of a 'reference' man and woman, and the effect of a very high, or very low, level of physical activity

Activity	Energy cost (kcal/min)	Reference man (Hours /day)	(kcal)	Very inactive man (Hours /day)	(kcal)	Very active man (Hours /day)	(kcal)
Lying	1.1	8	528	10	726	8	528
Sitting	1.5	6	540	10	900	4	360
Standing	2.5	6	900	2	300	2	300
Walking	3.0	2	360	2	360	2	360
Other	4.5	2	540	0	0	8	2160
		24	2868	24	2286	24	3708

Activity	Energy cost (kcal/min)	Reference woman (Hours /day)	(kcal)	Very inactive woman (Hours /day)	(kcal)	Very active woman (Hours /day)	(kcal)
Lying	1.0	8	480	10	600	8	480
Sitting	1.1	6	396	10	660	4	264
Standing	1.5	6	540	2	180	2	180
Walking	2.5	2	300	2	300	2	300
Other	3.0	2	360	0	0	8	1440
		24	2076	24	1740	24	2664

heavy work, so the difference in energy output depends partly on the actual pattern of activity, and partly on the body composition which goes with that pattern of activity.

(d) Energy cost of growth, pregnancy and lactation

Infants, and children during the adolescent growth spurt, have surprisingly high energy requirements. This is related to the energy cost of growth, which cannot easily be measured. The effect is seen most clearly in severely malnourished children who have been prevented by undernutrition from growing in the first year of life, and who are then fed at a level which permits catch-up growth. The metabolic rate of a severely malnourished child, aged 1 year, is quite low until it is refed, but when very high growth velocities are attained energy requirements may double[36].

During pregnancy energy requirements increase by about 200 kcal (0.8 MJ) per day[37]. During the early stages of pregnancy the extra energy is laid down as fat, and this subsidizes the greatly increased energy demands during the last few weeks of pregnancy[38].

The lactating woman, who is supplying the energy requirements of her infant with breast milk, obviously has to cover this extra route of energy loss either by sacrificing some of her fat stores, or by additional dietary energy. The energy requirement of a lactating woman cannot be defined in general terms: it must be calculated in the light of her output of breast milk, and the state of her fat stores.

Replication of results in individuals

There is little value in making very accurate measurements of energy expenditure by direct calorimetry if the energy output of individuals changes capriciously. Fortunately, replication of results is good on individuals measured under standard conditions. For example the six women whose daily energy losses are shown in Figure 2 were each measured twice, and the mean difference between duplicate measurements was 2% (Blaza, unpublished).

Variation between individuals

The task of assigning energy requirements to groups of individuals is very much easier than that of defining the requirements of an individual. Reports on dietary allowances, and national rationing policies in time of war, need only guess correctly the average requirement of a large group. In the case of most nutrients it does not matter if the guess is rather high, so long as most people get enough.

The problem of a clinician facing an individual patient is more exacting, specially if he is responsible for treating a condition of energy imbalance besity or cachexia) in this patient. The fact that the patient is not in energy nce may indicate that the requirements of this individual are not 'average', is important to recognise the range of individual variation.

As a first approximation, energy requirements can be adjusted for differences in body weight. Activities involving large body movements are harder work for bigger people, but this factor is trivial. Some tables of recommended allowances assume that 25% of energy expenditure is independent of body weight, while 75% is directly proportional to body weight. The effect of this calculation is to add or subtract 300 kcal/day for each 10 kg by which a man differs from the reference weight of 70 kg, and 250 kcal/day for each 10 kg by which a woman differs from the reference weight of 58 kg. However, a 'correction' of this sort does very little to reduce the scatter among individuals. Figure 3 shows the resting metabolic rate of 111 individuals ranging in weight from 55 to 160 kg. Certainly there is a significant increase in metabolic rate with increasing weight: the correlation coefficient is 0.79, which is statistically highly significant. However, at any given weight – say 80 kg – the observed oxygen uptake ranges from 200–300 ml/min, which is equivalent to a difference in resting energy expenditure of about 700 kcal/day, among individuals of the *same* weight.

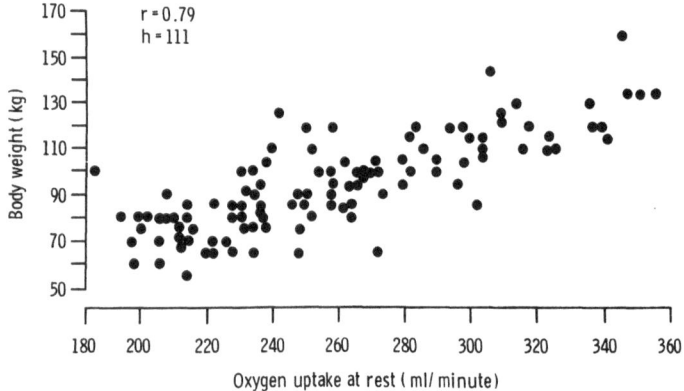

Figure 3 Resting metabolic rate, measured by indirect calorimetry, related to body weight in 111 normal and obese subjects.

More sophisticated correction standards have been proposed, of which the best known is that based on the observations of Boothby[39] and his colleagues at the Mayo Clinic. This involves a nomogram in which the subject's age, sex, weight and height are entered, to obtain an 'expected' basal metabolic rate. When the observed basal metabolic rate of 22 women (weight 90.2 ± 18.6 kg) was compared with the Mayo 'expected' metabolic rate, the correlation coefficient was 0.791, which was exactly the same as the correlation with simple body weight[40]. Thus corrections for age, sex and surface area do little to explain individual variation.

It is not only among obese patients well matched for age, sex and body weight that there are large differences in metabolic rate. A striking example of individual variation was given by Warwick[41] who studied two normal young women, both aged 23 years, both weighing 54 kg, and both with a surface area of 1.5 m². On direct calorimetry these two women showed differences in energy expenditure of 633 kcal/day, although each gave reproducible results on replicate measurements, and the difference could not be explained by any difference in the level or pattern of physical activity.

TECHNIQUES FOR MEASURING ENERGY STORES

If energy intake exactly matches requirements, the energy stores of the body will remain constant. It is easier to make accurate measurements of energy intake than of energy expenditure, especially under field conditions. Therefore, it would be convenient for those who try to estimate energy requirements if the energy stores of the body could be relied upon to remain constant or alternatively if the magnitude of the change in the stores could be accurately measured. In practice, neither of these helpful situations prevails.

The body composition of an average 70 kg man is shown diagrammatically in Figure 4. The components of body weight which are relevant to energy storage are fat (which is by far the main energy store), protein and glycogen. None of the other components has any significant energy value. Body weight is not a very reliable index of the state of the energy stores, since change in body water (which occurs for a variety of reasons) affects weight but not energy

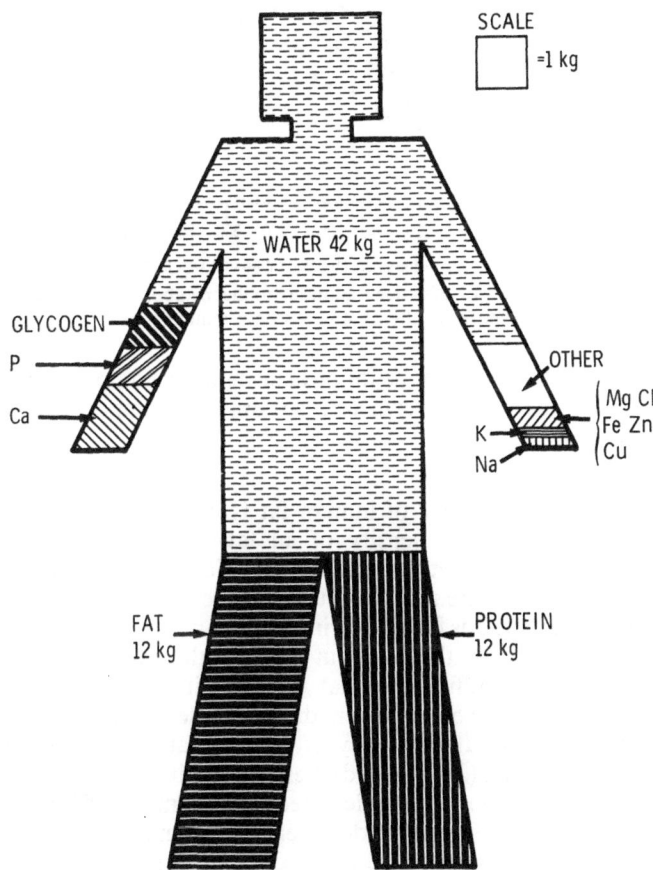

Figure 4 Diagrammatic representation of body composition in a normal adult male, weight 70 kg

stores. The man in Figure 4 is shown as having about 1 kg of glycogen, which is probably about the upper limit of possible storage[42]. If this man is starved for 24 hours much of this glycogen store will be used up, and body weight will fall sharply, because each gram of glycogen binds about 3–4 g water[42]. However, if the period of starvation continues the rate of weight loss will decrease[43], for when the glycogen stores are exhausted the energy deficit must be met from fat or protein. Lean tissue has a similar energy density to the glycogen:water pool, since the energy value of a gram of protein and a gram of glycogen are similar (4 kcal or 17 kJ), and each is associated with 3–4 g water. However, adipose tissue consists of about 83 % fat, 15 % water and 2 % protein, so each gram of adipose tissue stores about 7.5 kcal (31 kJ)[8].

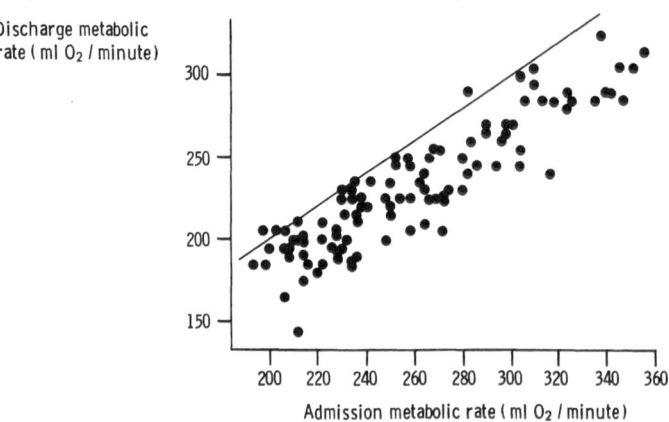

Figure 5 Resting metabolic rate of patients admitted to the metabolic unit, related to the resting metabolic rate of the same patients after 3–4 weeks on a reducing diet

The merits of various methods for measuring body composition have been reviewed in some detail elsewhere[8], so only the important points are summarized below.

(a) Body density
It is known that the density of human fat is close to $0.90 \, g \, cm^{-2}$. If it is assumed that the average density of all fat-free tissues in the body is $1.10 \, g \, cm^{-2}$, then it is evident that a determination of total body density will permit a calculation of the ratio of fat to fat-free tissue in the body[44,45].

Of the available methods for measuring body composition in living subjects, densitometry is probably the best, but it has both practical and theoretical difficulties. A practical difficulty is that, although it is easy to weigh a person with an accuracy of about 50 g, it is very difficult to determine the volume of the tissues with commensurate accuracy. If the true fat content of a man who weighed 70 kg was 14 kg (20 % of body weight), and if the volume of his tissues was overestimated by 500 ml, the calculated fat content would be 16.8 kg (24 % of body weight)[46]. Thus to provide a reliable estimate of fat content it is necessary to measure tissue volume very accurately. It is not simply a matter of submerging the subject in water and observing the displacement, or apparent weight loss, because the air in lungs and gut also displaces water, thus falsely increasing the apparent fat content. Another practical difficulty is that many people are unable, or unwilling, to submerge completely and calmly in water. Many attempts have been made to overcome these problems, and the most satisfactory solution so far has been to use a chamber in which the subject is submerged only up to the neck with the head enclosed in a clear plastic dome[46,47]. It is possible to measure the volume of air around the head, and in lungs and gut, by observing the pressure change for a given volume change within the dome. By this method replicate readings on individual subjects yield estimates of fat content which agree within about 0.3 kg.

However, even with technically accurate measurements a theoretical difficulty remains. The method depends on the assumption that fat-free tissue has a density of $1.10 \, g \, cm^{-2}$, this is not necessarily true, and certainly it is not true that the density of fat-free tissue lost or gained by subjects who are not in energy balance has a density of $1.10 \, g \, cm^{-2}$.

(b) Fat-soluble gases

Several gases, such as xenon, krypton and cyclopropane, are much more soluble in fat than in water, so if a person breathes an atmosphere containing a known concentration of one of these gases the amount taken up in the tissues at equilibrium should provide a measure of the amount of fat in the body[47,48]. This technique has been used to measure total body fat, and it has great theoretical attractions. However, it is not generally used because the gas is slowly transported in the blood to the fat depots, which are not perfused at a uniform rate, this attaining equilibrium is a slow and uncertain process.

(c) Skinfolds

Most of the fat in a normal, or obese, person is situated in a layer under the skin[49]. If the skin at sites such as the front or back aspect of the upper arm, at the angle of the scapula, or between the umbilicus and the iliac crest, is pinched up between the fingers, the thickness of the fold indicates the thickness of the layer of subcutaneous fat. Extensive studies, notably by Durnin and Womersley[50], have related the fat content of subjects, determined by density, to the thickness of the skinfolds at these four sites.

This method is very convenient for subjects of average build, but it requires considerable skill to obtain reproducible readings of skinfold thickness[51], and on very obese subjects it may be impossible to obtain a reading at all.

(d) Total body water

Recent advances in isotope mass spectrometry have made it possible to make very accurate measurements of the deuterium content of body fluids[52]. It is therefore possible to measure the deuterium content of the serum of a subject, administer a known dose of deuterium oxide (about 2 g) and, after allowing about 4 hours for equilibration, take another serum sample and measure the enrichment of deuterium (as a result of distribution of the tracer dose of deuterium in total body water). In this way estimation of the exchangeable deuterium pool (which is effectively total body water)[53] can be made with an error of about 0.5 %.

The measurement of water in itself throws no light on the energy stores of the body, but if the assumption is made that fat-free tissue contains 73 % water, and that all water is in fat-free tissue[54], it is easy to calculate the total mass of fat-free tissue, and hence of fat, from an estimate of total body water. The limitations of this approach are in the assumptions involved. It is obvious that although 73 % is a reasonable estimate of the water content of the fat-free component of most tissues, it is plainly incorrect for skin (which is drier) and for heart, kidney and adipose tissue (which have a higher ratio of water to fat-free weight)[55,56]. Furthermore, some of the water in the body is extracellular, and this compartment may increase without proportional increase in cell mass, thus causing clinical oedema and upsetting the assumed water to fat-free mass relationship[57,58]. Our own studies suggest that estimates of the fat content of obese patients, based on measurements of total body water, are likely to be in error by about 2 kg fat[59].

(e) Total body potassium

The naturally occurring radioactive isotope of potassium, ^{40}K, is uniformly distributed with the stable element, so potassium in human tissues can be measured by the characteristic high-energy gamma radiation coming from this endogenous label[60]. If the assumption is made that fat-free tissue contains a constant amount of potassium (68 mmol/kg for men, 60 mmol/kg for women)[8,59] then a measurement of total body potassium by gamma spectrometry of ^{40}K radiation provides an estimate of fat-free mass, and hence of fat.

This method has the same limitations as those mentioned above for water, namely that the assumed constant ratio of potassium to fat-free mass is not quite valid. To this must be added the disadvantage that measurement of potassium is less accurate than measurement of water: instead of achieving analytical accuracy of 0.5 %, it is reasonable to expect something around 3–5 %, depending on the design of the counter used. The effect of these limitations is that, using the same basis for comparison as that used for total body water[59], the error in fat content of obese patients, based on measurements of total body potassium, is about 3.5 kg.

CONSEQUENCES OF ENERGY IMBALANCE

Minor imbalances

Minor and transient imbalances between energy intake and expenditure are of no consequence whatever. Man is a meal eating animal, so energy intake occurs sporadically throughout the day, whereas energy expenditure is continuous. Thus one can only consider energy balance, or energy requirements, over a period of a day or more.

The energy stores shown in Figure 4 include about 1 kg of glycogen and 12 kg of fat. During a period of total starvation these could yield about 4000 kcal (17 MJ) and 108 000 kcal (452 MJ) respectively, so an energy imbalance of about 10 000 kcal (42 MJ) spread over a few weeks would hardly be noticed. This degree of imbalance probably occurs in most people during holidays, special festivities, or times of stress such as examinations, when food intake may be unusually high or low. The effect on body weight would be a change of perhaps 2 kg. Longitudinal surveys show that most normal people show fluctuations of body weight of about 10 kg over a period of several years[8,61], but tend to revert to a habitual weight by some mechanism which is not yet clearly understood.

Major excess – obesity

In the affluent countries of the world obesity is the most common and important nutritional problem[62]. The essential feature of obesity is an excessive fat store, and this cannot arise unless energy intake (from food) exceeds requirements. It has already been pointed out that transient errors of energy balance occur in almost everyone, so the factor which characterizes the obese person is that the cumulative error in energy balance is large and positive, and not automatically corrected by whatever mechanism maintains energy balance in 'normal' people.

Many attempts have been made to show that obese people eat more than normal, and although some do[63,64], many do not[64-69]. This is not surprising in view of the very large range of individual variation in energy requirements (see p. 10).

In the United Kingdom, the record for positive energy imbalance is held by one William Campbell who died in 1878 at the age of 22 years. In his short life he achieved a weight of 340 kg, which implies a storage of about 1 750 000 kcal (7315 MJ) in the form of excess adipose tissue. If this is expressed as an average daily positive imbalance it comes to 218 kcal (0.9 MJ) per day for 22 years. This imbalance, which produced record-breaking obesity, is small compared with the variations in energy expenditure which are observed between individuals of similar weight and body composition. Thus it is likely that some obese people, even while they are increasing in weight, must be eating less than some lean people of constant weight.

The disadvantages of being very obese are serious: life insurance companies[70,71] know that overweight people die younger, and hence are less profitable to insure, surgeons and anaesthetists know that they present difficult problems if they require surgical operations[72], they and their babies are at greater risk during childbirth[73], they are more prone to degenerative disease of weight-bearing joints[74], and to develop adult diabetes mellitus[75], and they also have social problems. In general, the disadvantages of obesity are reversible on weight loss[70].

With so much to gain from weight loss, it might be supposed the treatment of obese patients would present no problem: 'Since the immediate causes of obesity are overeating and under exercising, the remedies are available to all, but many patients require much help in using them'[76].

In fact, the situation is less simple than the above statement suggests. Probably, had William Campbell increased his energy expenditure by 218 kcal/day, and eaten the same as before, he would not have continued to gain weight. However, to lose weight it is necessary to generate a negative energy balance; typically about 800 kcal/day deficit will result in a rate of weight loss between 0.5 and 1 kg per week. If a diet is chosen which provides 800 kcal/day less than requirements, and it is strictly adhered to, the rate of weight loss will decrease as time goes on. In part this is due to a decrease in the mass of tissue on which energy requirements depend; it is obvious that a person who weighs 100 kg will have lower energy requirements when his weight is reduced to 70 kg. However, it has been known since the days of Benedict[77] that during undernutrition metabolic rate decreases more rapidly than can be explained merely by loss of weight. Figure 5 provides an example of this effect. The patients shown in Figure 3 were put on a reducing diet for 3 weeks which caused an energy deficit of about 25 000 kcal (100 MJ). On average the resting oxygen uptake rate fell by about 20 ml/minute *more* than would be expected on the basis of weight loss, but in some patients there was no decrease in metabolic rate, and in some the decrease was about 25 %. It will be seen from Figure 5 that the decrease is similar among those with a high or low initial metabolic rate. The cause of this adaptation to a reduced energy intake is not clear, but it is established that the initial metabolic rate is most closely linked to the initial lean body mass. Among the 19 patients cited earlier metabolic rate was no more closely related to the value predicted by the Mayo standards than it was to body weight (correlation coefficient 0.791 in both cases) but the best correlation (0.844) was with lean body mass[40]. Therefore, it is probable that weight loss associated with a large loss of lean tissue lowers energy requirements more than a similar weight loss in which there has been relative sparing of lean tissue, and loss predominantly of adipose tissue.

Major deficit – protein-energy malnutrition

Although obesity is the most important nutritional disease in affluent countries, in the world in general the main nutritional problem is undernutrition. Since young children have relatively high nutritional requirements, they are the section of the population which show most clearly the effects of nutritional deficit. At one stage the clinical syndrome of malnutrition in children was labelled either 'marasmus' if the child was grossly stunted in height and emaciated, or 'kwashiorkor' if the child had obvious oedema, depigmentation of the skin and hair, and sometimes fatty infiltration of the liver[78]. These terms have now given way to the more general term 'protein-energy malnutrition', since it was found that it was impossible to make any sharp distinction between the syndromes of marasmus and kwashiorkor: every shade of intermediate form of malnutrition has been found, and during the course of treatment a marasmic child may develop some of the features of kwashiorkor, and vice versa[79].

It is difficult enough to determine the food intake of people in normal circumstances, and virtually impossible to find out accurately the diet on which protein-energy malnutrition develops. The energy requirements of affected children can be determined from their response to treatment[36], and it can be assumed that while they were developing the disease they were not receiving these requirements. However, even this assumption is uncertain, because children on a marginal diet may be precipitated into malnutrition by infection, especially if it is associated with diarrhoea and vomiting[80].

In the treatment of protein-energy malnutrition it is important to distinguish two stages. In the severely ill child (e.g. one who weighs 5 kg at the age of 1 year, or half the normal weight for age) the first task is to restore fluid and electrolyte abnormalities towards normal, and to treat infections. In this early stage too vigorous attempts to refeed the child may be fatal[81]: the objective is to give enough food to prevent the malnutrition becoming worse. When this first phase is over (which may take 2–14 days, depending on the state of the child) the second stage is reached, in which the objective is to provide the child with enough food, and particularly energy, to enable it to catch up with the growth which was lost as a result of undernutrition. In this phase of treatment the energy intake is limited by what the child can take, but increased rates of growth, and a more strongly positive nitrogen balance, are observed with energy intakes up to about 200 kcal (0.8 MJ) per kg body weight per day[81]. This is considerably greater than the 'normal' requirements even of a newborn child.

CONCLUSION – 'OPTIMUM' ENERGY INTAKE

At the start of this paper it was pointed out that the best one can do is to recommend an energy intake which is appropriate for an average person of a given age, sex, weight and lifestyle. If the individual slavishly follows this advice it is quite likely that there will be an imbalance between energy intake and expenditure of some 15 %, because such is the variation in energy requirements of individuals of similar age, sex, weight and lifestyle. An error of energy balance of this magnitude would be disastrous, say 100 000 kcal (400 MJ) or 150 kg of adipose tissue gained or lost in a year!

This calculation illustrates that it is as absurd to try to lay down recommended energy intakes for individuals, as it is to say how much an individual ought to budget to spend on travel each year; the requirements of

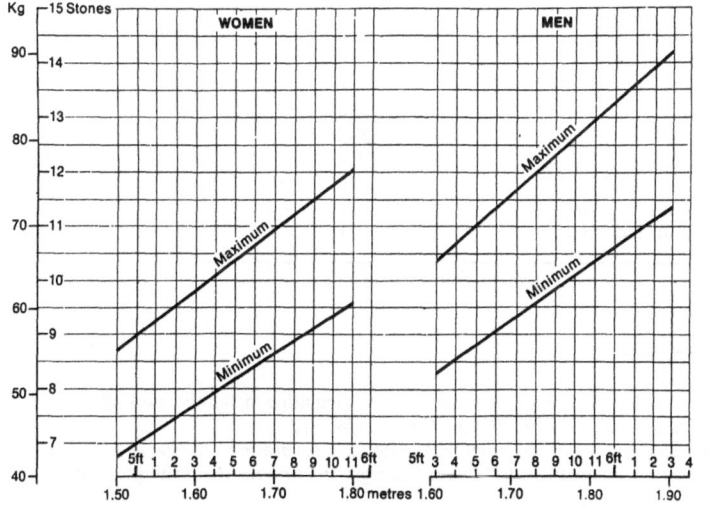

Figure 6 Range of 'desirable' weight-for-height in men and women: life insurance statistics show that individuals within this range have better life expectancy than those outside it

individuals differ in both cases. Fortunately it is quite easy for an individual to know if his or her energy intake is optimal by consulting Figure 6. This indicates the 'desirable' range of weight-for-height, according to the experience of life insurance companies. Individuals within the range tend to live longer, and are more profitable to insure, than individuals outside the range. Therefore, a person whose weight is within the range, and stable, can reasonably assume that he or she has about the right energy intake. This figure does not apply to children, in whom a weight-for-height calculation is complicated by changing growth and weight velocities, especially during puberty, so it is necessary to consult the appropriate growth centile charts to see if the weight of a child is appropriate for its age and height.

A person who is outside the desirable range of weight probably has too much, or too little, fat. There are exceptions to this rule, since professional athletes, such as weightlifters and boxers, may be so heavily muscled that they are 'overweight', although they do not carry excess fat. Conversely, post-menopausal women may lie within the normal weight range despite an excess of fat[48], because their lean body mass is so small. However, as a practical guide to energy requirements of individuals the use of weight-for-height criteria is more reliable, and easier to use, than a prescribed energy intake.

It is interesting to study trends in recommended energy intakes over the past decade. Table 3 shows values extracted from the US reports of 1964 and 1974, and the UK report of 1969. There is broad agreement between the reports, but there is also a trend to reduce recommended intakes for adults and teenagers. It is really over this period of time that the problem of obesity has been generally recognised.

Table 3 Recommended average energy intakes

	1964		1969		1974	
Age, sex, weight of subject	(kcal)	(MJ)	(kcal)	(MJ)	(kcal)	(MJ)
Men, 18–35 y, 70 kg	2900	(12.1)	2700	(11.3)	2700	(11.3)
Women, 18–35 y, 58 kg	2100	(8.8)	2200	(9.2)	2000	(8.4)
Children 1–2 y, 11 kg	1300	(5.4)	1200	(5.0)	1300	(5.4)
7–9 y, 25 kg	2100	(8.8)	2100	(8.8)	2400	(10.0)
Boys, 12–15 y, 45 kg	3000	(12.5)	2800	(11.7)	2800	(11.7)
Girls, 12–15 y, 45 kg	2500	(10.4)	2300	(9.6)	2400	(10.0)
Addition for pregnancy	200	(0.8)	200	(0.8)	300	(1.3)
Addition for lactation	1000	(4.2)	500	(2.1)	500	(2.1)

References

1. Weir, J. B. de V. (1949). New methods for calculating metabolic rate with special reference to protein metabolism. *J. Physiol. (Lond.)*, **109**, 412
2. Atwater, W. O. and Benedict, F. G. (1905). *A respiration calorimeter with Appliances for the Direct Determination of Oxygen*. Carnegie Institution of Washington, Washington, D.C., Publication **42**, 193
3. Blaxter, K. L., Brockway, J. M. and Boyne, A. W. (1972). A new method for estimating the heat production of animals. *Q. J. Exp. Physiol.*, **57**, 60

4. Spinnler, G., Jequier, E., Favre, R., Dolivo, M. and Vanotti, A. (1973). Human calorimeter with a new type of gradient layer. *J. Appl. Physiol.*, **35**, 158

5. Webb, P., Annis, J. F. and Troutman, S. J. (1972). Human calorimetry with a water-cooled garment. *J. Appl. Physiol.*, **32**, 412

6. Atwater, W. O., and Benedict, F. G. (1899). Experiments on the metabolism of matter and energy in the human body. *Bull. US. Dept. Agric.*, **69**, 112

7. Garrow, J. S., Murgatroyd, P., Toft, R. and Warwick, P. (1977). A direct calorimeter for clinical use. *J. Physiol. (Lond.)*, **267**, 16

8. Garrow, J. S. (1978). *Energy Balance and Obesity in Man.* 2nd edn. (Amsterdam: Elsevier-North Holland Biomedical Press)

9. De Looy, A. E. (1974). Socially acceptable methods for measuring energy expenditure in man. *PhD. Thesis*, University of London.

10. Booyens, J. and Hervey, G. R. (1960). The pulse rate as a means of measuring metabolic rate. *Can. J. Biochem.*, **38**, 1301

11. Moss, A. J. and Wynar, B. (1970). Tachycardia in house officers presenting cases at grand rounds. *Ann. Intern. Med.*, **72**, 255

12. Boothby, W. M. and Sandiford, I. (1929). Normal values for standard metabolism. *Am. J. Physiol.*, **90**, 290

13. Aschoff, J. and Pohl, H. (1970). Rhythmic variations in energy metabolism. *Fed. Proc.*, **29**, 1541

14. Garrow, J. S. and Hawes, S. F. (1972). The role of amino acid oxidation in causing 'specific dynamic action' in man. *Br. J. Nutr.*, **27**, 211

15. Kaplan, M. L. and Leveille, G. A. (1976). Calorigenic responses in obese and non-obese women. *Am. J. Clin. Nutr.*, **29**, 1108

16. Rubner, M. (1902). *Die Gesetze des Energieverbrauchs bei der Ernährung.* Leipzig & Vienna.

17. Krebs, H. A. (1964). The metabolic fate of amino acids. In Munro, H. N. and Allison, J. B. (eds.). *Mammalian Protein Metabolism.* pp. 125–176. (New York: Academic Press)

18. Neumann, R. O. (1902). Experimentelle Beiträge zur Lehre von dem täglichen Nahrungsbedarf des Menschen unter besonderer Berücksichtigung der notwendigen Eiweissmenge. *Arch. Hyg. (Berl.)*, **45**, 1

19. Gulick, A. (1922). A study of weight regulation in the adult human body during overnutrition. *Am. J. Physiol.*, **60**, 371

20. Miller, D. S., Mumford, P. and Stock, M. J. (1967). Gluttony. 2. Thermogenesis in overeating man. *Am. J. Clin. Nutr.*, **20**, 1223

21. Apfelbaum, M., Bostsarron, J. and Lacatis, D. (1971). Effect of caloric restriction and excessive caloric intake on energy expenditure. *Am. J. Clin. Nutr.*, **24**, 1405

22. Passmore, R., Meiklejohn, A. P., Dewar, A. D. and Thow, R. K. (1955a). Energy utilization in overfed thin men. *Br. J. Nutr.*, **9**, 20

23. Strong, J. A., Shirling, D. and Passmore, R. (1967). Some effects of overfeeding for four days in man. *Br. J. Nutr.*, **21**, 909

24. Glick, Z., Shvartz, E., Magazanik, A. and Modan, M. (1977). Absence of increased thermogenesis during short-term overfeeding in normal and overweight women. *Am. J. Clin. Nutr.*, **30**, 1026

25. Garrow, J. S. (1978). Regulation of energy expenditure in man. In Bray, G. A., (ed.) *Second International Congress on Obesity.* (London: Newman)

26. Buskirk, E. R., Thompson, R. H. and Whedon, G. D. (1960). Human energy expenditure studies in the National Institute of Arthritis and Metabolic Diseases Metabolic Chamber. 1. Interaction of cold environment and specific dynamic action. 2. Sleep. *Am. J. Clin. Nutr.*, **8**, 602

27. Quaade, F. (1963). Insulation in leanness and obesity. *Lancet*, **2**, 429

28. Wyndham, C. H., Williams, C. G. and Loots, H. (1968). Reactions to cold. *J. Appl. Physiol.*, **24**, 282

29. Rochelle, R. H. and Horvath, S. M. (1969). Metabolic responses to food and acute cold stress. *J. Appl. Physiol.*, **27**, 710

30. Goldman, R. F. (1975). Introduction to bioenergetics. In Bray, G. (ed.). *Obesity in Perspective.* p. 119. Washington DC: US Govt. Printing Office

31. Jung, R. T., Shetty, P. S. and James, W. P. T. (1979). The effects of beta-adrenergic blockage on basal metabolism and peripheral thyroid metabolism. *Proc. Nutr. Soc.*, **38**, 57A

32. Landis, C. (1925). Studies of emotional reactions. IV. Metabolic rate. *Am. J. Physiol.*, **74**, 188
33. Passmore, R. and Durnin, J. V. G. A. (1955). Human energy expenditure. *Physiol. Rev.*, **35**, 801
34. Edholm, O. G., Fletcher, J. G., Widdowson, E. M. and McCance, R. A. (1955). The energy expenditure and food intake of individual men. *Br. J. Nutr.*, **9**, 286
35. Garry, R. C., Passmore, R., Warnock, G. M. and Durnin, J. V. G. A. (1955). Studies on Expenditure of Energy and Consumption of Food by Miners and Clerks (1952). Medical Res Council. Fife, Scotland, *Sp Rep Ser 289*, pp. 70. London: HMSO
36. Ashworth, A. (1974). Ad lib. feeding during recovery from malnutrition. *Br. J. Nutr.*, **31**, 109
37. Blackburn, M. W. and Calloway, D. H. (1976). Energy expenditure and consumption of mature, pregnant and lactating women. *J. Am. Diet. Assoc.*, **69**, 29
38. Hytten, F. E. and Leitch, I. (1971). *Physiology of Human Pregnancy.* 2nd Edn., (Oxford: Blackwell Scientific Publications)
39. Boothby, W. M. and Berkson, J. (1933). In Bray, G. A. (ed.), *Obesity in Perspective*, Appendix 4, Table 7. Washington DC: DHEW
40. Halliday, D., Hesp, R., Stalley, S. F., Warwick, P., Altman, D. G. and Garrow, J. S. (1979). Resting metabolic rate, weight, surface area and body composition in obese women. *Int. J. Obesity*, **3**, 1
41. Garrow, J. S., Durrant, M. L., Mann, S., Stalley, S. F. and Warwick, P. M. (1978). Factors determining weight loss in obese patients in a metabolic ward. *Int. J. Obesity*, **2**, 429
42. Olsson, K. -E. and Saltin, B. (1970). Variation in total body water with muscle glycogen in man. *Acta. Physiol. Scand.*, **80**, 11
43. Forbes, G. B. (1970). Weight loss during fasting: implications for the obese. *Am. J. Clin. Nutr.*, **23**, 1212
44. Allen, T. H., Krzywicki, H. J. and Roberts, J. E. (1959). Density, fat water and solids in freshly isolated tissues. *J. Appl. Physiol.*, **14**, 1005
45. Behnke, A. R., Feen, B. G. and Welham, W. C. (1942). The specific gravity of healthy men: body weight and volume as an index of obesity. *J. Am. Med. Assoc.*, **118**, 495
46. Irsigler, K., Heitkamp, H., Schlick, W. and Schmid, P. (1975). Diet and energy balance in obesity. In Jequier, E. (ed.), *Regulation of Energy Balance in Man.* pp. 72–83. (Geneva: Editions Médecine et Hygiene
47. Diethelm, R., Garrow, J. S. and Stalley, S. F. (1977). An apparatus for measuring the density of obese patients. *J. Physiol. (Lond.)*, **267**, 14P
48. Lesser, G. T., Deutsch, S. and Markofsky, J. (1971). Use of independent measurement of body fat to evaluate overweight and underweight. *Metabolism*, **20**, 792
49. Alexander, M. K. (1964). The postmortem estimation of total body fat, muscle and bone. *Clin. Sci.*, **26**, 193
50. Durnin, J. V. G. A. and Womersley, J. (1974). Body fat assessed from body density and its estimation from skinfold thickness: measurement on 481 men and women from 16–72 years. *Br. J. Nutr.*, **32**, 77
51. Ruiz, L., Colley, J. R. T. and Hamilton, P. J. S. (1971). Measurement of tricepts skinfold thickness. An investigation of sources of variation. *Br. J. Prev. Soc. Med.*, **25**, 165
52. Halliday, D. and Miller, A. G. (1977). Precise measurement of total body water using trace quantities of deuterium oxide. *Biomed. Mass. Spectrom.*, **4**, 82
53. Culebras, J. M., Fitzpatrick, G. F., Brennan, M. F., Boyden, C. M. and Moore, F. D. (1977). Total body water and exchangeable hydrogen. II. A review of comparative data from animals based on isotope dilution and desiccation, with a report of new data from the rat. *Am. J. Physiol.*, **232**, R60
54. Pace, N. and Rathbun, E. N. (1945). Studies on body composition. III. Water and chemically contained nitrogen content in relation to fat content. *J. Biol. Chem.*, **158**, 685
55. Dickerson, J. W. T. and Widdowson, E. M. (1960). Chemical changes in skeletal muscle during development. *Biochem. J.*, **74**, 247
56. Widdowson, E. M. and Dickerson, J. W. T. (1960). The effect of growth and function on the chemical composition of soft tissues. *Biochem. J.*, **77**, 30
57. Pierson, R. N., Wang, J., Yang, M. U., Hashim, S. A. and Van Itallie, T. B. (1976). The assessment of body composition during weight reduction: evaluation of a new model for clinical studies. *J. Nutr.*, **106**, 1694
58. Womersley, J., Durnin, J. V. G. A., Boddy, K. and Mahaffy, M. (1976). Influence of muscular development, obesity and age on the fat-free mass of adults. *J. Appl. Physiol.*, **41**, 223

59. Garrow, J. S., Stalley, S. F., Diethelm, R., Pittet, Ph., Hesp, R. and Halliday, D. (1979). A new method for measuring the body density of obese adults. *Br. J. Nutr.*, **42**, 173
60. Burch, P. R. J. and Spiers, F. W. (1953). Measurement of the γ radiation from the human body. *Nature (London)*, **172**, 519
61. Gordon, T. and Kannel, W. B. (1973). The effects of overweight on cardiovascular diseases: *Geriatrics*, **28**, 80
62. DHSS/MRC Study Group (1976). In James, W. P. T., (ed.), *Research on Obesity*. 94 pp. (London: HMSO)
63. Beaudoin, R. and Mayer, J. (1953). Food intakes of obese and non-obese women. *J. Am. Diet. Assoc.*, **29**, 29
64. Ries, W. (1973). Feeding behaviour in obesity. *Proc. Nutr. Soc.*, **32**, 187
65. Johnson, M. L., Burke, B. S. and Mayer, J. (1956). Relative importance of inactivity and over-eating in the energy balance of obese high school girls. *Am. J. Clin. Nutr.*, **4**, 37
66. Stefanik, P. A., Heald, F. P. and Mayer, J. (1959). Calorie intake in relation to energy output of obese and non-obese adolescent boys. *Am. J. Clin. Nutr.*, **7**, 55
67. McCarthy, M. C. (1966). Dietary and activity patterns of obese women in Trinidad. *J. Am. Diet. Assoc.*, **48**, 33
68. Lincoln, J. E. (1972). Calorie intake, obesity and physical activity. *Am. J. Clin. Nutr.*, **25**, 390
69. Thomson, A. M., Billewicz, W. Z. and Passmore, R. (1961). The relation between calorie intake and body weight in man. *Lancet*, **1**, 1027
70. Dublin, L. I. (1953). Relation of obesity to longevity. *N. Engl. J. Med.*, **248**, 971
71. Donald, D. W. A. (1973). Mortality rates among the overweight. In Robertson, R. F. (ed.), *Anorexia and Obesity*. pp. 63–70. Edinburgh: Royal College of Surgeons
72. Fisher, A., Waterhouse, T. D. and Adams, A. P. (1975). Obesity: its relation to anaesthesia. *Anaesth.*, **30**, 633
73. Maeder, E. C., Barno, A. and Mechlenburg, F. (1975). Obesity: a maternal high risk factor. *Obstet. Gynecol.*, **45**, 669
74. Leach, R. E., Baumgard, S. and Broom, J. (1973). Obesity: its relationship to osteoarthritis of the knee. *Clin. Orthop.*, **93**, 271
75. Rimm, A., Werner, L. H., Van Yserloo, B. and Bernstein, R. A. (1975). Relationship of obesity to disease in 73 522 weight conscious women. *Publ. Hlth Rep.*, **90**, 44
76. Davidson, S. and Passmore, R. (1969). *Human Nutrition and Dietetics*, 4th edn., p. 385. (Edinburgh: Livingstone)
77. Benedict, F. G., Miles, W. R., Roth, P. and Smith, M. (1919). *Human Vitality and Efficiency under Prolonged Restricted Diet*. Carnegie Institution, Washington, D.C., Publication 280, 701 pp.
78. Waterlow, J. C., Cravioto, J. and Stephen, J. M. L. (1960). Protein malnutrition in man. *Adv. Protein Chem.*, **15**, 131
79. Alleyne, G. A. O., Hay, R. W., Picou, D. I., Stanfield, J. P. and Whitehead, R. G. (1977). *Protein-energy Malnutrition*. (London: Edward Arnold)
80. Whitehead, R. G., Rowland, M. G. M. and Cole, T. J. (1976). Infection, nutrition and growth in a rural African environment. *Proc. Nutr. Soc.*, **35**, 369
81. Waterlow, J. C., Golden, H. N. and Patrick, J. (1978). Protein-energy malnutrition: treatment. In Dickerson, J. W. T. and Lee, H. A. (eds.) *Nutrition in the Clinical Management of Disease*, pp. 49–71. (London: Edward Arnold)

2
Fluoride and the fluoridation of water

G. N. JENKINS

MOTTLED ENAMEL

In the early years of this century a dentist in Colorado, Frederick McKay, observed that the permanent teeth of many of his patients showed either white chalky patches or lines which, in more severe cases, had a rough surface and, some years after eruption, became an unsightly yellow or brown. The condition was uncommon in the deciduous teeth. McKay collected a great deal of descriptive data and studied the histology of what came to be known as 'mottled enamel'[1-4], but only one fact about its aetiology emerged, namely, that it was associated with certain drinking waters taken during the years of tooth formation (i.e. up to the age of 8, or 12 if the third molars are included). McKay also drew attention to the unexpected fact that in spite of their enamel being 'more corrugated and rougher than normal', the mottled enamel 'does not seem to increase the susceptibility of the teeth to decay'[5] an unfortunate inversion of emphasis. Ainsworth[6] discovered a similar condition in Maldon, Essex, England, and stated[7] that 7.9 % of permanent teeth of schoolchildren were carious in this town compared with 13.1 % in the country as a whole, the first suggestion that mottling was associated with fewer cavities. In the late 1920s it became clear that children born and bred in Bauxite, Arkansas, a town built for employees of the Aluminum Company of America, had mottled enamel which led to the finding by the company chemists that the only unusual constituent of its water was 13.9 parts per million (ppm) of fluoride[8]. Analyses of other waters which were associated with mottling showed that they contained at least 2 ppm of fluoride, and there was a reasonable correlation between the severity of the mottling and the fluoride concentration. The administration to rats of water which induced mottling in children had no effect, but when this water was concentrated tenfold, its ingestion resulted in the rat's continuously-growing incisor becoming 'strikingly dull, white in appearance and pitted'[9] an effect produced by adding fluoride to their water. This confirmed the dental effects of fluoride and showed that rats are less sensitive than man to fluoride. The explanation is not known but may be related to the short time during which rat's teeth are forming and thus able to accumulate fluoride, or to differences in the effective concentration in blood as a result of binding mechanisms[10].

23

A comprehensive survey relating fluoride levels in water to mottling was undertaken by Dean[11] who was familiar with the possibility that mottled enamel might be less prone to caries. He eventually extended his survey to include the caries experience among 7257 12 to 14-year-old children living in areas where the fluoride concentration ranged from 0 to about 3 ppm[12–14]. This survey demonstrated unequivocally that concentrations of fluoride up to 1 ppm (too low to produce mottling) were associated with a lower caries experience (Figure 1). The data in Dean's diagram are somewhat ambiguous on the optimal intake as, at about 1 ppm, the points for the caries score are scattered. Later work, including that in England[15,16] (Figure 2) has shown that the optimum concentration for caries prevention is about 2 ppm. But as this produces an unacceptably high prevalence of mottling, 1 ppm has been adopted as the most desirable concentration in temperate climates (reduced to 0.6 ppm in warmer climates to allow for the greater water intake)[17,18].

In Figure 2 the caries score is higher at 6 ppm than at the optimum. Recent work has confirmed that excessive fluoride intake increases caries (for review, see Forsman[19]).

Final proof that fluoride itself, and not some substance associated with it in the water, prevents caries followed from the numerous studies showing the effectiveness of the addition of fluoride to water[20–25] (reviewed by McClure[26] and Murray[27]). Unfortunately, the fluoridation of water has been bitterly opposed by some individuals and organized groups so that its effectiveness and safety have become political as well as scientific questions. Arguments have tended to become polarized into 'pro' and 'anti' positions with unfortunate effects on scientific accuracy and objectivity.

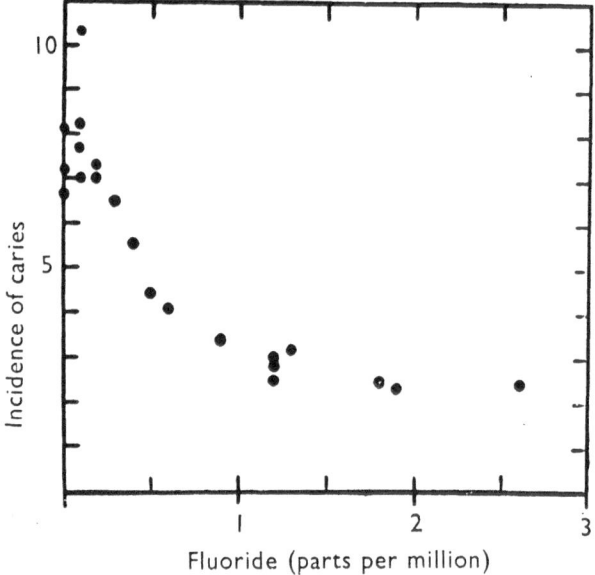

Figure 1 The relationship between the fluoride concentration of the water and average number of decayed, missing and filled DMF teeth in 12–14 year old children in the USA (after Dean[14])

24

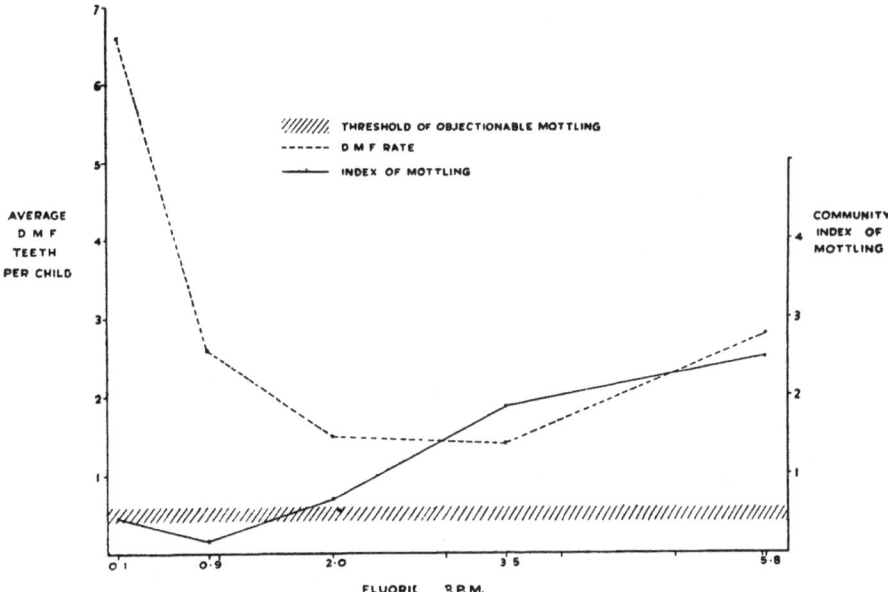

Figure 2 The relationship between fluoride in water, caries (upper curve) and mottling (lower curve) in England[16]. Note that the index of mottling is higher at 0.1 ppm F (idiopathic opacities) than at 0.9 ppm, and the threshold for the objectionable value is about 1.8 ppm. (Courtesy of Miss J. F. Forrest and the *Br. Dent. J.*)

The nature of mottled enamel

Histological sections of mottled enamel stained with silver nitrate show that the permeability of the outer third is greater than normal[28] and microradiographs show that this region of the mottled enamel is unusually radiolucent[29]. Electron micrographs reveal that enamel prisms are surrounded by large gaps free of minerals, and there are more intercrystalline spaces than usual, which explain the increased permeability[30]. The slight hypomineralization would, by affecting the optical properties of the enamel, account for the chalkiness present in mottled teeth at eruption. The increased permeability could account for both the pigmentation which, in severe cases, gradually develops some years after eruption presumably by the entry of oral fluids. The increased permeability can also account for the increased caries associated with severe mottling, by the diffusion of more sugar or acid. Mottled enamel is not an entirely suitable name for a defect which may consist of either chalky or pigmented patches: 'fluorosis' is to be preferred.

THE MECHANISM OF FLUOROSIS

Fluorosis might be produced either by affecting the matrix formed in the early stages of enamel development or be concerned with its later mineralization, or both (reviewed in Ref. 31). Single doses of fluoride equivalent to 7, 3 and 0.1 mg fluoride/kg body weight injected into 4-day-old rats[32] caused vacuolation of the rough endoplasmic reticulum in the ameloblasts – the cells producing the enamel matrix – an effect which was just detectable with 0.1 mg F/kg body weight (equivalent to 0.35 mg in a newborn baby, and comparable to the daily dose in fluoride-containing water drunk by babies who are not breast-fed[33]). All three doses had a detectable effect in reducing the uptake of tritiated proline by the ameloblasts[34]. A further experiment on a lower range of doses (3, 0.05 and 0.01 mg F/kg), with tritiated serine as a marker, confirmed the smaller uptake with 3 mg but showed an increased uptake with 0.01 mg[35]. Stimulation of cell metabolism by very low doses of fluoride has been previously reported[36]. With larger and more prolonged doses to adult rats (50 ppm fluoride in drinking water for 10 days) reduction in the amount, and change in the amino acid composition, of the protein in the enamel of the continuously-growing incisor were reported[37]. These experiments show that protein synthesis by ameloblasts is affected by low doses of fluoride, thus suggesting an explanation for mottling.

Mineralization of enamel, unlike mineralization in bone, involves the removal of most of the original protein and water of the matrix and its replacement by hydroxyapatite (HA). Low concentrations of fluoride tend to favour the deposition of HA from saturated solutions *in vitro*. The hypomineralized areas of enamel in clinical fluorosis cannot therefore be explained as a result of physico-chemical changes in mineralization (the reverse would be expected). Possibly the abnormal protein matrix apparently laid down may not be so readily removed, thus obstructing crystal growth.

The available limited evidence suggests a defect in matrix formation, especially in the area between the enamel prisms, leading secondarily to imperfect mineralization.

The sensitivity of ameloblasts

Because enamel is the first site of a detectable adverse effect of fluoride it has been supposed that ameloblasts are more sensitive to fluoride than other cells. But it has also been argued that other cells may be affected but the results are not visible. This question could be answered by injecting low doses of fluoride into young rats and examining cells from many tissues for vacuolation similar to that in the ameloblasts, or any other abnormality.

An alternative explanation of the apparent sensitivity of ameloblasts (and osteoblasts, as bone is the first site of unfavourable reaction to fluoride in older people[40]), is that they are near mineralized tissues which contain the highest concentrations of fluoride in the body. Some of this fluoride may diffuse, or be released, into the tissue fluid bathing the cells[41]. It is not known why mottling is patchy and affects only parts of the enamel surface, nor why it varies in severity in different people drinking the same water. These differences may be related either to variations in the amount of water, and therefore of fluoride, ingested at different times or by different individuals but variation in sensitivity to fluoride cannot be ruled out.

Idiopathic mottling

High fluoride intake is not the only cause of chalky patches on the enamel. Some teeth developed in low fluoride areas show chalky patches ('idiopathic' mottling or opacities) which may, in the past, have been confused with mild fluorosis, especially by individuals who are opposed to water fluoridation and wish to exaggerate its possible disadvantages. Among the many suggested causes of these blemishes are:

(1) infection of the permanent tooth germs spreading from abscessed deciduous teeth arising from caries[42]; evidence against this hypothesis is that the distribution of caries in the deciduous teeth does not correspond with that of idiopathic mottling on the permanent successors

(2) general childhood diseases causing systemic upset

(3) blows in the mouth region[43] during the early years when the permanent teeth are developing.

It has been stated that one difference between fluoride blemishes and idiopathic opacities is that the former are bilaterally symmetrical which would be expected for an effect produced systemically, like fluorosis, whereas the latter are not[42,44]. This distinction has not been confirmed in a recent study[45]. Idiopathic opacities are *less* prevalent in areas with about 1 ppm fluoride in the water (illustrated in Figure 2) but the explanation is still speculative. In towns with approximately 1 ppm of fluoride in their water ('F areas'), most probably the higher concentrations of fluoride in the mouth fluids may lead to the deposition of some calcium phosphate from saliva into the hypomineralized areas thus, at least partly, sealing them up[38,39]. The association of fluoride with fewer idiopathic opacities could be readily explained if this condition were caused by infection from carious deciduous teeth, because fluoride will, of course, prevent caries and reduce its severity in these teeth. Thus, 1 ppm of fluoride, although not giving optimum protection against caries is the best compromise; a very substantial protection against both caries and idiopathic mottling and the absence of fluoride mottling. The aesthetic unimportance of mottling in areas containing optimum fluoride was well illustrated by Al Alousi *et al.*[45]. They arranged for five postgraduate dental students and five lay observers to look at 50 randomly selected transparencies of teeth from an 'F area' and 50 from a control 'non-F area'. The observers were asked to decide, from the appearance of each tooth, which came from the 'F area' and whether its structure was perfect, imperfect but acceptable, or so imperfect as to be unacceptable. Neither group of observers distinguished clearly between the two sets of teeth, from which it may be concluded that mottling from 1 ppm of fluoride does not present a practical aesthetic problem.

THE CLINICAL EFFECT OF FLUORIDE IN CARIES

The measurement of caries

Caries is not easy to measure, especially in the very early stages of the disease in fissures, and comparisons of caries scores reported by different workers are not in good agreement. The commonest scoring method is to count the number of decayed, missing and filled teeth (DMFT): this ignores the severity of caries so that in a more refined measure the numbers of tooth surfaces affected are counted (DMFS). Neither score differentiates between teeth missing for reasons other than caries, so that the score can be extremely inaccurate in older people. Both methods assume that all fillings are inserted as treatment for existing caries although some dentists fill fissures before caries begins, as a prophylactic measure. Most studies on the effect of fluoride suffer from the deficiencies of these scoring methods.

The effect of fluoride on DMF values

The average DMFT score in 5–15-year-old children in an 'F area' is about 50% less than in controls[12,15,16,20–25]. The effect is not exerted equally on all surfaces of the teeth, however, but smooth surfaces and the contact points between the teeth (approximal surfaces) are protected much more (about 80%) than pits and fissures (about 40%). This means that molars receive less protection than incisors and the premolars are in an intermediate position. Since caries occurs more frequently in pits or fissures, the absolute number of molars protected exceeds that of the anterior teeth. For example, in the Dutch fluoridation scheme[23,46] 88% reduction of smooth surface cavities at age 15 saved an average of three cavities, whereas 43% reduction of caries in pits and fissures saved over five cavities per subject. The molar fissures are easier to fill compared with the less accessible areas between the incisors so, in practice, the more favourable effect on incisors greatly reduces the need for difficult filling procedures[46]. If the distribution of the DMF score among the population of towns with and without fluoride is compared, it becomes clear that in those with fluoride there are more individuals with low DMF scores and fewer or none with the higher scores[23,47]. This leads to the important practical conclusion that those who have a natural tendency for high DMF (say 10 at age 15) will benefit more from fluoridation (saving 5 teeth) than those with a low DMF (say two who will save only one tooth). Survey data[46,47] show that the contribution of missing teeth to the DMF score is smaller in 'F areas' than in controls (i.e. more teeth are capable of being filled rather than requiring extraction), and radiological studies indicate that carious lesions are shallower in the 'F areas'[48]. These data indicate that the severity and rate of development of cavities are reduced by fluoride as well as the number of cavities. Since all enamel and dental plaques (see later) contain some fluoride the differences in caries experience between populations in high F or low F areas measures only the effect of the additional fluoride obtained from the water. The full effect of fluoride can never be measured in man because the control groups are presumably already obtaining some benefit from the 'basal' concentration of fluoride.

THE AGE GROUPS WHICH BENEFIT

The limited effect of fluoride during pregnancy and lactation

Several lines of evidence show that the placenta acts as a partial barrier to fluoride (reviewed in reference 49). Autoradiographs of sections of pregnant mice injected with radioactive fluoride (^{18}F with a half-life of 110 min) show that fluoride accumulates in the placenta (in the same locations as does labelled calcium) and that comparatively little enters the fetus[50,51]. Nevertheless, the bones and teeth of the newborn do contain some fluoride and the concentration of fluoride in human fetal blood at term has been reported to be similar to that of maternal blood[52], so the barrier is incomplete. Some analytical figures on maternal and fetal blood from subjects on a low fluoride intake suggest little obstruction by the placenta. With fluoridated water or fluoride tablets, however, the fluoride of fetal blood was less than the maternal[53] implying a control occurring at higher intakes. All the figures in this work[53], carried out before the advent of the fluoride ion selective electrode, were much higher than more recent results (see later) and must be accepted with caution. Studies of the DMF of children from mothers who have received fluoride supplements during pregnancy have usually failed to show any effect when compared with controls[54,55]. It may be concluded that insufficient fluoride crosses the placenta to effect a consistently detectable reduction in caries, but the difficulty of measuring small differences in caries has already been emphasized.

The fluoride concentration of human milk, measured by gas liquid chromatography, is extremely low, in the neighbourhood of 0.05 ppm, 90 % of this is bound and only slightly increased by drinking fluoridated water[56]. The free ionic fluoride, measured by the specific ion electrode, is reported to be as low as 0.004 ppm in a low F area and 0.008 ppm in a high F area[56]. The concentration reported in cows' milk is somewhat higher, about 0.1 ppm[56].

Clearly breast-fed babies receive very little fluoride until they are weaned, but those on dried milk made up with fluoridated water may receive up to 50 times more as its concentration will approach the 1 ppm of the water. Teeth from a group of children fed with dried milk in 'F areas' contained 2–3 times more fluoride than breast-fed children[57]. This increased fluoride level was associated with a very slightly higher non-significant, prevalence of mottling but did not influence the caries score[58]. The low dose of fluoride received before birth probably explains the relative rarity of mottling in deciduous teeth, although these teeth do receive sufficient fluoride in 'F areas' to give protection from caries.

Effect of fluoride on caries in adults

Caries surveys on large populations show that the effect of fluoride is still apparent well into middle age[59–61] although two small scale studies[62,63] suggested the contrary. Murray[64–66] attempted to differentiate between loss of teeth from caries and loss for other reasons, by the following method[67]. Murray asked dentists to collect teeth from different age groups of life-long residents of York (low fluoride) and Hartlepool (fluoride then 1.9 ppm), the teeth were classified into morphological types and examined for caries. It was then possible to estimate what proportion of extracted incisors, molars, etc., were removed for caries at different ages. A correction factor could then be applied to the 'missing' component of the DMF score, so that the observed values could be converted to the values related only to caries. He then reported a lower caries score in Hartlepool up to the age of 65.

The fluoride concentration in Hartlepool until recently has been higher (1.9 ppm) than that recommended for fluoridation (mottling has been higher than the acceptable level). There are no DMF figures for an adequate sample of an elderly population on 1 ppm fluoride in Britain, although a survey in the USA in a town with 1.2 ppm showed a marked effect up to the age of 49[61]. The rate of caries falls almost to zero after the fifth decade (Figure 3) although loss of teeth from periodontal disease continues, and this is not reduced by fluoride. Consequently, if the DMF (for caries only) is lower than average at age 50, it is likely to remain lower throughout life as shown in Figure 3.

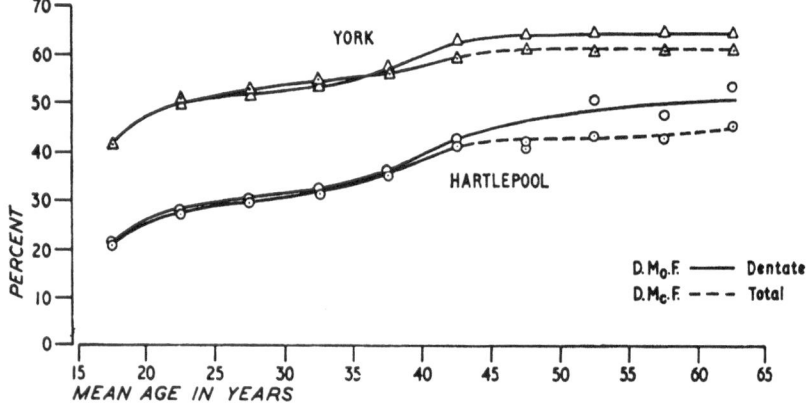

Figure 3   The effect of fluoride in Hartlepool (1.9 ppm) on the percentage of decayed, missing or filled (DMF) teeth compare with York (fluoride 0.1 ppm) over the age range 15–65 years. The full line is based on the observed DMF values and excludes edentulous subjects, the broken line represents the values for the whole population corrected for loss of teeth for reasons other than caries. (Courtesy of Prof. J. J. Murray and the *Br. Dent. J.*)

Comparisons of the caries scores of children who have received fluoride throughout their lives with those who were first exposed to it after their permanent teeth were already erupted, show that for the full effect, fluoride must be ingested during tooth formation[25], and continued after eruption. Nevertheless, there is some protection in teeth in young people whose first contact with fluoridated water occurs after eruption[68,69] and this resembles the situation mentioned above, with the deciduous teeth of breast-fed babies. Evidently the fully formed tooth is influenced by additional fluoride, either by a direct uptake by the enamel or by inhibitory influences on the bacteria responsible for caries, suggesting that continued exposure to booster doses of fluoride is necessary for maximum protection[70]. This is certainly true of other fluoride vehicles such as dentifrices and mouthrinses[71,72]

EFFECTS ON ERUPTION

Suggestions have been made that fluoride delays the eruption of the permanent teeth; and that the reduction in caries is more apparent than real, arising simply because the duration of exposure to sugar is shorter. Animal experiments and clinical data show that high fluoride intakes do delay eruption slightly, the effect having been detected in water containing 1.6 ppm[73], but populations exposed to 1 ppm fluoride show either no significant effect[74] or even a slightly accelerated eruption[75]. Some of the delayed eruption with the higher intakes is associated with a longer retention of the deciduous teeth (perhaps because fewer were extracted prematurely for caries[75,76]), and is not necessarily an interference with growth processes. It is clear that delays in eruption, if present, are far too small to explain the lower caries scores among older children in the 'F areas' (although this claim is still made by opponents of fluoridation), and even if there were a few months' delay it could not possibly account for a lower DMF at age 65!

THE BIOCHEMISTRY OF DENTAL PLAQUE AND CARIES

When a tooth, cleaned of all deposits, is exposed to saliva the first event is the formation of the 'pellicle'. This is a bacteria-free layer of salivary protein which is adsorbed onto the hydroxyapatite of the enamel surface, and penetrates some distance into the outer enamel in the space between the crystals[77]. This layer is not removed by toothbrushing but is removed by a 'scale and polish' with an abrasive. It reforms within a few hours of removal, and is believed to protect the enamel against acid[78]. The next stage is the formation outside the pellicle of the 'dental plaque', the much thicker layer of protein matrix containing tightly packed bacteria (estimated at 400×10^6 per mg) and with a texture which makes it removable by toothbrushing. The exact source of the protein matrix, and the factors responsible for its deposition, and its invasion by bacteria are still controversial[77] but its composition is that of a calcium phosphate–protein complex[77–79]. Contrary to popular belief it contains very little food debris.

Following access of sugar (which unlike solid food debris does diffuse readily into plaque) the plaque forms acid extremely rapidly, and reduces the pH from the normal, near neutral, fasting value to about 5.5 (Figure 4) or even lower in the sheltered sites where caries occurs[80,81]. Saliva and the fluid phase of fasting plaque are, like the plasma, saturated with calcium phosphate at pH values of 6.0 or higher so that the enamel surface does not dissolve[82,83]. But as the pH falls the solubility of apatite increases (because PO_4^{3-} in the aqueous phase is converted to HPO_4^{2-} thus lowering the common ion effect) and at some critical pH, the concentrations of calcium and phosphate in the plaque fluid cease to saturate it and some enamel will tend to dissolve[83,84]. The dissolving of enamel is believed to be restricted by the pellicle surrounding the apatite crystals. Consequently, the acid tends to diffuse past the pellicle into the deeper enamel, which is one of the suggested explanations for the fact that caries is a slowly penetrating lesion, slightly damaging a considerable depth of enamel before causing a frank cavity[85]. A further prerequisite for the development of caries, in addition to a pH low enough to make the environment of the tooth unsaturated with calcium phosphate, is believed to be a concentration gradient of unionised lactic acid sufficient to ensure its diffusion inwards, as only the unionised molecule is thought to penetrate the enamel[85,86].

When the sugar is used up and acid production in the plaque slows, the pH begins to rise and may take 20–30 min to return to its fasting level, the sequence of pH changes being referred to as a 'Stephan Curve' (Figure 4)[80,81]. In addition to forming acid from sugar, the bacteria synthesize several types of polysaccharide from sucrose and continue slowly to form acid from them, which delays the rise in pH. The rise in pH occurs partly because the acid diffuses out, and partly because bicarbonate from saliva diffuses in and neutralizes the acid. A polypeptide present in saliva, known as sialin or the 'pH rise factor', may also enter plaque and, by encouraging base production, play a part in raising the pH[87]. As the pH rises, a value will be reached at which the plaque fluid again becomes saturated with calcium phosphate and above this value some of the apatite dissolved from the enamel may be precipitated. Caries is thus the alternate demineralization during the acid phase followed by some remineralization when the pH has risen. The progress of caries presumably depends on the relative rates of these two opposing processes.

THE MECHANISM OF THE PREVENTION OF CARIES BY FLUORIDE

The much greater success of fluoridation in reducing caries, compared with other procedures, may arise from its action at many stages of the caries process. There is good, although controversial, evidence for three main effects, which complement each other in reducing the progress of caries. They are (1) a decreased solubility of the enamel in acid, (2) a reduction in the bacterial attack, and (3) a reduction in the size of the teeth and in the depths of their fissures.

A contrast must be drawn between the overwhelming clinical evidence for the effectiveness of fluoride in reducing caries – probably the best attested fact in the whole of preventive dentistry – and the question of its mode of action which is still uncertain and controversial.

INTERACTIONS OF FLUORIDE WITH APATITE

Fluoride has a powerful affinity for hydroxyapatite (HA) with which it reacts in several ways, even at concentrations as low as 0.1 ppm[88]. It can exchange with the hydroxyl ion, it can occupy vacancies in the apatite structure[89] and with concentrations above 100 ppm it forms calcium fluoride which becomes adsorbed on the apatite crystal[90], but in an aqueous medium, as in the mouth, is dissolved within a few days. Fluoride uptake by HA is favoured by acid pH values. Although the concentration of fluoride in biological fluids is extremely

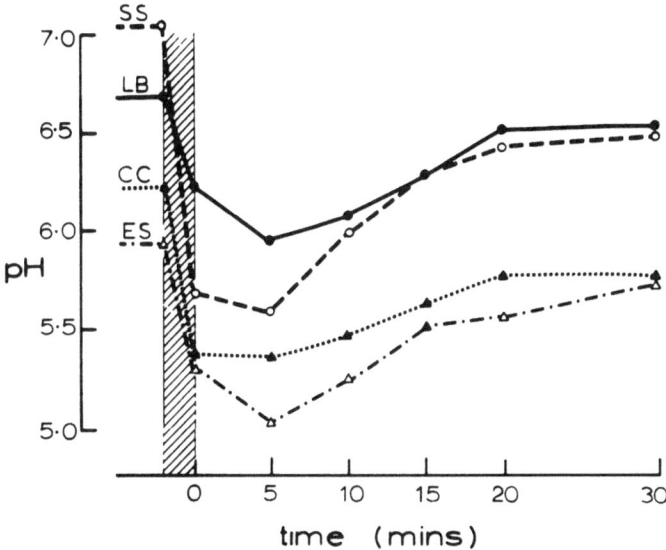

Figure 4 The pH changes in plaque 30 min after a glucose rinse (a 'Stephan curve'). Hatched area indicates period of glucose rinsing. Subject LB was free from caries and the pH values of his plaque were higher than in E. S. who was highly caries prone. (Courtesy of Dr W. M. Edgar)

low (about 0.1 ppm), of which only a small fraction is present as free ions (see later), nevertheless the bones and teeth can take it up and may acquire concentrations of several thousand parts per million in old age[91].

DISTRIBUTION OF FLUORIDE IN THE MINERALIZED TISSUES

The fluoride is not uniformly distributed in the hard tissues. In newly erupted enamel the concentration on the outer surface is up to 10 times greater than that within (Figure 5) and the concentration is related to the amount of fluoride ingested[92–94], which with most diets, is influenced more by the concentration in water than in food.

Early studies based on the analysis of successive layers of enamel, ground or dissolved off the whole tooth surface, suggested that there was a gradual build up of inorganic fluoride with age[93]. The analysis of many small areas of enamel from anterior teeth (dissected off by an etching technique developed by Weatherell and Hargreaves[94]) has shown the tremendous variation in fluoride concentration, and that the outer fluoride-rich layer is lost over much of the enamel with increasing age, presumably by attrition from coarse foods and toothbrushing (Figure 6)[95]. The high fluoride layer on the surface is so thin that little enamel need be removed to cause a marked drop in the surface fluoride concentration. With increasing age, the fluoride concentration tends to rise near the gum line by a process discussed later[95]. The apparent conflict between these results showing a fall in enamel fluoride with age, and the earlier once suggesting a steady increase, probably arose because dissection

33

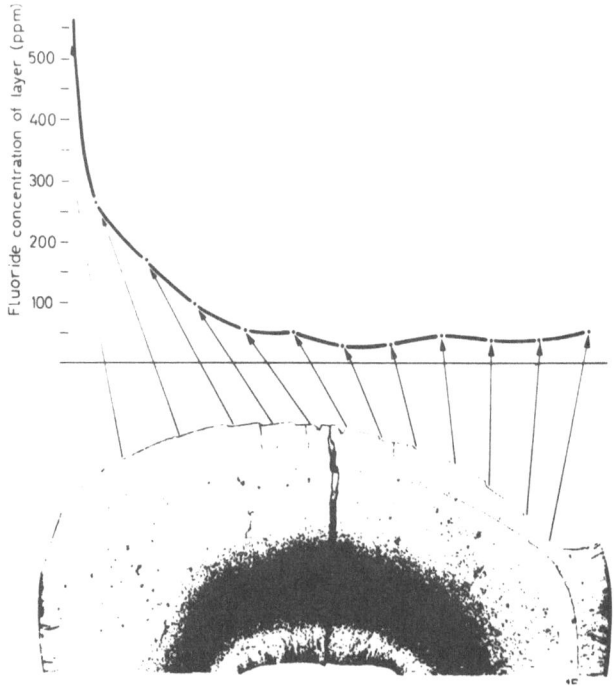

Figure 5 The steep fall in fluoride concentration from the outer surface to the enamel within (upper curve). The lower part of the figure indicates the sites from which the samples were dissolved off for analysis. (Courtesy of Dr J. A. Weatherell and Pergamon Press)

techniques show that the age changes vary in different regions of the tooth, whereas the earlier results applied to the enamel as a whole.

Little *et al.*[96] produced evidence of the accumulation of an organic fluoride on the outer surface of enamel during ageing, especially in discoloured sound enamel and in early carious lesions, which would not have been detected by Weatherell's technique. Its existence has been confirmed (Jenkins unpublished) although in lower concentration than reported by Little *et al.* It is tempting to speculate that the organic fluoride in old teeth resembles the bound fluoride of plaque (discussed later) some of which might be expected, over a lifetime, to become firmly attached to the outer enamel.

REASONS FOR DISTRIBUTION OF FLUORIDE

The high concentration of fluoride on the outer enamel has usually been explained on the assumption that the fluoride was acquired from tissue fluid, by ionic exchange in the apatite crystals. As the inner enamel mineralizes, each layer of apatite would take up some fluoride from the tissue fluid but would be rapidly sealed off by the next layer of crystals. However, before it erupts the outer surface remains in contact with tissue fluid for long periods, even up to

34

several years with some teeth, during which time fluoride could be acquired without any interruption. Even after eruption a tooth continues for some time to acquire minerals, presumably including fluoride. Animal experiments have shown that the resistance to caries increases immediately after eruption, a process, probably of great practical importance, known as 'post-eruptive maturation'[97]. Uptake of fluoride by the enamel is probably one of the factors involved.

Studies on rat, bovine[98] and pig[99] teeth have, however, surprisingly shown that at one early stage in enamel formation, when mineral is entering, the fluoride concentration falls. As this coincides with the removal of organic matter, it seems likely that the fluoride removed is organically bound.

Several techniques have shown that early carious lesions, before cavitation occurs, contain a fluoride concentration two or three times higher than that of adjacent sound enamel[100-102]. Presumably this occurs due to the increased permeability following the dissolving of some apatite, and the exposure of more crystal surfaces to fluoride from oral fluids at the low pH value associated with caries, which favours fluoride uptake by apatite.

Study of the effect of fluoride on enamel has been greatly clarified by biopsies – and two techniques have been developed. In one, enamel is ground off and the powder collected and analysed for fluoride and, in order to estimate

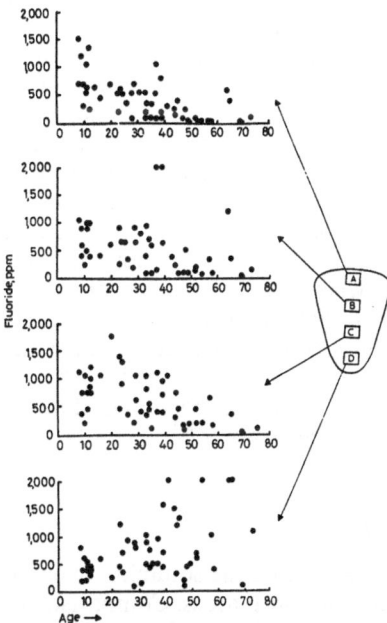

Figure 6   The fluoride concentration on different part of the surfaces of anterior teeth at different ages. In areas A, B and C (the occlusal and central surface of the enamel) the average concentration falls with increasing age, but at D (near the gum line) the concentration tends to rise. (Courtesy of J. A. Weatherell and of *Caries Research*)

sample size, also for calcium[103,104]. In the other method, acid is placed on the enamel either in a filter paper disc or as a drop of 4 or 6 μl of perchloric acid, and after 3–6 s the acid is withdrawn and analysed[105,106]. Owing to the steep gradient of fluoride concentration, control of the depth of the sample is of great importance.

EFFECT OF FLUORIDE ON SOLUBILITY

Fluoride and the solubility of apatite

When an intact tooth or powdered enamel is shaken with a sodium fluoride solution, fluoride is taken up and the solubility of enamel is reduced[107]. This very simple experiment, repeatedly confirmed in many laboratories, suggested that the effect of fluoride in caries prevention is to reduce enamel solubility, presumably by increasing the proportion of fluorapatite, a crystal containing 3.4 % of fluoride and believed on theoretical grounds to be more stable and less soluble than hydroxyapatite.

Biopsies show that a typical concentration of fluoride in the outer 0.5 μm of enamel formed in an 'F area', and enjoying maximal protection from caries, is 2500 ppm (0.25 %) or only about 7 % of the possible substitution of the hydroxyl groups[108]. Moreno et al.[109] found with a series of synthetic apatites containing different percentages of fluoride that the minimum solubility occurred with a substitution of about 50 % of the hydroxyls by fluoride, and that less than 10 % substitution hardly affected solubility. However, the extreme outer crystals of enamel (forming too thin an outer layer for separate analysis) may contain a much higher concentration than the 0.25 % found by biopsy. Another suggestion was that the additional fluoride in enamel found in 'F areas' might not be exchanged with hydroxyl ions but might fill the vacancies known to exist in apatite. The hydroxyl groups of hydroxyapatite are placed within one set of calcium atoms arranged as triangles in the unit cell structure (Figure 7). The number of hydroxyl ions 'pointing above' the triangles is thought to be identical with the number 'pointing down' (Figure 7) so that there must be points where the orientation of the hydroxyls change. For spatial reasons two hydroxyls cannot be orientated in opposite directions in adjacent calcium triangles, so there is a vacancy at changeover points and this might be expected to introduce an instability into the crystal. If fluoride enters these vacancies, and only a small proportion of fluoride might be needed for this, the instability would be removed[89].

Solubility of enamel

The practical question is whether the solubility of enamel formed in a high F area is lower than that from low F areas. Comparison of the solubility in vitro of the outer enamel of teeth from high and low F areas have consistently shown a tendency for a lower solubility of enamel from high F areas but the differences are small with borderline statistical significance (Table 1)[110–114]. In most of these experiments, the rate of dissolution has been measured (i.e. the

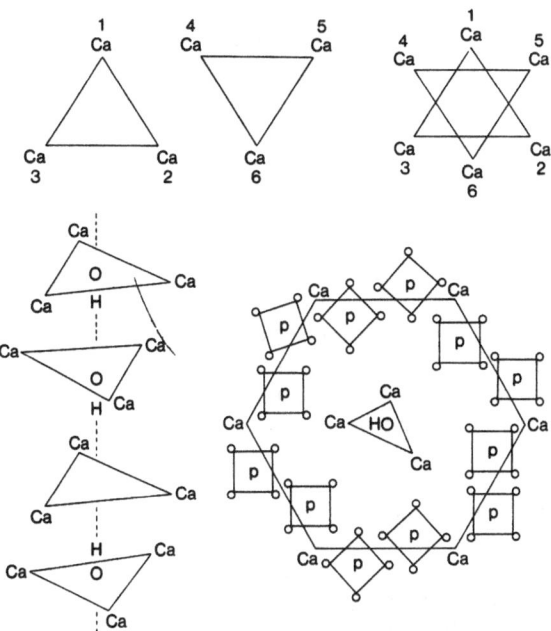

Figure 7 Diagrammatic representation of hydroxyapatite. On the left are the calcium triangles with the hydroxyl groups contained inside them. Vacancies occur where the orientations of the hydroxyl groups change, making the crystal unstable. Fluoride atoms may enter the vacancies and stabilize the apatite. Adjacent calcium triangles are staggered, so that when viewed longitudinally along the C axis they appear as a series of hexagons (top right). The calcium triangles are placed inside hexagons of calcium atoms associated with the phosphate groups (bottom right) (Courtesy of Blackwell Scientific Publications)

amount of enamel dissolving in a fixed volume of buffer solution in a short time) and not the true solubility (the amount dissolved at equilibrium). Dissolution rate is probably relevant to caries, at least in its early stages, as very small amounts of enamel are dissolving in too short a time (the 5–10 min during which the pH is below the critical level) to reach equilibrium. Later,

Table 1 Mean solubility rates (μg/ml P dissolving in acetate buffer in 10 min) of outer enamel from subjects with varying F concentrations in the drinking water

	Approx. ppm F in water			
	0	1	2	% diff
Deciduous teeth	10.4	9.2	—	11.5 (not sig.)
Deciduous teeth	12.0	—	9.5	21 (sig. at 5% level)
Permanent teeth (intact)	12.7	—	12.1	5 (not sig.)
Permanent teeth (carious)	8.2	—	6.7	18 (sig. at 5% level)

Data from Jenkins[115]

when a true cavity has formed, food debris is present and the pH remains low most of the time[115] but the outward diffusion of calcium and phosphate ions probably prevents the establishment of equilibrium.

PHYSICO-CHEMICAL CRITICISM OF SOLUBILITY STUDIES

The validity of these solubility experiments has been questioned by Brown *et al.*[116] who emphasize that simple gravimetric comparison of solubility may give misleading results. They point out that when enamel is exposed to acid, the hydroxyapatite (HA) may not only dissolve but may be partly converted into one of the several other crystalline forms of calcium phosphate (brushite, whitlockite, octa calcium phosphate) each differing in solubility. The solvent may be under-saturated with respect to one crystal, which dissolves, but saturated with respect to another, which crystallizes out. Fluoride is known to play a part in controlling these interconversions[39] so that when fluorapatite (FA) dissolves, the fluoride released may alter the nature of the crystals precipitating out, and thus alter the composition of the liquid phase: such alterations might erroneously suggest that less of the more heavily fluorosed apatite was dissolving. An additional complication is that when HA dissolves, OH^- is released so the pH tends to rise, but when FA dissolves HF is released and the pH may fall. When amounts of HA or FA are dissolved such that equal concentrations of calcium and phosphate are present in the liquid phase, the pH of the FA solution will be lower than that of the HA. Therefore, the effect of the fluoride in the apatite is to ensure that no more dissolves in spite of the lower pH which normally would be expected to dissolve more apatite. In a buffered medium, such as plaque with its high protein content, it is doubtful whether the amounts of apatite dissolving at any one time would be sufficient to affect pH in this way.

Brown *et al.* also point out that the lower pH in the presence of dissolving FA, mentioned above, would tend to reduce the activity of $Ca(OH)_2$ and increase that of unionized H_3PO_4, thus lowering the concentration gradients for the outward movement of calcium and phosphate ions and favouring their inward diffusion. Brown thinks that these effects on diffusion may be more influential than the effect, in the opposite direction, of the reduced common ion. This author, however, questions the applicability of these theoretical considerations to the plaque-enamel environment which is more complicated than the *in vitro* conditions of the experiments of Brown *et al.*

INFLUENCE OF CARBONATE AND MAGNESIUM IN ENAMEL

The apatite in enamel contains carbonate (about 2%) and citrate (about 0.1%) and many trace elements in much lower concentrations. During the mineralization of enamel there is evidence of a reciprocity between the concentrations of fluoride and carbonate entering, and the ratio between the two has been reported to be related to the caries susceptibility of the tooth[117,118] (Table 2). Though more data on this are urgently required, the widespread use of fluoride dentifrices has made it difficult to study the original fluoride content of enamel. It is known that the first mineral to be lost from the enamel in caries is a mixture of calcium and phosphate ions along with a much higher proportion of carbonate and magnesium than is present throughout the enamel[119]. In other words, the carbonate appears to be a vulnerable part of the enamel structure and it might be expected that anything, e.g. fluoride, tending to lower its concentration would reduce the number of sites especially vulnerable to acid.

Table 2 Relationship between fluoride and carbonate on outer surface of enamel to fluoride in drinking water and the presence of caries

	1 ppm in water	0.1 ppm in water
Non-carious teeth		
$CO_3\%$	1.90 ± 0.077	2.07 ± 0.063
F ppm	375 ± 93.6	136 ± 20.6
Ratio	0.53	1.52
Carious teeth		
$CO_3\%$	2.13 ± 0.045	2.03 ± 0.014
F ppm	22.9 ± 50	83 ± 13
Ratio	0.93	2.45

Data from Nikiforuk[117,118]

All the differences in F concentration are significant. The differences between the CO_3 of the teeth from the high and low F areas are not significant, but those between the carious and non-carious are significant in the high F area

There is also evidence that carbonate reduces the size and crystallinity of apatite, i.e. poisons the surface of developing apatite crystals and prevents their growth, whereas fluoride has the opposite effect. Larger crystals have been detected in bone of animals fed high concentrations of fluoride[120] but the data on enamel are contradictory[121,122]. The apatite crystals of enamel are normally about 10 times larger than those in bone and dentine[123] so that there may not be much scope for further increase in size.

EFFECT OF FLUORIDE ON THE PRECIPITATION OF APATITE

Concentrations of fluoride, even as low as 0.1 ppm, in an acid solvent reduce the amount of enamel dissolving[88] and similar additions to a saturated solution of apatite lead to its precipitation. These effects have been independently observed by different workers but they may, of course, be two aspects of the same phenomenon: an apparent reduction in solubility may arise from a precipitation of some of the apatite previously dissolved. When enamel with a high concentration of fluoride dissolves, either into the fluid phase of the innermost layer of plaque, or into the small amount of water in carious enamel, the fluoride released will presumably act in the same way and tend to increase the remineralization of the enamel when the pH rises.

Fluoride favours the deposition of apatite, rather than other less stable crystalline forms from saturated solutions of calcium phosphate, also some fluoride enters the apatite and thus in two ways it increases the resistance of the remineralized enamel. The effect on mineralization is thought by some workers to be the main action of fluoride in caries although conclusive proof is lacking.

SUMMARY

The position on solubility may be summarized as follows: the solubility of apatite is too complicated to decide with certainty whether it is reduced by fluoride, and when remineralization of enamel in the saturated environment of plaque is considered the position is even more complicated. However, fluoride does interact in this system in several ways and if, as seems likely, they are relevant to caries, they would tend to reduce the number and progress of the lesions.

ANTI-ENZYME ACTION OF FLUORIDE IN THE DENTAL PLAQUE

In order to decide the effectiveness of fluoride as an inhibitor of the bacterial enzymes in plaque, and the contribution which such inhibition might make to the reduction of caries, two pieces of information are needed: (1) the concentration of fluoride required to produce significant inhibition of plaque bacteria, and (2) the concentration of fluoride in the plaque, in a form capable of inhibiting bacteria.

THE SENSITIVITY OF SALIVARY BACTERIA TO FLUORIDE

Bibby and van Kesteren[124] reported in 1940 that concentrations of fluoride as low as 1 ppm reduced acid production during the incubation of various oral streptococci and lactobacilli with sugar. Much higher concentrations (250 ppm) were needed to inhibit growth. Similar results were obtained in experiments on the pH fall during the incubation of the mixed organisms in saliva with sugar[125]: 10 ppm produced a marked inhibition (Figure 8) and 1 ppm was the lowest concentration producing a statistically significant inhibition, although non-significant trends were detected with even lower concentrations.

Borei[126] reviewed a number of factors which influenced the inhibition of yeast by fluoride. Sensitivity was increased by a low pH, by anaerobiosis, the fasting state and by increased concentrations of magnesium and phosphate. Lilienthal[127] investigated the importance of these factors in the fluoride inhibition of salivary organisms incubated in a bicarbonate buffer at pH 6.8

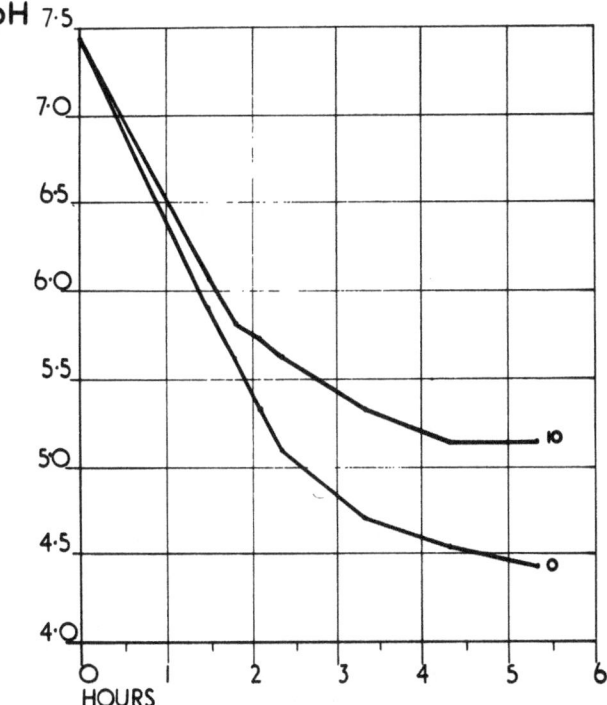

Figure 8 The effect of 10 ppm of fluoride on the pH changes during the incubation of salivary bacteria and glucose. Note that this inhibition is not significant until the pH falls below 6 (Courtesy of Pergamon Press)

(conditions which precluded a study of the effect of pH) and concluded that a minimum of 19 ppm was required for inhibition. Similar experiments were carried out on saliva–glucose mixtures with particular reference to the effect of pH (the point which Lilienthal was unable to test). The results confirmed previous findings on other organisms that fluoride inhibition is greatly increased at pH values of about 5.0[128]. At this pH, incubation of saliva with 10 ppm of fluoride results in a *rise* in pH instead of the usual fall (Figure 9). An analysis of this result showed that lactic acid production was completely stopped while the removal of any lactic acid present was accelerated, and other reactions which raise the pH (ammonia and amine production) were slightly stimulated[129].

THE NATURE OF THE pH SENSITIVITY·

Borei[126] suggested that the greater sensitivity of yeast to fluoride at low pH values might be explained because, as the pH fell, a higher proportion of fluoride was present as HF and that the cell wall was more permeable to HF than to fluoride. Experiments in the author's laboratory (Katayama,

41

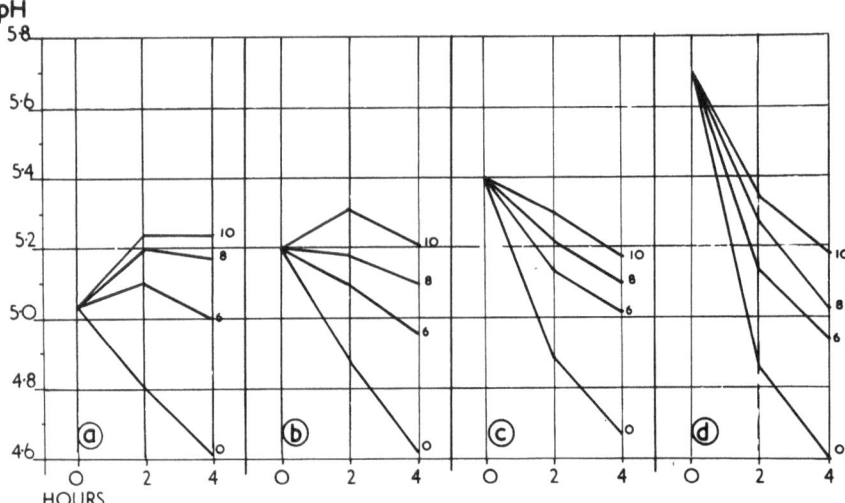

Figure 9 The effect of 6, 8 and 10 ppm of fluoride on the pH changes of incubated saliva–glucose mixtures adjusted to pH values between 5 and 5.7. At 5.05 the pH rises during the incubation with 8 and 10 ppm F. (Courtesy of Pergamon Press)

unpublished) have detected an increased entry *in vitro* of fluoride into oral organisms as the pH is reduced to 5.0 but, having entered the cell at 5.0, the increased fluoride exerted little inhibitory effect when the medium was adjusted back to pH 7. Increased uptake of fluoride at lower pH values does not seem, therefore, to explain the greater sensitivity at pH 5.0.

An alternative explanation for pH sensitivity is that the conformation of enolase (the enzyme thought to be the most sensitive to fluoride) at pH 5.5 might be more susceptible to inhibition by fluoride than at 7.0. However, tests on this in the author's laboratory[141] showed the opposite, the enzyme was more sensitive at pH 7.2 ($K_I = 4.7 \times 10^{-4}$ mol l^{-1}) than at pH 5.5 ($K_I = 8 \times 10^{-4}$ mol l^{-1}). The greater fluoride sensitivity of oral organisms at lower pH values cannot yet be explained.

THE CONCENTRATION OF FLUORIDE IN PLAQUE

These data on the inhibitory concentrations of fluoride tended to discount the importance of enzyme inhibition because concentrations in saliva were reported to be about 0.1 ppm – too low for inhibition, and direct contact of the bacteria with the 1 ppm in the drinking water was assumed to be of too short a duration to affect the bacteria. No attempts were made to investigate the fluoride concentration of plaque until about 1960, when Hardwick and Leach[130] reported their astonishing finding that plaque samples collected randomly from dental patients contained between 6 and 180 ppm of fluoride on a wet weight basis (estimated by colorimetric methods) and exceeded the concentration in the saliva bathing by a factor of several hundred.

Comparison of the fluoride concentration in plaque from residents in high and low F areas showed that fluoride in the plaque was related to that in the water[131], although the values obtained at first were higher than more recent findings (Table 3) (see later).

Table 3 Comparison of fluoride concentration in water and in plaque (ppm dry weight)

	ppm fluoride		
In water	0.1	1.0	1.0
In plaque	13.5 ± 8.3	22.6 ± 16.8	25.6 ± 16.4

From Agus *et al.*[133]

Clearly, the plaque must bind the fluoride in some way, as it is inconceivable that such a concentration gradient could be otherwise maintained. Shortly after the discovery of these high concentrations, the method of estimating fluoride – previously difficult and with low accuracy when present within biological material – was revolutionized by the introduction of the fluoride specific ion electrode[132]. This made the estimation of concentrations of ionic fluoride down to about 0.1 ppm relatively easy (although still full of pitfalls and requiring caution in interpreting the results), but unfortunately the concentration in biological fluids is considerably less than this and is very near the limits of accuracy even of this method. Estimation of the ionic fluoride in plaque by the electrode showed that it represents at most only a few per cent of the total. The total fluoride of plaque estimated with the electrode, after its release by various procedures, gave results of about 5–10 ppm, considerably lower than those first obtained by colorimetric methods[133]. But, as the concentration in saliva was also found to be lower (about 0.02 ppm) than previously thought[134,135] the ratio of hundreds to one is still valid.

THE NATURE OF PLAQUE FLUORIDE

Three possibilities arose to explain the high concentration of fluoride in plaque: it could be bound to calcium phosphate (although the existence of this salt in plaque *in vivo* is uncertain), to the organic matrix or within or on the surface of the bacteria. Birkeland[136] concluded that the fluoride was present as fluorapatite because he found that when saliva is allowed to stand its fluoride concentration falls, due to the formation of precipitates of calcium phosphate which incorporate the fluoride. If the precipitation is prevented by the addition of acid or citrate, the fluoride concentration did not fall.

The present reviewer accepts Birkeland's results on saliva *in vitro*, but doubts whether they are relevant to the whole of the fluoride plaque *in vivo*. The matrix of plaque is a calcium phosphate–protein complex but it is doubtful whether apatite exists as such in plaque. Kaufman and Kleinberg[137] detected apatite by X-ray diffraction but the plaque has to be dried before examination by this method, and it seems likely that apatite might crystallize during the processing even if it were not present in the original plaque *in vivo*. Extracts of plaque with neutral buffers which removed calcium and phosphate (although not in the calcium/phosphate ratio of apatite) did not contain fluoride, as would be expected if it were bound to the apatite[138].

Singer *et al.*[139] reported that when plaque was diluted, its fluoride was readily diffusible so they favoured a binding mechanism to a small molecule. However, if the plaque is suspended in a small volume of water the fluoride does not diffuse – apparently the great dilution used by Singer *et al.* released the fluoride in a diffusible form. If the constituents of plaque matrix are shaken with fluoride there is no evidence of binding[140] thus disproving the second possibility and leading to the third hypothesis, that the plaque fluoride is associated with the bacteria.

THE EFFECT OF FLUORIDE ON PLAQUE BACTERIA

This was tested by growing a pure culture of various oral organisms in media containing fluoride, then washing and estimating the fluoride in the bacteria. Some species were found to be capable of taking up fluoride to concentrations many times greater than those of the medium, provided it contained less than a ceiling of about 50 ppm – above which no further concentration occurred: the value obtained depended on the method of analysis[141]. Bacteria grown on a medium without added fluoride contained concentrations up to 5 ppm, taken up from the 0.2 ppm present in the medium as a contaminant (Table 4A) but higher concentrations were needed for the bacteria to build up levels comparable with those in plaque. Many bacteria grown in the laboratory on synthetic media probably contain higher concentrations of fluoride than has

Table 4 (A) Estimation by two methods of fluoride stored in mixed plaque bacteria grown with or without fluoride in their medium

F added to medium (ppm)	Analysis by method A*	method B†
0	0.6	5.6
1	1.3	7.1
10	8.8	20.4
50	28.3	47.3

(B) Typical estimations of fluoride in pooled plaque

method A*	method B†
4.1	8.3

* diffused with 0.5 mmol/l $HClO_4$ at room temperature.
† diffused with 50% H_2SO_4 at 60°C.
Data from Edgar and Jenkins[141] and unpublished data.

been realized. Analysis of cultures of several species chosen at random all contained higher concentrations than the media on which they were grown[142]. Analysis of extracts of the bacteria with cold perchloric acid ('ionisable' fluoride) gave values about half those obtained with more destructive methods involving hot, concentrated acids, thus suggesting that two forms of fluoride are present, one much more firmly bound than the other[141,143]. Analysis of plaque by the same two methods also gave higher values with the hot acid thus strengthening the probability that plaque fluoride was associated with the bacteria (Table 4B).

The cells, after washing (to remove any free fluoride adhering to them from the medium) and occasionally overnight storage, were suspended in fresh medium containing glucose but no fluoride, and any pH change measured. Some mixed cultures of oral organisms and some species in pure culture were inhibited, others produced virtually as large a pH drop when their fluoride concentration was high whilst some species gave no consistent pattern (Table 5)[142]. There was no clear relationship between the degree of inhibition and the concentration of fluoride taken up in either the ionisable or bound form[142]. Non-growing cells of some species (*Strep. sanguis*, *Lactobacillus casei*) take up fluoride when exposed to a solution for 30–60 min, the uptake being slightly enhanced at pH 5.5 compared with pH 7[143]. However, when non-growing cells took up fluoride it inhibited their ability to form acid from glucose only slightly, if at all.

pH CHANGES IN PLAQUE FROM HIGH AND LOW F AREAS

Plaque was collected from children resident in high and low F areas who had been requested not to clean their teeth for 24 h previously, and samples from three to four children with similar numbers of decayed teeth were pooled, weighed portions were incubated with sugar and the pH measured in a one-drop glass electrode after 15 min[144]. The results (Table 6) of two series of tests were in agreement in showing a slightly smaller fall in pH of the plaque from

Table 5 Uptake of total F (ppm wet weight) and final pH after 24 h incubation with glucose by selected bacteria grown with and without F in the media

	F in bacteria grown in media containing:		pH after incubation of bacteria in F-free medium after growth in:	
	0	10 ppm	0	10 ppm
Strep. mutans LM7	5.2	16.9	3.50	3.52
Staph. albus	4.3	27.2	3.53	4.18
Mixed salivary organisms	10.5	24.8	4.18	4.94
Mixed plaque	9.3	14.6	4.65	4.85

All the organisms took up fluoride to concentrations greater than in the media, but the fluoride did not always inhibit acid production (e.g. *Strep. mutans*).

From Reference 142 and unpublished data.

Table 6 *In vitro* pH changes in plaques from high and low fluoride towns
(20 mg plaque and 20 µl sucrose solution)

| F of water | Mean pH | | Mean diff | No. of expts | p |
	Initial	15 min			
0	6.28	4.89			
			0.15 ± 0.12	34	<0.001
1.8	6.32	5.04			
0	6.30	4.88			
			0.05 ± 0.09	13	between 0.1 and 0.05
1.0	6.38	4.93			

Data from Jenkins *et al.*[144]

the high F areas which was statistically significant in Hartlepool (fluoride concentration of water then 1.9 ppm), but failed to reach conventional levles of significance in Watford (artificially fluoridated at 1 ppm). Although these results seemed to indicate that the higher fluoride concentrations in the plaque from the F areas had a direct effect in inhibiting acid production, other interpretations were possible. Subjects free from caries tend to have higher plaque pH values in the fasting state and they fall to a smaller extent after sugar than do plaques from subjects with a high caries activity[145-147] (Figure 4) an observation usually taken to support the causal nature of the pH changes in caries. In the 'F areas' (especially in Hartlepool with 1.9 ppm) there are many more children free from caries and with lower DMF values than in North Shields, the low F area chosen. The differences in pH might arise as a secondary result from the different caries prevalence of the two towns. It was possible to test this because the plaques were pooled on the basis of donors with similar DMF values. The results (Table 7) confirmed that the effect was related to fluoride rather than caries, because when groups with low or medium DMF were compared the pH differences were still present. The groups with high DMF did not show this but the number in the high F population was small.

Similar tests on the effect of fluoride on plaque pH were made on students in Newcastle upon Tyne and Durham City before and 2 months after the introduction of fluoridation in the former city[148]. The pH changes *in vitro* of

Table 7 pH in plaques classified on basis of caries after 15 min incubation with sucrose

| | F in water | |
	0	1.8
DMF <2	4.82 (6)	5.00 (29)
DMF 2-8	4.56 (37)	4.76 (28)
DMF >8	4.67 (16)	4.60 (7)

No. of observations in brackets

the plaques from the two cities were identical before fluoridation, but the Newcastle plaques after fluoridation did not fall quite so far, the differences being statistically significant (Table 8). For reasons beyond control, comparison of the 'before' figures with the 'after' figures for each city is not valid, but scrupulous care was taken to make the figures from the two cities comparable on each of the six occasions when the plaques were collected.

Although several lines of evidence suggest therefore that plaque fluoride reduces acid production, the effect is admittedly small. However, if it is real and we accept the concept of a 'critical pH' above which no enamel dissolves, small differences in the pH change occurring near the critical values may be of considerable practical importance.

Table 8 Mean plaque pH values after 15 min incubations with sucrose

| City | pH | |
	Before Fluoridation	After Fluoridation
Newcastle	5.21 ± 0.44 (27)	5.07 ± 0.20 (22)
Durham	5.21 ± 0.26 (17)	4.94 ± 0.24 (32)
	Sig. ($p < 0.01$)	

No. of observations in brackets.
Data from Edgar et al.[148]

THE POSSIBLE SITES OF FLUORIDE INHIBITION IN PLAQUE BACTERIA

It was naturally assumed that fluoride inhibited glycolysis in oral bacteria at the enolase stage following the discovery by Warburg and Christian (1941) of the high fluoride sensitivity of this enzyme[149]. Early attempts to detect the accumulation of 2-phosphoglyceric acid (2-PGA) in bacteria incubated with fluoride (which might be expected if enolase were inhibited) failed, suggesting that some other site might be affected. However, after the application of 50 ppm at pH 5.8 a rise in 2-PGA was detected in *Strep. salivarious*[150]. The synthesis of intracellular polysaccharides by oral bacteria and the formation of acid from this endogenous source were also inhibited by fluoride[150,151]. Acid formation from these polysaccharides may continue in the plaque after ingested sugar has been diluted by saliva and swallowed. This prolonged source of acid is believed to be one of the factors responsible for the slowness of the return of the pH to fasting levels in the 'Stephan curve' after its rapid drop following contact with sugar so that its inhibition – by reducing the duration of time when the pH is below the critical figure – could be important in reducing caries.

Although acid production and the synthesis of these polysaccharides from exogenous sugar are equally sensitive, the breakdown of the polysaccharides is much less sensitive[150]. The site common to exogenous acid production and polysaccharide synthesis is glucose uptake by the cell and the effect of fluoride upon it became clear with the discovery of the phosphoenolpyruvate (PEP) phosphotransferase system[152]. This system functions in many oral streptococci and requires PEP for the uptake of glucose. If enolase is inhibited, there will be insufficient PEP generated to phosphorylate the glucose so the cell will be starved of glucose (or other sugars on which the system also operates).

Van Houte *et al.*[153] reported that the number of plaque bacteria synthesizing intracellular polysaccharides was significantly lower in an 'F area' than in its control. But whether fluoride reduces the synthesis by individual organisms or the number of organisms able to synthesize polysaccharides was not determined. The proportion of cells producing these polysaccharides was higher (56.9 %) in the caries-active compared with caries-free children (39.0 %). When plaque from sound caries-free teeth from the high and low F areas were compared, no difference was found, which again raises doubts as to whether fluoride was the cause of the lower proportion of polysaccharide-storing organisms or whether this was an indirect effect of lower caries prevalence.

FLUORIDE AND PLAQUE WEIGHT

The concentration of fluoride in an individual plaque has been stated to be inversely related to the weight of plaque collected from that individual, i.e. the larger the amount of plaque present the lower its fluoride concentration[133,154,155]. It is also known that in thicker plaques the pH after sugar falls to lower values[155-157]. The sequence of events could conceivably be: if small deposits of plaque are present, the pH drop is decreased and at the same time the fluoride concentration tends to be high: this might be misinterpreted as a direct effect of fluoride on pH drop. Some *in vitro* studies have suggested that a high fluoride concentration in enamel reduces the tendency for it to adsorb salivary proteins[158,159]. Others[160,161] have found the opposite – that FA adsorbs more macromolecules than HA and also that fluoride influences the type of protein adsorbed, suggesting that the composition of pellicle might vary with different proportions of fluoride[161]. There are no satisfactory data on the amount of plaque or the composition of pellicle in populations in high and low F areas. Such measurements however are extremely difficult owing to great individual variation in, for example, the thoroughness of toothbrushing. There are reports that fluoride mouthrinses reduce plaque formation in children[162] but they involve very high concentrations of fluoride and are of doubtful relevance to the concentrations available from drinking water. No attempt appears to have been made to compare specifically the plaque weights in high and low fluoride areas, but when such plaques have been collected and weighed for other determinations, there has been no suggestion that their weights differed. Although the correlation of fluoride with plaque weight is still a conceivable explanation of what appears to be differences in pH changes, there are no firm grounds for believing this.

SUMMARY OF THE ACTION OF FLUORIDE IN PLAQUE

Although there is considerable and varied evidence for a direct inhibitory effect of plaque fluoride on the bacteria, none of it is conclusive because alternative explanations are possible, if not particularly likely. Some apparent inhibition may arise from other effects of fluoride (e.g. changes in weight). However, plaque fluoride does have other actions which tend to reduce caries. The ionic fluoride of plaque, even at its very low concentration, might be expected to reduce the demineralizing effect of the acid formed by the bacteria as the addition of fluoride in concentrations as low as 0.1 ppm to an acid buffer certainly does[88]. This fluoride is also likely to increase remineralization during the phase of rising pH of the 'Stephan curve'[81]. It will also enter the apatite of the enamel, especially when the plaque pH is low and is probably the source of the increased enamel fluoride found in plaque-covered parts of the tooth surface shown in Figure 6. The higher uptake in early lesions probably also arises from the plaque. The bound fluoride of plaque may enter the enamel to form the organic fluoride reported in old and slightly carious enamel, although the effect of this material on enamel, if any, is unknown.

The finding that fluoride needs to be taken after eruption to exert its full effect, and the many observations with rinses that frequency of dosing is more important than concentration, all point to an effect on plaque. Because plaque forms every day on individuals who brush their teeth, plaque fluoride requires constant replenishment unlike enamel fluoride which, contrary to earlier beliefs, does not seem to be taken up readily in a stable form except via plaque.

THE SOURCE OF PLAQUE FLUORIDE

Three possible sources of fluoride suggest themselves: (1) saliva or gingival fluid (the fluid seeping from the gingival crevices surrounding the teeth), (2) food and drink, (3) the outer surface of enamel. Although a constant source of fluoride is necessary to maintain plaque levels, the absolute amount required is very small. About 10 mg of plaque (wet weight) is formed each day and if it contains, say 10 ppm of fluoride, the amount of fluoride entering the plaque is only 0.1 μg per day. Experiments on bacteria grown in culture suggest that concentrations greater than 0.2 ppm are necessary before they can build up levels similar to those in plaque. The concentration of fluoride in saliva is usually less than 0.05 ppm and values below 0.01 ppm have been recorded, i.e. below the required level. The fluoride concentration of gingival fluid does not appear to have been estimated in man but when ^{18}F was injected into dogs within a few minutes the concentration in gingival fluid equalled that of plasma (MacFadyen *et al.*, personal communication) but would be expected to be too low to be used by the bacteria. In view of its intimate contact with plaque in the gingival region it could be one source, but is probably insufficient in quantity to account for the whole. It is tempting to speculate that plaque must contain some substance(s) which can bind fluoride and later release it under certain conditions, e.g. a reduced pH forming local concentrations higher than in saliva, and thus allowing the uptake and accumulation of fluoride by the bacteria. Apatite has these properties although as mentioned above, our evidence does not support its presence in plaque. The fluoride in saliva is only very slightly affected by the ingestion of 1 mg (in one dose)[163,164], of fluoride as sodium fluoride so that the effects of the much smaller amounts of fluoride taken at any one time in drinking water would be even less[165] and are thus unlikely to explain the higher plaque fluoride in high F areas. The most likely source of this extra fluoride in plaque from high F areas seems to be the direct contact of plaque with water during drinking. Although the contact time of drinks with the tooth is short, a certain amount of water probably lingers in the vicinity of the tooth – perhaps sufficiently to increase the concentration in plaque. The 0.1 μg of fluoride entering the average plaque daily is equivalent to the fluoride content of as little as 10 ml of saliva or 0.1 ml of fluoridated water.

Enamel seems an unlikely source of plaque fluoride because, if its fluoride were transferred to the plaque, calculation shows that it would soon lose its high concentration and cease to be a source. The evidence shows that plaque-covered enamel slowly gains fluoride[95,156], rather than loses it, and is almost certainly taking it up from the plaque.

EFFECT OF FLUORIDE ON THE MORPHOLOGY OF THE TOOTH

When sodium fluoride solution containing approximately 0.1 mg F was injected into rats, at an age when their teeth were developing, it resulted in slightly smaller teeth with much wider fissures than normal being produced[166]. Such changes might be expected to make the teeth more self-cleansing and therefore less liable to caries.

Careful measurements of the size of cusps and depths of fissures in human teeth formed in high or low F areas have shown a favourable effect of fluoride[167,168] but, although most of the differences were statistically significant, they were small and of doubtful practical value in protecting against caries. Some observers[168,169] found that fluoride is associated with larger teeth while others[167,170] reported that the teeth were smaller in 'F areas'. Thus the small effects of fluoride on the shape of the teeth may contribute slightly to the anti-caries action but the reports on the effects on size are inconsistent.

THE METABOLISM OF FLUORIDE

Fluoride intake

The concentration of fluoride in most foods is between 0.5 and 1 ppm (wet weight)[171]. Early analyses (collected by McClure[172]) suggested that fish were high in fluoride but the material analysed appears to have included the skin and bones, and more recent analyses show that the edible flesh contains less than 1 ppm[173,174]. Typical fish skin contains 8 ppm (wet weight) possibly taken up from the sea water which averages 1.4 ppm F and only the bones are a really rich source. Even when edible, as in tinned sardines and salmon, the total amount of bone in an average helping would not provide more than 1 or 2 mg of fluoride. The only rich source of fluoride in the British diet is tea[175,176]. For unknown reasons, the tea plant has the capacity for taking up fluoride from the soil (normally containing fluoride in concentrations up to several hundred ppm) and transferring it to the leaves so that when they are dried the concentration ranges from 100 to 260 ppm. The concentration in the infusion varies from 0.1 to 3.4 ppm (in low F areas) depending on the brand and strength of the tea: the practice of 'watering the pot' usually means that second and subsequent cups are about half the concentration of the first brew[177]. In an 'F area' with 1 ppm these values are, of course, 1 ppm higher.

In a low F area, the fluoride intake is dominated by the amount of tea drunk, and in an 'F area' the total volume of fluid, and the proportion taken as tea, virtually determines the intake. In one American survey, the total average intake of non-fluoridated water was 0.86 mg (range 0.73–0.94) and of fluoridated water 1.96 mg (range 1.23–2.41)[171]. An estimate of intake under British conditions is given in Table 9.

Table 9 Estimated fluoride intake (mg) in Britain

	No F in water	F in water
Food	0.5–1.0	1–2 (?)
Tea (5 cups)	1–3.0	2–4
Other drinks (5 cups)	0	0.8
Total	1.5–4.0	3.8–6.8
Without tea	0.5–1.0	2.6–3.6

It has been stated[178] that with extensive fluoridation of water the fluoride content of cooked and processed foods tends to rise. This seems likely, but the USA is the only large country where fluoridation is sufficiently widespread for a significant rise to occur in processed foods, but some fluoride also enters foods when cooked in fluoridated water.

Absorption

The absorption of fluoride is rapid and begins in the stomach[179] and continues in the upper intestine almost to completion, as the fluoride in the faeces is normally only about 5–10 % of intake. Experiments with everted gut sacs show that absorption does not occur against a concentration gradient[180] so there is no evidence for active transport.

The calcium and phosphate in the diet can affect the absorption of fluoride. In rats, addition of phosphate alone to the diet increased fluoride absorption (the explanation is unknown) and calcium reduced it (presumably by forming calcium fluoride with a solubility of only 16 ppm)[181]. Phosphate given simultaneously with calcium reduced the absorption more than calcium alone[182], as calcium phosphate is precipitated at neutral pH it would take up more of the fluoride. If calcium and phosphate were given 15 min after the fluoride their effect was smaller, presumably some fluoride was absorbed in the stomach before the calcium and phosphate was given. Fluoride is not well absorbed if given as calcium fluoride or with calcium phosphate, as in bone meal[183] (which has been recommended as a caries preventive) or in the bone of tinned fish. The limited absorption from bones probably occurs in the stomach when some of the bone dissolves and releases its fluoride.

NATURAL VERSUS ARTIFICIAL FLUORIDE

This raises the question of whether other constituents of a water supply can affect the metabolism of fluoride. It has been widely believed by laymen that the actions of 'natural' and 'artificial' fluoride may differ, especially in toxicity. This was based on the idea that 'natural' fluoride was present as calcium fluoride (non-toxic as a solid, owing to its low solubility), whereas in artificial fluoridation usually sodium fluoride (very soluble and with a lethal dose of about 5 g) or sodium fluorosilicate is added to water. In this form, the argument is, of course, absurd but the more general question of the effect of other elements in water on the metabolism and action of fluoride requires consideration; most waters with 'natural' fluoride are hard, well waters derived from chalk or magnesium limestone, whereas the hardness is quite irrelevant to artificial fluoridation.

The effects of several ions, at concentrations likely to be present in the gut, on the activity of fluoride were tested with the fluoride electrode[184]; calcium reduced F activity by 2%, magnesium by 6.6%, and aluminium was the only powerful complexer, 0.3 ppm complexed 35.5% of 1 ppm of fluoride. A small scale experiment in the author's laboratory showed that 3 mg of aluminium (as $AlCl_3$) along with 3 mg of fluoride (as NaF) reduced the urinary excretion by less than 20%, but whether this was caused by reduced absorption or increased storage was not determined. The proportion of aluminium to fluoride was much higher than would occur in a water supply (usually less than 0.2 ppm) so even this small difference would not be expected. Therefore, in practice, aluminium in water is unlikely to interfere with the metabolism of fluoride, although the much higher concentrations in food might do so[184].

It may be concluded that the ions normally present in hard water are unlikely to influence fluoride metabolism, and this is confirmed by the experiments in which naturally fluoridated water (1 ppm and 8 ppm from Bartlett, Texas) was fed to rats and the fluoride storage was compared with that of distilled water containing the same added concentration as NaF[185]. There was a small non-significant tendency for less fluoride to be stored in the skeleton from the natural source than from the controls. This experiment has been repeated on mice in the present author's laboratory on water from Hartlepool (natural fluoride now 1.5 ppm), Newcastle and deionised water (artificially made up to 1.5 ppm). The experiment is still in progress but results so far suggest no significant difference.

Another point relevant to the hardness of water is sometimes raised. What is the effect of boiling the water down, either absent mindedly or in soups or stews which are slowly simmered? Marked differences in the behaviour of Hartlepool and Newcastle water have been found[174] confirming other studies on hard water[186]. The presence of the high magnesium concentration in Hartlepool water results in a cloudy precipitate appearing when the volume is reduced to about 75% of the original. Further reduction of the volume increases the precipitate and the concentration of fluoride rises to about 3 ppm but does not exceed it. On the other hand, in Newcastle water with a similar calcium but a much lower magnesium concentration, the fluoride concentration rises to 14 ppm before reaching a ceiling[174]. It seems most unlikely that a dangerous concentration would be reached repeatedly in the same household, if only because of the cost of the wasted fuel. Highly concentrated Newcastle water is dark brown and so uninviting that its ingestion is unlikely.

EXCRETION AND SKELETAL STORAGE

After absorption, fluoride is either rapidly taken up by the skeleton or excreted in the urine. The fluoride concentration in bone of lifelong residents of Britain increases steadily with age, reaching 2000–3000 ppm by age 80 in the compact bone and, because of its greater contact with blood, about double this figure in cancellous bone[91]. Bone storage occurs at all levels of intake, contrary to early statements by McClure[183,187] that in waters containing less than 5 ppm, excretion was complete. The proportion stored in bone tends to fall with increasing age, presumably because the higher the fluoride concentration in the bone crystals the more difficult it becomes for them to take up more. Similarly, when fluoride is introduced into a water supply, the urinary excretion rises to a constant value within weeks in adults but may take several years to reach a steady state in children[188]. Other changes in the composition of bone, when its fluoride content rises following increased ingestion, are a fall in sodium, carbonate and citrate and a rise in magnesium[189]. Similar changes probably occur as the fluoride concentration increases with ageing.

When the fluoride in the water of Bartlett, Texas, was suddenly reduced from 8 to about 1 ppm, the average urinary concentration fell within 1 week from 7.7 ppm to 5.1 ppm, but even 2 years later was still considerably higher (2.5 ppm) than that of the drinking water[190]. There was no apparent relation between the age of the adults and the pattern of excretion, but the children (aged 7–16) mobilized rather more fluoride than did the adults. The loss from the adult skeleton was probably from recently acquired fluoride on the surface of apatite crystals, but in the younger skeletons some additional fluoride might be lost in the course of the remodelling associated with growth.

About half the daily input is excreted in the urine, much of it within a few hours of ingestion. The proportion of the daily output in the urine is increased by diuresis, so that more is lost when fluoride is taken in water rather than as tablets or other concentrates[191]. The renal clearance of fluoride is greatly increased if the pH of urine falls. Between 35 and 45% of the fluoride in the glomerular filtrate is reabsorbed in the proximal tubule irrespective of the pH, but in acidosis most of the reabsorption occurs in the distal tubule probably in the non-ionic form of HF[192]. If the fluoride of urine is studied under conditions of constant intake either (1) by allowing the urine to remain in the bladder for several hours or (2) by collecting urine at frequent intervals so that none of it remains in the bladder for long, the amount excreted is slightly higher in the latter case. This suggests some absorption from the bladder (Jenkins and Edgar, unpublished).

Sweat

Some fluoride is lost in the sweat, concentrations of 0.3 to 1.8 ppm[183,187] having been reported. Although these values were obtained long before the development of accurate micro-methods of analysis, their trend was confirmed by the finding of a sharp fall in urine concentration when experimental subjects on a controlled fluoride intake were placed in hot, moist conditions[188,193].

The fluoride of blood plasma

The rapidity of the uptake by bone and the excretion by the kidney results in very low and fairly constant levels in the body fluids (about 0.1 ppm or 5 μm/l total fluoride). As methods of analysis have improved, the published values for the concentration in blood have fallen. Until the introduction of the specific ion electrode, it had not been possible to detect any relation between the fluoride levels in plasma and drinking water unless the latter exceeded 2.5 ppm[194]. Slightly higher concentrations of ionic fluoride have now been detected with water at 1 ppm compared with controls, with a daily peak in the afternoon[195,273]. The plasma concentration rises slightly with advancing age especially in high F areas[196,197], probably because it is in equilibrium with bone fluoride which, as mentioned above, increases with age[196]. It falls steadily throughout pregnancy[197].

Taves[198,199,273] found that ionic fluoride concentrations in serum were much lower than those obtained either by ashing or by diffusion techniques involving strong acids and colorimetric methods, an observation later confirmed by direct reading with the fluoride electrode[200,201]. This suggests that serum contains two forms of fluoride, the majority being bound and about 20% existing as free ion (approximately 0.02 ppm or 1 μmol/l). Taves[202] carried out electrophoresis of plasma to which ^{18}F had been added, and found that the mobility of 80% coincided with that of albumin.

Singer and Armstrong[203] confirmed that a high proportion of serum fluoride was bound, but concluded that it was not to albumin but to a constituent with a molecular weight not greater than 25 000. Fractionation on Sephadex of human sera to which ^{18}F had been added also failed to show any binding to macromolecules[204].

Venkateswarlu[205] concluded that colorimetric methods on diffusates of serum were in serious error as an unidentified volatile substance interfered with the colorimetric test greatly increasing the reading. He concluded that all the inorganic fluoride in serum is ultrafiltrable and ionic. Patterson et al.[206]

compared the results obtained by six methods of analysis on serum collected from sheep, rabbits and rats before, and at intervals after, injection of 3 mg/kg body weight of fluoride as sodium fluoride. Ashing or diffusion with acid gave results about four times higher than direct measurements with the electrode. They showed marked species differences in that fluoride was released by perchloric acid from the sera of sheep and rabbits but was released from rat sera by perchloric acid only after ashing.

No conclusion is yet possible about the nature of serum fluoride. There is wide, but not universal, agreement that there are two forms and it is now considered unlikely that the bound form is attached to protein and its nature is still uncertain. At one time, Taves[202] speculated that it might be fluorocitrate or fluoroacetate derived in traces from vegetable foods. Later, after fractionation[201] of plasma, he concluded that it was present as perfluorooctanoic acid derived from the atmosphere contaminated with the fluoridated hydrocarbons widely used as propellants in sprays[273].

THE RELATIVE IMPORTANCE OF CONCENTRATION V. AMOUNT OF INGESTED FLUORIDE

It would seem fundamentally unsound, although convenient, to compare the effect of fluoride on populations on a basis of concentration in their water ('1 ppm' compared with '2 ppm', etc.) although this is usual in the dental literature. It would be expected that total intake would be relevant, so that a child consuming, say, 1 litre of water containing 1 ppm would be affected in the same way as another consuming 500 ml with 2 ppm. The clear correlation between the average DMF in large populations and the concentration of fluoride in a water arises because in large populations the average fluid intakes will be similar.

Ruzicka et al.[207] posed the question whether the concentration or total intake of fluoride was the more important in determining the biological effects. They compared the storage of fluoride in mouse bone on intakes of, e.g. 6 ml of 60 ppm or 2.4 ml of 150 ppm (i.e. both groups received 0.36 mg per day). With these very high doses they found that the storage was much greater from the small volume with higher concentration than from the same absolute amount of fluoride contained in a larger volume of lower concentration (Table 10). A higher concentration in drinking water would presumably raise plasma concentrations much more, be more likely to affect storage and produce enzyme effects than the divided dose. This finding may favour the practice of taking fluoride as 1 mg or 0.25 mg tablets, or even in school milk (about one fifth of a child's fluid intake) in which the concentration would need to be about 5 ppm to provide the same amount ot fluoride as fluoridated water. This work is being repeated, by the present reviewer, on a range of doses and results so far confirm that with high concentrations (3 ml of 50 ppm or 1 ml of 150 ppm) the storage of fluoride in bone is affected more by the concentration than by the total amount ingested. This difference did not occur when bone storage from 1 ml of water containing 30 ppm fluoride exposure was compared with that from 3 ml with 10 ppm. Therefore, there would seem to be no

Table 10   Comparison of the effect of concentration of fluoride versus total intake on bone structure in mice

Conc. of F in drinking water (ppm)	Daily Intake (mg)	% of F in ash		Degree of Fluorosis
		Tibiae	Incisors	
60	0.36	0.73	0.33	1.24
150	0.36	0.84	0.59	2.53
150	0.90	0.94	0.58	2.15
375	0.90	1.09	0.93	2.89

Data from Ruzicka et al. (1973)[207].

The results show that on equal intakes (0.36 mg) the high concentration of 150 ppm leads to more storage of F in bone and teeth and more severe fluorosis; widely different intakes (0.36 and 0.90 mg), but at the same concentration (150 ppm) produce similar storage and fluorosis.

contraindications to the fluoridation of milk from the metabolic point of view, but there is some slight risk of mottling from fluoride tablets which, for a short time, raise blood levels to a greater level than does fluoridated water.

IS FLUORIDE AN ESSENTIAL ELEMENT?

The widespread distribution of trace amounts of fluoride in foods, and the problem of removing it, has made it extremely difficult to provide an acceptable and adequate experimental diet completely free from fluoride. Several early attempts were made with highly purified dietary constituents but they were technically unsatisfactory and will not be described (reviewed by Muhler[208]). One method of overcoming the difficulties[209,210] is to make up a diet based on plants grown on fluoride-free nutrient solutions. Rats died after a few months on this diet; the cause was stated to be starvation following the destruction of their teeth by caries. This was prevented in some animals by giving 1 μg of fluoride in milk but whether their survival was due to the milk or the fluoride is uncertain. Although on too small a scale and with an unsatisfactory control, this work suggests that fluoride is essential.

A contrary result was obtained in a further application of this technique in which soybeans and sorghum, grown by hydroponics, gave a diet with less than 0.005 ppm of fluoride[211]. No significant differences were found in growth rates of rats receiving this diet compared with controls on the same diet supplemented with 2 ppm of fluoride, although their bones contained only 2.92 ppm of fluoride contrasting with 34.6 ppm found in the rats with the 2 ppm fluoride supplement. The activities of some enzymes were studied but only isocitric dehydrogenase was affected; this was increased in the serum and decreased in the liver of the fluoride-deficient rats[211]. In another investigation suggesting that fluoride was not essential, a diet was prepared from four exhaustively purified constituents with a fluoride concentration too low to be estimated but from the amount stored in the body the diet was calculated to contain 0.007 ppm, this was fed to rats over three generations[212]. The animals, including their teeth, seemed normal compared with controls receiving a fluoride supplement, but as the diet used is not cariogenic in rats, their resistance to caries was not tested. Muhler[208] fed a purified diet containing only 0.1 ppm to rats and reported that they 'were extremely nervous and irritable, their coats were thin, and the epithelial structures were denuded and edematous'. Reproduction was poor. Addition of fluoride to the diet improved the animals' condition, but it was not clear that all the defects were caused by fluoride deficiency, purification of the diet may have altered it in other ways. Schwartz[213], on the other hand, did find that 2.5 ppm of fluoride added to a purified diet increased growth rate by 30 % in experiments with rats living in a 'more or less trace element sterile isolation'. The reasons for these contradictory results are not clear, but may arise from the uncontrolled dietary concentration of those ions which affect fluoride absorption (such as calcium or phosphate).

Experiments by Messer et al.[214] first suggested that fluoride deficiency impaired reproduction in mice, the number of litters being reduced and the young being anaemic, although the growth and litter size were not affected. Later, the basal diet was found to be only marginally adequate in iron and copper for normal growth, but inadequate for repeated pregnancies. This implies that fluoride may be necessary only when these other elements are deficient, but the explanation is unknown. Variations in the adequacy of other constituents of the diets, fed in other experiments, may explain the discrepant results.

Evidence from a quite different field[39], indicating that, in vitro, calcium phosphate precipitates as apatite only in the presence of fluoride, suggests that fluoride might be essential for the normal structure of bone. However, apart from the results of McClendon[209,210] showing defective teeth in a fluoride deficiency, no evidence has emerged that the skeleton is affected by diets low in fluoride.

While it seems premature to conclude that fluoride is essential (although this is often stated) there certainly are indications that this is so, at least under certain conditions but more experiments are needed to clarify this technically difficult question.

OBJECTIONS TO FLUORIDATION

Objections to the artificial fluoridation of water have followed three arguments: (1) that it is ineffective, benefits only children, or is not sufficiently effective to justify the cost and alleged risks, (2) that it is not safe, or that its safety has not been sufficiently investigated, and (3) that it interferes with the liberty of the subject.

THE EFFECTIVENESS OF FLUORIDE

The claim that fluoride is ineffective in reducing caries is supported only by selecting atypical DMF figures. As explained earlier, the protective effect of fluoride on molars is much less than that on incisors. Opponents of fluoridation in Britain quote DMF figures for age groups (e.g. 11 y) in which most of the caries is in the molars, so minimizing the effect (apparently to a postponement of caries in one tooth for 1 year). This was probably an honest misunderstanding at first, but the propagandists have continued to make this statement after the error has been repeatedly pointed out to them, and after many sets of data throughout the world confirmed the results of Dean[13,14]. For example, for artificially fluoridated Anglesey among the 15-year-old groups and its controls the average DMF values are 6.4 and 11.4, respectively (i.e. a saving of 5 teeth or a 44 % reduction). The corresponding figures for the naturally fluoridated area of Hartlepool and its control York are 4.96 and 8.95, respectively[27].

To receive the full benefit, fluoride must be taken throughout the 8 years during which the teeth are forming, as well as being continued indefinitely. The emphasis on fluoride uptakes during childhood may have confused some people into thinking that the benefits were confined to children, and the small protection found among adults in some of the earlier studies encouraged this belief. But, as shown above, the data on the effect of fluoride on caries in adults, taken as a whole, show a lifelong protection.

BIOCHEMICAL ASPECTS OF THE SAFETY OF FLUORIDATION

Fluoride and the prevalence of major diseases

Much of the data on the safety of fluoridation is based on epidemiology rather than on nutrition or biochemistry, and although beyond the scope of this review has been critically appraised elsewhere[215–219]. The critics suggest that the additional fluoride intake from 1 ppm in water may increase some diseases, including some of the killer diseases, and they support their case with vital statistics. The most recent controversy suggests a higher incidence of cancer in American fluoridated cities[220,221]. This study has been challenged on the grounds that the populations concerned were inadequately matched for changes in age and race[222], and when these differences are allowed for the cancer rates become slightly lower in the high F areas[223] although these criticisms are not accepted by the original authors[224].

Epidemiological evidence that the populations of long established natural fluoride areas enjoy as good a health record as in low F areas is sometimes challenged on the grounds that artificial fluoride is more toxic than natural fluoride, a point discussed above.

Fluoride and minor ill-health

A much more plausible objection, and one much more difficult to test, is the possibility that fluoridation may lead to minor complaints, and as fluoride accumulates in the skeleton, the bones would seem the most likely sites of undesirable effects. The question can be approached by collecting data on fluoride intake in a population known to be near the threshold of toxic effects.

This seems particularly important in Britain which, as a tea drinking country, has a higher basal intake of fluoride than the USA or other European countries. Assurances of the safety of fluoridation under American conditions were adopted in Britain, with very little detailed study of the contribution of tea to fluoride intake. Figures based on a small-scale survey by Longwell[225] suggested average intakes but it is those who consume the largest volumes of fluid which set the safety limit rather than the general average. Two main problems require investigation. At what age do children begin to drink tea, how much fluoride do they receive from it, and does this increase the risk of mottling when water is fluoridated? No effect more serious than mottling would be expected in children. A subsidiary question is whether sufficient fluoride is taken in tea to reduce caries. The second question is whether lifelong body storage of fluoride from fluoridated water and from other sources, such as tea, could adversely affect metabolism.

TEA DRINKING IN CHILDREN

Surveys of tea drinking among children in Manchester and Newcastle revealed that this habit begins at a very early age, although it is difficult to obtain data on volume consumed or, as the tea is diluted with milk, its fluoride concentration. A small survey was conducted in Newcastle based on questionnaires filled in by parents of children under the care of health visitors (Table 11). The Manchester survey[226] related the number of cups of tea drunk by children aged 15 to their DMF values and found a significant negative correlation (implying that sufficient fluoride was taken in tea to reduce caries). This was not confirmed among 5-year-old children in Newcastle[227] probably because in this age group the tea was taken too late to exert a systemic effect on the deciduous teeth and was too weak for a topical effect. The low incidence of fluoride mottling in Britain even in areas with fluoridated water suggests that tea is not leading to excessive fluoride intake.

Table 11 Tea drinking habits of 83 children

Age	No. children	No. taking tea	Av. no. of cups
0–11 m	7	3	2
1 y	10	8	2.4
2 "	11	11	2.6
3 "	12	12	3.5
4 "	11	11	2.6
5 "	8	7	2.4
6 "	13	12	2.5
7 "	11	11	1.9

Totals: 83 children from 29 families.

Taking tea: 75 (virtually all the children over 2 y old).

Data from Jenkins (unpublished).

FLUORIDE INTAKE BY ADULTS

A radiologically detectable thickening of bone produced by a larger quantity of, usually undermineralized, bone[228] is the first sign of chronic fluorosis followed by stiffness of joints beginning in the spine leading, in severe cases, to complete ankylosis ('poker back'). In severe fluorosis, both in experimental animals and in man, areas of resorption alternate with the formation of thicker bone with disorientation of the Haversian system and exostoses[229]. These changes which involve matrix production cannot be explained by the known effect of fluoride, i.e. of favouring the precipitation of apatite from saturated solutions. The cause of these changes is unknown but it might be speculated that the fluoride reaches high concentrations in the mineral, thus raising the equilibrium concentration in tissue fluid to levels which affect the metabolism of the bone cells. There is evidence that the exostoses and increased bone formation are primary, and the resorption is secondary, as exostoses have been found without signs of resorption but resorption was never seen in the absence of bone formation[229]. Possibly the resorption occurs in response to the mineral requirement for rapid formation of new bone. Is it possible in an 'F area' to store sufficient fluoride in the skeleton to bring about the earliest stage of these changes?

The range of intake of fluoride by adults in fluoridated Newcastle was studied by two procedures. Questionnaires were sent to organizations which held frequent meetings requesting members to find out, by a show of hands at a meeting, how many normally drank 0–5, 5–10, 10–15 or over 15 cups of tea daily. Needless to say, no precision is claimed for the results but they give some indication of the distribution of intake. The results from about 800 people showed that 40 % drank fewer than 5 cups, 52 % between 5 and 10 cups and 8 % more than 15 cups daily.

Some of the individuals who claimed to be drinking many cups of tea were personally contacted and were mostly found to have very small cups of very weak tea, providing fluoride intakes of only 3–4 mg, but a few did take up to 8 or 9 mg daily[174] (and unpublished data).

The second method of contacting heavy tea drinkers was through health visitors who put us in touch with suitable patients. The highest intake recorded was by a man who drank 22 cups of tea and 4 pints of beer daily. One daily output of urine (4.76 litres) contained about 7 mg of fluoride and, making a generous allowance of 25 % for skeletal storage in an elderly man, his intake was approximately 9 mg.

THE THRESHOLD INTAKE FOR ADVERSE EFFECTS

Two estimates may be made about the threshold intake for the first signs of adverse effects. One hundred and sixteen of the longterm inhabitants of Bartlett, Texas (fluoride 8 ppm) were given a thorough medical examination in 1943 and 1953[230-232] along with 121 from neighbouring Cameron (fluoride 0.4 ppm). Among the 40 tests carried out, no significant medical differences were found between the two localities, except for mottled enamel in Bartlett and slight bony changes detected radiographically among 10–15% of the Bartlett residents. The bony changes were not accompanied by any subjective symptoms. This suggests that bone is the most sensitive tissue in the elderly. The death rate of subjects over 65 was higher in Bartlett (9 out of 21) than in Cameron (3 out of 16) during the ten years between the examinations, but it was stated that the differences between the age-corrected death rates were not statistically significant. It may be concluded that water containing 8 ppm in Texas (with a hot climate) is on the borderline of a completely safe dose. The fluid intake was not measured, but it might be expected, in that climate, to be at least 1.5 litres and probably more, providing 12–16 mg of fluoride daily. Although the proportion of fluid intake using local water was not recorded, it is reasonable to suppose that most of it was made from or consisted of Bartlett water. It is perhaps unfortunate that the second series of medical examinations was carried out 18 months after the Bartlett water supply had been reduced to 1 ppm but it was assumed that adverse effects would not have regressed in that time. This is reasonable, as urine levels (and therefore presumably plasma levels), although falling during the 18 months, had still not reached control values so that the tissues remained in contact with a higher concentration of fluoride than did the controls.

The second estimate of the threshold dose of fluoride for adverse effects comes from the results of a survey published in 1949[233], where the workers were exposed to fluoride-containing fumes for an average of 15 years in the aluminium smelting plant at Fort William, Scotland. Skeletal changes were detected radiographically in 25% of the most exposed workers in the furnace room but, as in Bartlett, they were not accompanied by any disability. The fluoride contents of the 24 h urines ranged between 3 and 23 mg and averaged 9 mg. Allowing for the profuse sweating and bone storage the intake seems likely to have averaged about 15–18 mg, possibly exceeding 25 mg in the 9% who excreted more than 16 mg. There was no significant correlation between the urinary output and the presence of abnormal radiographs. It has to be conceded that these workers were, in a sense, self-selected, as had they recognized any undesirable results from their work, they would presumably have left. The maximum intake from tea, by a small number of people in a fluoridated area, of about 9 mg is therefore within the safe limit, as suggested by these two surveys.

THE EFFECT OF FLUORIDE ON ADENYLATE CYCLASE

The well known effect of fluoride at 100–200 ppm (5–10 mmol/l) in stimulating adenylate cyclase in broken cell preparations[234] has not been observed in intact cells, and it was therefore expected that the dietary intake of fluoride would not influence levels of cyclic AMP in tissues and body fluids. However, elevated levels of cAMP in urine and tissues of rats receiving 50 ppm fluoride in their diet have been reported, in spite of the insensitivity of the rat to fluoride, mentioned above[235,236]. Human subjects excreted 25% more cAMP in the urine during the 6 h after receiving single doses of 3.75 mg fluoride (as NaF) than on control days when no fluoride was given[237]. Re-investigation of this latter finding in human subjects in my laboratory showed a similar tendency, but when fluoride (5 mg/day) was administered in divided doses taken with meals for 7 days, simulating the effect of fluoridated water, urinary cAMP output was raised by only 12–15 % in comparison with pre-dosage output, an increase which is within normal variation and is not statistically significant.

Although no comparisons appear to have been made of urinary excretion of cAMP in high and low F areas or in heavy tea drinkers, the existing data do not suggest that differences are likely.

None of the recognized toxic effects of high doses of F (mottled enamel, stiffened joints, exostoses) have been attributed to increased activity of adenyl cyclase.

THE POSSIBILITY OF HYPERSENSITIVITY

Although the safety of fluoridation seems assured as far as chronic skeletal and other reactions are concerned, the possibility has been raised that some people may be hypersensitive to fluoride and that even the small doses obtained from fluoridated water may produce unfavourable reactions. Waldbott[239–241] and Grimbergen[242] have suggested that some non-specific symptoms, e.g. stomatitis, gastritis, visual disturbances and headaches occurred in their patients in 'F areas' in the USA and the Netherlands, respectively, were caused by the fluoride. Waldbott stated that symptoms disappeared when the patients were given fluoride-free water. A variety of tests, some described as 'blindfold', were set up and gave results incriminating fluoride, but all involved doses higher than would be obtained at any one time with water containing 1 ppm fluoride. Grimbergen organized a 'double-blind' test in which patients were given bottles containing either distilled water or a solution of sodium fluoride apparently of 0.5 % (his paper is unclear on this point), with instructions to dilute it to 1 ppm and to try to distinguish between the two. The patients were apparently able to do this, although the procedure is obviously unsatisfactory as the patients had access to a concentrated solution which they might identify by taste or by the white residues left from evaporating drops. Therefore, the existence of the condition cannot be regarded as proved.

In Britain, as a tea-drinking nation, the population has been exposed to moderate doses of fluoride and has therefore been at risk of hypersensitivity for centuries, if this danger is real. The recent report[243] of rare but severe reactions to tea, coffee and even tomatoes and potatoes has increased the range of foods associated with hypersensitivity, and therefore increased the possibility that hypersensitivity to fluoride may exist. It is not suggested that these cases were caused by fluoride (which is not high in coffee or in the foods mentioned above): caffeine was suggested as the active substance in tea and coffee, the hypersensitivity being perhaps due to lack of some enzyme concerned in its metabolism. Conceivably, if an individual is already deficient in an enzyme sensitive to fluoride, increased fluoride ingestion might reduce its activity below some critical level.

Although it is logically impossible to prove a negative, in this case to *prove* that fluoridated water cannot cause any harm to individuals, the evidence makes the possibility of such harm very remote. Nevertheless, vigilance should be continued and when adverse effects are suspected it is important that they should be thoroughly investigated.

THE ETHICAL OBJECTION

The third objection to the fluoridation of water is that it interferes with the liberty of the individual, but this is a value judgement outside the scope of a scientific article.

THE ADMINISTRATION OF FLUORIDE BY ROUTES OTHER THAN THE COMMUNAL DRINKING WATER

Other vehicles for ingestion

The opposition to water fluoridation has prevented its introduction into some countries, restricted its application in Britain, led to its abandonment in Sweden and The Netherlands and has encouraged research on other methods of providing fluoride.

In the USA, the water supplies of some schools have been fluoridated at concentrations varying from 2.3 to 5.0 ppm[244,245]. The higher concentration compensates for the relatively small proportion of total fluid consumption taken at school on school days only, and its introduction at the later age of 5–6 compared with communal fluoridation (reviewed in reference 246). The concentration now recommended is 5 ppm and this has been shown to be effective[247].

The addition of fluoride to salt and milk has been proposed and tested. Salt fluoridation (250 mg F/kg) has been used in Switzerland[248] and Hungary[249] for some time, and a reduction in caries has followed. The fluoridation of milk has been tested in two small-scale surveys[250,251] and several larger ones are now in progress[252]. The fluoride in milk is utilized only slightly less efficiently than from water, and clearly involves much smaller quantities of sodium fluoride for a given population than the fluoridation of water (only about 1 % of a water supply is used for drinking). However, the main difficulty (apart from the fact that some children dislike milk) is that of providing it at a sufficiently early age to influence the composition of the teeth (though it is uncertain how much of its effect is topical rather than systemic). Also it is unlikely to be taken after leaving school, whereas there is evidence that to derive the full benefit, fluoride should be taken continuously[70–72].

Tablets containing 1 or 0.25 mg F[253,254] are available and effective. If they are sucked the fluoride released into saliva may reach over 100 ppm and provide a local effect, as well as a systemic one after the dissolved tablet is swallowed. Topical application and rinses have a detectable effect even in areas with fluoridated water (reviewed in reference 27), so that the action of fluoride from different sources is to some extent additive. However, it is doubtful whether the magnitude of the effect of these additional measures is sufficient in areas with fluoridated water to justify their cost. Tablets are contra-indicated in 'F areas' as the risk of mottling is too high.

LOCAL APPLICATION OF FLUORIDE NOT INVOLVING INGESTION

Since fluoridation of water at 1 ppm gives a reduction in DMF of about 50% in children, it was hoped that the much higher concentrations of fluoride in dentifrices (1000 ppm is usual) might have a larger effect or might greatly supplement the effect of fluoridated water. Among the many methods tried for providing fluoride, other than by drinking water, are dentifrices containing sodium or stannous fluoride, sodium monofluorophosphate or amine fluorides; mouthrinses of sodium fluoride (in neutral or acid solution) or stannous fluoride, and 'topical applications' i.e. painting the teeth 2 or 3 times a year with solutions or gels of 2% NaF or 8% SnF_2 or 1.23% NaF in 0.1 mmol/l H_3PO_4 ('APF') (reviewed below and in references 27, 255–257).

Fluoride-containing dentifrices (about 90% of dentifrices now sold in Britain contain fluoride) have been shown repeatedly in clinical trials to reduce caries by about 20%, or up to 30% in the teeth erupting during the trials, usually of 3 years' duration[258]. A decline in caries has been reported among children in England during the last decade, and the widespread use of fluoridated dentifrices seems the most likely explanation[258a].

COMPARISON OF DIFFERENT FLUORIDES IN DENTIFRICES

Sodium fluoride has not been widely used in dentifrices, because the fluoride becomes unavailable by reacting with the more usual abrasives (chalk, dicalcium phosphate). Stannous fluoride is used in various preparations following *in vitro* tests showing that it reduced enamel solubility more powerfully than sodium fluoride[259], and because the stannous ion also forms a very stable complex with enamel[260]. The results of the many clinical trials have not, as a whole, shown that it is more powerful than sodium fluoride in preventing caries, and it has the disadvantage in some subjects of causing a yellow stain after prolonged use[261].

Topical application is effective in its original form of painting neutral solutions of sodium fluoride on the tooth surface, but needs the use of expensive dental manpower once or twice a year.

Apatite takes up fluoride more readily from acid than from neutral solution[262], but if acids were applied they might dissolve some of the enamel. A compromi e was reached by using a solution of 1.23% sodium fluoride in 0.1 M phosphoric acid (known as acid phosphate fluoride, or APF) which would provide the acid conditions favouring uptake but, by a common ion effect, would be expected to be less damaging than other acids[262]. In spite of some very high reductions of caries in the early experiments[263], the results as a whole seem very similar to those obtained with neutral sodium fluoride[264], although there are indications that APF produces a more prolonged effect continuing after the cessation of treatment[264].

Of the methods of self-application of fluoride other than dentifrices, mouthrinsing is the most widely used; e.g. most Scandinavian children regularly rinse with fluoride solutions in school. The usual regime is 0.2 % NaF weekly but greater prevention has been obtained with 0.05 % and 0.025 % NaF on a daily basis[265]: this stresses the importance of frequency of application.

To be effective, rinsing, along with the chewing of fluoride tablets, has to be supervised, and is thus only practicable during the school years.

The effect of rinses and dentifrices is rather short lived as, if they are discontinued, the DMF values 2 years later are only slightly lower than in controls[71,72].

INGESTION OF FLUORIDE FROM DENTRIFICES AND RINSES

Because overdoses of fluoride in children up to 8 years of age cause mottling, the ingestion of fluoride from dentifrices and mouthrinses has been measured[266]. Children aged 2–3, tested with various volumes of water, were found to have difficulty in spitting it out and tended to swallow it. Children aged 3 and 4 could usually keep 7 ml of fluoride in their mouths for about 30 seconds, but there was considerable individual variation. Older children could rinse for 1 minute. When tests were repeated with 0.05 % sodium fluoride solutions an average of only 75 % and 80 % was recovered in the expectorate in the two age groups, indicating retention of about 0.4 and 0.35 mg F, respectively.

Another investigation in which the expectorate, after the use of a dentifrice, was filtered, washed and dried and the insoluble abrasive particles weighed as a measure of the recovery, confirmed that pre-school children behave erratically in spitting out their dentifrice, and many children tended to swallow some of it on occasion but none did so habitually.

Ericsson and Forsman[266] concluded that even in areas with fluoridated water, weekly rinses of 0.025 % F were completely safe for children over 4 years of age. In 'non-F areas', twice daily use of fluoridated dentifrice with proper supervision is satisfactory for children over 4, but under this age the authors recommended that the amount should not be larger than the size of a pea. In 'F areas', the same quantity should be used only once a day for children under the age of 4.

Similar experiments with dentifrices containing 0.1 % F showed average retentions of slightly more than 0.1 mg[267]. For the maximum effect of a fluoridated dentifrice on caries prevention it would be expected that rinsing should be avoided, but this point does not appear to have been tested clinically.

CONCLUSION

Fluoride, in the various methods of its application to the teeth, is by far the most effective means known at present for preventing caries. Fluoridated water has the great advantage over other methods of application of not requiring any co-operation on the part of the public. Some other methods such as frequent use of mouthrinses or tablets are comparable in activity but, in general, do need supervision and are therefore limited in application. Topical applications require skilled manpower and are therefore expensive, and dentifrices provide a useful protection though less than that of fluoridated water.

NOTE ADDED NOVEMBER 1981

The ability of certain bacteria to concentrate fluoride (p. 44) has been confirmed and two further explanations have been offered for the greater F-sensitivity of bacteria at low pH values (p. 41). One suggestion is that at pH 5 more F is released from bound forms within the cell and is thus made available for enzyme inhibition[268]. The other explanation is based on the concept that 'cytoplasmic pH is generally more alkaline than the environment pH[269], so that if unionized HF permeates the cell wall it meets a higher pH within and dissociates, so maintaining a concentration gradient of HF favouring uptake[269]. The two hypotheses are not mutually exclusive.

By adding ^{18}F to the cytoplasm, released after disrupting oral streptococci and separation on Sephadex G-100, at least 11 binding peaks have been detected. These included enolase, although it had a low affinity for F compared with other constituents[270]. The uptake in the living cells may, of course, be different from that of the substances released after cell destruction.

When *Strep. mutans* has been grown in a chemostat at various pH values, the cultures grown at pH 5.5 were, surprisingly, less sensitive to F than those grown at pH 6 or 6.5[271]. It was suggested that the former are less dependent for their glucose uptake on the PEP phosphotransferase system, but utilize some other transport mechanism relatively insensitive to F[271].

In the USA analyses with the electrode for F in foods, bone and urine have failed to confirm any substantial increased intake, and data suggesting an increase following extensive fluoridation (p. 51)[178,272] were based on unreliable colorimetric methods.[273]

The absorption of F from the kidney tubules is greatly increased if the pH falls, probably because HF, rather than the charged and hydrated F ion, is absorbed[274]. Absorption from the urinary bladder (which is suspected to occur in man) has been proved in the rat by injecting ^{18}F into the bladder with the ureters ligated, and this mechanism is also pH dependent[ ].

A review of enzyme inhibition by F reveals that the concentrations required, even of those most sensitive to F, far exceeds those in normal plasma[276].

ACKNOWLEDGEMENTS

I am extremely grateful to my colleagues, Dr W. M. Edgar and Dr A. J. Rugg-Gunn for much helpful discussion during the preparation of this review.

References

1. McKay, F. S. (with Black, G. V.) (1916). *Dent. Cosmos.*, **58**, 477
2. McKay, F. S. (1916). *Dent. Cosmos.*, **58**, 627
3. McKay, F. S. (1916). *Dent. Cosmos.*, **58**, 781
4. McKay, F. S. (1916). *Dent. Cosmos.*, **58**, 894
5. McKay, F. S. (1928). *J. Am. Dent. Assoc.*, **15**, 1429
6. Ainsworth, N. J. (1933). *Br. Dent. J.*, **60**, 233
7. Medical Research Council (1925). *Med. Res. Counc. Spec. Rep. Ser.*, (Lond.) No. 97
8. Churchill, H. V. (1931). *Ind. Eng. Chem.*, **23**, 996
9. Smith, M. C. and Lantz, E. M. (1933). *Univ. Zriz. Tech. Bull.*, No. **45**, 327
10. Patterson, C. M., Kruger, B. J. and Daley, T. J. (1977). *Arch. Oral Biol.*, **22**, 419
11. Dean, H. T. (1933). *Publ. Hlth Rep. Washington*, **48**, 703
12. Dean, H. T. (1938). *Publ. Hlth Rep. Washington*, **53**, 1443
13. Dean, H. T., Jay, P., Arnold, F. A. Jr and Elvove, E. (1941). *Publ. Hlth Rep. Washington*, **56**, 761
14. Dean, H. T., Arnold, F. A. Jr. and Elvove, E. (1942). *Publ. Hlth Rep. Washington*, **57**, 1155
15. Weaver, R. (1950). *Br. Dent. J.*, **88**, 231
16. Forrest, J. R. (1956). *Br. Dent. J.*, **100**, 195
17. Galagan, D. J. (1953). *J. Am. Dent. Assoc.*, **47**, 159
18. Galagan, D. J. and Vermillion, J. R. (1957). *Publ. Hlth Rep. Washington*, **72**, 491
19. Forsman, B. (1974). *Community Dent. Oral Epidemiol.*, **2**, 32
20. Arnold, F. A., Likins, R. C., Russell, A. L. and Scott, D. B. (1962). *J. Am. Dent. Assoc.*, **65**, 780
21. Brown, H. K. and Poplove, M. (1965). *J. Can. Dent. Assoc.*, **31**, 505
22. Department of Health (1969). *Rep. Publ. Hlth. Med. Subj. Lond.*, **122**
23. Kwant, G. W., Houwink, B., Backer Dirks, O., Groenveld, A. and Jager, W. (1973). *Neth. Dent. J.*, **80**, suppl. 9
24. Ludwig, T. G. (1971). *N.Z. Dent. J.*, **67**, 155
25. Ministry of Health, Scottish Office, Ministry of Housing and Local Government. (1962). *Rep. Publ. Hlth. Med. Subj.*, **105**
26. McClure, F. J. (1970). *Water Fluoridation. The Search and the Victory*. US Department of Health, Education and Welfare, Bethesda, Maryland
27. Murray, J. J. (1976). *Fluorides in Caries Prevention*. Dental Practitioner Handbook No. 20. (Bristol: John Wright & Sons Ltd)
28. Williams, J. L. (1923). *J. Dent. Res.*, **5**, 117
29. Newbrun, E. and Brudevold, F. (1961). *Arch. Oral Biol.*, **2**, 15
30. Fejerskov, O., Johnson, N. W. and Silverston, L. M. (1974). *Scand. J. Dent. Res.*, **82**, 357
31. Fejerskov, O., Thylstrup, A. and Joost Larsen, M. (1977). *Scand. J. Dent. Res.*, **85**, 510
32. Kruger, B. J. (1970). *Arch. Oral Biol.*, **15**, 109
33. Ericsson, Y. and Ribelius, U. (1971). *Caries Res.*, **5**, 78
34. Kruger, B. J. (1970). *Arch. Oral Biol.*, **15**, 103
35. Kruger, B. J. (1972). *Arch. Oral Biol.*, **17**, 1389
36. Hodge, H. C. and Smith, F. A. (1968). *Ann. Rev. Pharmacol.*, **8**, 395
37. Patterson, C. M., Basford, K. E. and Kruger, B. J. (1976). *Arch. Oral Biol.*, **21**, 131
38. Brudevold, F., McCann, H. G. and Grøn, P. (1965). In Wolstenholme, G. E. W. and O'Conor, M. (eds.) *Caries-Resistant Teeth*. p. 121. (London: Churchill)
39. Newesley, H. (1970). *Adv. Oral Biol.*, **4**, 11
40. Wilkie, J. (1940). *Br. J. Radiol.*, **13**, 213
41. Weatherell, J. A. (1969). In Barltrop, D. and Burland, W. L. (eds.) *Mineral Metabolism in Paediatrics*. p. 53. (Oxford: Blackwell Scientific Publications)
42. Jackson, D. (1961). *Arch. Oral Biol.*, **5**, 212

43. Andreason, J. D. and Ravn, J. J. (1973). *Scand. J. Dent. Res.*, **81**, 203
44. Zimmerman, E. R. (1954). *Publ. Hlth Rep. Washington*, **69**, 1115
45. El-Alousi, W., Jackson, D., Crompton, G. and Jenkins, O. C. (1975). *Br. Dent. J.*, **138**, 9
46. Backer Dirks, O. (1974). *Caries Res.* **8**, (Suppl. 1), 2
47. Dean, T. H., Jay, P., Arnold, F. A. Jr. and Elvove, E. (1941). *Publ. Hlth Rep. Washington*, **56**, 761
48. Hayes, R. L., McCauley, H. B. and Arnold, F. A. Jr. (1956). *Publ. Hlth Rep. Washington*, **71**, 1228
49. Gedalia, I. (1970). In *Fluorides and Human Health*. p. 128. World Health Organisation Monograph Series No. 59. Geneva
50. Ericsson, Y. and Ullberg, S. (1958). *Acta. Odontol. Scand.*, **13**, 363
51. Ericsson, Y., Ullberg, S. and Appelgren, L. E. (1960). *Acta Odontol. Scand.*, **18**, 253
52. Armstrong, W. D., Singer, L. and Makowski, E. L. (1970). *Am. J. Obstet. Gynecol.*, **107**, 432
53. Gedalia, I., Brzezinski, A., Zukerman, H. and Mayersdorf (1964). *J. Dent. Res.*, **43**, 699
54. Carlos, J. P., Gittelson, A. and Haddon, W. Jr. (1962). *Publ. Hlth Rep. Washington*, **77**, 658
55. Lilienthal, O. C. M. and Lang, L. P. (1971). *Med. J. Aust.*, **2**, 821
56. Backer Dirks, O., Jongeling-Eijndhoven, J. M. P. A., Flissebaalje, T. D. and Gedalia, I. (1974). *Caries Res.*, **8**, 181
57. Ericsson, Y. (1973). *Caries Res.*, **7**, 56
58. Ericsson, Y. and Ribelius, U. (1971). *Caries Res.*, **5**, 78
59. Adler, P. (1970). In *Fluorides and Human Health*, p. 338. World Health Organisation Series No. 59, Geneva.
60. Russell, A. L. and Elvove, E. (1951). *Publ. Hlth. Rep. Washington*, **66**, 1389
61. Englander, H. R. and Wallace D. A. (1962). *Publ. Hlth Rep. Washington*, **77**, 887
62. Weaver, R. (1944). *Br. Dent. J.* **77**, 185
63. Forrest, J. R., Parfitt, G. J. and Bransby, E. R. (1956). *Mon. Bull. Minist. Health, London*, **10**, 104
64. Murray, J. J. (1971a). *Br. Dent. J.*, **131**, 391
65. Murray, J. J. (1971). *Br. Dent. J.*, **131**, 437
66. Murray, J. J. (1971). *Br. Dent. J.*, **131**, 487
67. Jackson, D. (1961). *Arch. Oral Biol.*, **6**, 80
68. Hayes, R. L., Littleton, N. W. and White, C. L. (1957). *Am. J. Public Health*, **47**, 192
69. Arnold, F. A. Jr., Dean, H. T., Jay, P. and Knutson, J. W. (1956). *Publ. Hlth Rep. Washington*, **71**, 652
70. Way, R. M. (1964). *J. Dent. Child.* **31**, 151
71. Koch, G. (1969) *Odontol. Revy*, **20**, 323
72. Koch, G. (1970). *Caries Res.*, **5**, 343
73. Short, M. E. (1944). *J. Dent. Res.*, **23**, 247
74. Scheinin, A., Kalijarvi, E., Harjola, O. and Heikkinen, K. (1964). *Acta Odontol. Scand.*, **22**, 229
75. Künzel, W. (1976). *Caries Res.*, **10**, 96
76. Adler, P. (1970). In *Fluorides and Human Health*, p. 349. World Health Organisation Monograph Series No. 59, Geneva
77. Jenkins, G. N. (1978). *Physiology and Biochemistry of the Mouth*. 4th edn. (Oxford: Blackwell)
78. Meckel, A. H. (1965). *Arch. Oral Biol.*, **10**, 585
79. Kleinberg, I. (1970). *Adv. Oral Biol.*, **4**, 43
80. Stephen, R. M. (1940). *J. Am. Dent. Assoc.*, **27**, 718
81. Kleinberg, I. (1961). *J. Dent. Res.*, **40**, 1087
82. Various authors in a symposium (1974). *J. Dent. Res.*, **53**, 162
83. Fosdick, L. D. and Starke, A. C. (1939). *J. Dent. Res.*, **18**, 417
84. Ericsson, Y. (1949). *Enamel-Apatite Solubility*, (Stockholm: A. B. Thule)
85. Gray, J. A. and Francis, M. D. (1963). In Sognnaes, R. F. (ed.) *Mechanisms of Hard Tissue Destruction*, Am. Assoc. Adv. Sci. Washington
86. Featherstone, J. D. B., Duncan, J. F. and Cuttrass, T. W. (1978). *Arch. Oral Biol.*, **23**, 397, 405
87. Kleinberg, I., Craw, D. and Komiyama, K. (1973). *Arch. Oral Biol.*, **18**, 787
88. Manly, R. S. and Harrington, D. P. (1959). *J. Dent. Res.*, **39**, 910
89. Young, R. A. and Elliott, J. C. (1966). *Arch. Oral Biol.*, **11**, 699

90. McCann, H. G. and Bullock, F. A. (1955). *J. Dent. Res.*, **34**, 59
91. Weatherell, J. D. (1969). In Barltrop, D. and Barland, W. L. (eds.). *Mineral Metabolism in Paediatrics*. p. 53. (Oxford: Blackwell Scientific Publications)
92. Jenkins, G. N. and Speirs, R. L. (1953). *J. Physiol.*, **121**, 21P
93. Brudevold, F., Gardner, D. E. and Smith, F. A. (1956). *J. Dent. Res.*, **35**, 420
94. Weatherell, J. D. and Hargreaves, J. A. (1965). *Arch. Oral Biol.*, **10**, 139
95. Weatherell, J. D., Robinson, C. and Hallsworth, A. S. (1971). *Caries Res.*, **6**, 312
96. Little, M. F., Cooper, H. C. and Rowley, J. (1971). In Fearnhead, R. W. and Stack, M. V. (eds.). *Enamel II*. p. 100. (Bristol: Wright)
97. Fanning, R. J., Shaw, J. H. and Sognnaes, R. F. (1954). *J. Am. Dent. Assoc.*, **49**, 668
98. Weatherell, J. D., Deutsch, D., Robinson, C. and Hallsworth, A. S. (1975). *Nature. (London)* **256**, 230
99. Speirs, R. L. (1976). *Caries Res.*, **10**, 139
100. Myers, H. M., Hamilton, J. G. and Becks, H. (1952). *J. Dent. Res.*, **31**, 743
101. Dowse, C. M. and Jenkins, G. N. (1957). *J. Dent. Res.*, **36**, 816
102. Weatherell, J. D., Deutsch, D. and Robinson, C. (1977). *Caries Res.* **11**, (Suppl. 1), 85
103. Brudevold, F., McCann, H. G. and Grøn, P. (1968). *Arch. Oral Biol.*, **13**, 877
104. Wei, S. H. Y. and Schalz, E. M. Jr. (1975). *Caries Res.*, **9**, 50
105. Hotz, P., Mühlemann, H. R. and Schait, A. (1970). *Helv. Odontol. Acta*, **14**, 26
106. Munksgaard, E. C. and Bruun, C. (1973). *Arch. Oral Biol.*, **18**, 735
107. Volker, J. F. (1939). *Proc. Soc. Exp. Biol. Med.*, **42**, 725
108. Aasenden, R., Allukian, M., Brudevold, F. and Wellock, W. D. (1971). *Arch. Oral Biol.*, **16**, 13399
109. Moreno, E. C., Kresak, M. and Zahradnik (1977). *Caries Res.*, **11**, (Suppl. 1), 142
110. Jenkins, G. N., Armstrong, P. A. and Speirs, R. L. (1952). *Proc. R. Soc. Med.*, **45**, 517
111. Jenkins, G. N. (1963). *J. Dent. Res.*, **42**, 444
112. Isaac, S., Brudevold, F., Smith, F. A. and Gardner, D. E. (1958). *J. Dent. Res.*, **37**, 254
113. Healy, W. B. and Ludwig (1966). *N.Z. Dent. J.*, **62**, 276
114. Cuttress, T. W. (1972). *Arch. Oral Biol.*, **17**, 93
115. Dirksen, T. R., Little, M. F., Bibby, B. G. and Crump, S. L. (1962). *Arch. Oral Biol.*, **7**, 49
116. Brown, W. E., Gregory, T. M. and Chow, L. C. (1977). *Caries Res.*, **11**, (Suppl. 1), 118
117. Nikiforuk, G. (1961). In Mühlemann, H. R. and König, K. G. (eds.). *Caries Symposium, Zurich.* p. 62. (Berne: Huber)
118. Nikiforuk, G. and Grainger, R. M. (1965). In Stack, M. V. and Fearnhead, R. W. (eds.). *Tooth Enamel II*. p. 26. (Bristol: Wright)
119. Hallsworth, A. S., Weatherell, J. A. and Robinson, C. (1973). *Caries Res.*, **7**, 345
120. Zapanta-Legeros, R., Legeros, J. P. and Trautz, O. R. (1964). *J. Dent. Res.*, **43**, 775
121. Frazier, P. D., Little, M. F. and Casciani, F. S. (1967). *Arch. Oral Biol.*, **12**, 35
122. Sundstrom, B., Jongebloed, W. L. and Arends, J. (1978). *Caries Res.*, **12**, 329
123. Rönholm, E. (1962). *J. Ultrastruc. Res.*, **6**, 249
124. Bibby, B. G. and Van Kesteren, M. (1940). *J. Dent. Res.*, **19**, 391
125. Wright, D. E. and Jenkins, G. N. (1954). *Br. Dent. J.*, **96**, 30
126. Borei, H. (1945). *Arch. Kemi. Mineral. Geol.*, **20**, 1
127. Lilienthal, B. (1956). *J. Dent. Res.*, **35**, 197
128. Jenkins, G. N. (1959). *Arch. Oral Biol*, **1**, 33
129. Jenkins, G. N. (1960). *J. Dent. Res.*, **39**, 684
130. Hardwick, J. L. and Leach, S. A. (1962). *Arch. Oral Biol. Suppl.* 151
131. Dawes, C., Jenkins, G. N., Hardwick, J. L. and Leach, S. A. (1965). *Br. Dent. J.*, **119**, 164
132. Frant, M. S. and Ross, J. W. (1966). *Science*, **154**, 1553
133. Agus, H. M., Schamschula, R. G., Barmes, D. E. and Bunzel, M. (1976). *Community Dent. Oral Epidemiol.*, **4**, 210
134. Grøn, P. (1968). *Arch. Oral Biol.*, **13**, 203
135. Shannon, I. (1977). *Caries Res.*, **11**, (Suppl. 1), 206
136. Birkeland, J. M. (1973). *Caries Res.*, **7**, 11
137. Kaufman, H. W. and Kleinberg, I. (1973). *Calc. Tiss. Res.*, **11**, 97
138. Edgar, W. M. and Jenkins, G. N. (1972). *Proc. Int. Assoc. Dent. Res. Abs.*, 173
139. Singer, L., Jarvey, B. A., Venkateswarlu, P. and Armstrong, W. D. (1970). *J. Dent. Res.*, **49**, 455

140. Birkeland, J. M. and Rölla, G. (1972). *Arch. Oral Biol.*, **17**, 455
141. Jenkins, G. N. and Edgar, W. M. (1977). *Caries Res.*, **11**, (Suppl. 1), 226
142. Edgar, W. M., Cockburn, M. and Jenkins, G. N. (1981). *Arch. Oral Biol.*, **26**, 615
143. Kashket, S. and Rodriquez, V. M. (1976). *Arch. Oral Biol.*, **21**, 459
144. Jenkins, G. N., Edgar, W. M. and Ferguson, D. B. (1969). *Arch. Oral Biol.*, **13**, 105
145. Stephen, R. M. (1944). *J. Dent. Res.*, **23**, 257
146. Englander, H. R., Carter, W. J. and Fosdick, L. S. (1956). *J. Dent. Res.*, **35**, 792
147. Edgar, W. M. (1976). *Caries Res.*, **10**, 241
148. Edgar, W. M., Jenkins, G. N. and Tatevossian, A. (1970). *Br. Dent. J.*, **128**, 129
149. Warburg, O. and Christian, W. (1942). *Biochem. Z.*, **310**, 384
150. Weiss, S., Kirby, W. I., Kestenbaam, R. C. and Donohue, J. J. (1965). *Ann. N.Y. Acad. Sci.* **131**, 839
151. Hamilton, I. R. (1977). *Caries Res.*, **11**, (Suppl. 1), 262
152. Kaback, H. R. (1970). *Ann. Rev. Biochem.*, **39**, 561
153. Van Houte, J., Backer Dirks, O., de Stoppelaar, J. D. and Jansen, H. M. (1969). *Caries Res.*, **3**, 178
154. Hardwick, L. J. (1970). In McHugh, W. D. *Dental Plaque*. p. 171. (Edinburgh: Livingstone)
155. Rugg-Gunn, A. J., Edgar, W. M., Cockburn, M. A. and Jenkins, G. N. (1981). *Arch. Oral Biol.*, **26**, 61
156. Charlton, G., Blainey, B. and Schamschula, R. (1974). *Arch. Oral Biol.*, **19**, 139
157. Clarke, N. G. and Fanning, E. A. (1971). *Aust. Dent. J.*, **16**, 1
158. Ericsson, T. and Ericsson, Y. (1967). *Helv. Odontol. Acta*, **11**, 10
159. Rölla, G. and Melsen, B. (1975). *Caries Res.*, **9**, 66
160. Moreno, E. C., Kresak, M. and Zahradnik, R. T. (1977). *Caries Res.*, **11**, (Suppl. 1), 150
161. Moreno, E. C., Kresak, M. and Hay, D. I. (1978). *Arch. Oral Biol.*, **23**, 525
162. Birkeland, J. M. (1972). *Scand. J. Dent. Res.*, **80**, 82
163. Grøn. P., McCann, H. G. and Brudevold, F. (1963). *Arch. Oral Biol.*, **13**, 203
164. Shannon, I. and Edmonds, E. J. (1973). *Arch. Oral Biol.*, **17**, 1303
165. Ericsson, Y. (1969). *Caries Res.*, **3**, 159
166. Kruger, B. J. (1962). *J. Dent. Res.*, **41**, 215
167. Cooper, V. K. and Ludwig, T. G. (1965). *N.Z. Dent. J.*, **61**, 33
168. Simpson, W. J. and Castaldi, C. R. (1969). *Odontol. Revy*, **20**, 1
169. Wallenius, B. (1959). *Odontol. Revy*, **10**, 76
170. Lovius, B. B. J. and Goose, D. H. (1969). *Br. Dent. J.*, **127**, 322
171. Osis, D., Kramer, L., Wiatrowski, E. and Spencer, H. (1974). *J. Nutr.*, **104**, 1313
172. McClure, F. J. (1949). *Publ. Hlth Rep., Washington*, **64**, 1061
173. Stones, H. H., Forrest, J. R., Thompson, A. M. and Longwell, J. (1955). *Br. Med. J.*, **1**, 667
174. Jenkins, G. N. and Edgar, W. M. (1973). *J. Dent. Res.*, **52**, 984
175. Cook, H. A. (1969). *Lancet*, **2**, 329
176. Singer, L., Armstrong, W. D. and Vatassery, G. T. (1967). *Econ. Bot.*, **21**, 285
177. Harrison, M. F. (1949). *Br. J. Nutr.*, **3**, 162
178. Marier, J. R. and Rose, D. (1966). *J. Food Sci.*, **31**, 941
179. Wagner, M. J. (1960). *J. Dent. Res.*, **39**, 670
180. Stookey, G. K., Dellinger, E. L. and Muhler, J. C. (1964). *Proc. Soc. Exp. Biol. Med. N.Y.*, **115**, 298
181. Weddle, D. A. and Muhler, J. C. (1957). *J. Dent. Res.*, **36**, 386
182. Wagner, M. J. and Muhler, M. J. (1960). *J. Dent. Res.*, **39**, 49
183. McClure, J. F., Mitchell, H. H., Hamilton, T. S. and Kinser, A. C. (1945). *J. Ind. Hyg. Toxicol.*, **27**, 159
184. Brudevold, F., Moreno, E. and Bakhos, Y. (1972). *Arch. Oral Biol.*, **17**, 1155
185. Wagner, M. J. and Muhler, J. C. (1957). *J. Dent. Res.*, **36**, 552
186. Fremlin, J. H. and Mathieson. (1967). *Arch. Oral Biol.*, **12**, 61
187. McClure, F. J. and Kinser, C. A. (1944). *Publ. Hlth Rep. Washington*, **59**, 1575
188. Zipkin, I., Likins, R. C., McClure, F. J. and Steere, A. C. (1956). *Publ. Hlth Rep. Washington*, **71**, 767
189. Zipkin, I., McClure, F. J. and Lee, W. A. (1960). *Arch. Oral Biol.*, **2**, 190
190. Likins, R. C., McClure, F. J. and Steere, A. C. (1956). *Publ. Hlth Rep. Washington*, **71**, 217

191. Carlson, C. H., Armstrong, W. D. and Singer, L. (1960). *Proc. Soc. Exp. Med. Biol. N.Y.*, **104**, 235
192. Whitford, G. M., Pashley, D. H. and Stringer, G. I. (1976). *Am. J. Physiol.*, **230**, 527
193. Crosby, N. D. and Shepherd, P. A. (1957). *Med. J. Aust.*, **2**, 341
194. Singer, L. and Armstrong, W. D. (1960). *J. Appl. Physiol.*, **15**, 508
195. Ekstrand, J. (1978). *Caries Res.*, **12**, 123
196. Ericsson, Y., Gydell, K. and Hammarskjold, T. (1973). *J. Int. Res. Commun.* **1**, 333
197. Hanhijarivi, H. (1974). *Proc. Finn. Dent. Soc.*, **70**, (Suppl. 3)
198. Taves, D. R. (1966). *Nature (London)*, **211**, 192
199. Taves, D. R. (1967). *Nature (London)* **218**, 1380
200. Singer, L. and Armstrong, W. D. (1969). *Arch. Oral Biol.*, **14**, 1343
201. Taves, D. R. (1968). *Nature (London)* **217**, 1050
202. Taves, D. R. (1968). *Nature (London)* **220**, 582
203. Singer, L. and Armstrong, W. D. (1973). *Biochem. Med.*, **8**, 415
204. Ekstrand, J., Ericsson, Y. and Rosell, S. (1977). *Arch. Oral Biol.*, **22**, 229
205. Venkateswarlu, P. (1975). *Biochem. Med.*, **14**, 368
206. Patterson, C. M., Kruger, B. J. and Dalu, T. J. (1977). *Arch. Oral Biol.*, **22**, 419
207. Ruzicka, J. A., Mrklas, L. and Rokytova, K. (1973). *Caries Res.*, **7**, 166
208. Muhler, J. C. (1960). In Muhler, J. C. and Hine, M. K. (eds.) *Fluorine and Dental Health.* (London: Staples)
209. McClendon, J. F. (1944). *Feder. Proc.*, **3**, 94
210. McClendon, J. F. and Gershon-Cohen, J. (1953). *J. Agr. Food Chem.*, **1**, 464
211. Doberenz, A. R., Karwick, A. A., Kurtz, E. B., Meninerer, A. R. and Reid, B. L. (1964). *Proc. Soc. Exp. Biol. Med. N.Y.*, **117**, 689
212. Maurer, R. L. and Day, H. G. (1957). *J. Nutr.*, **62**, 56
213. Schwarz, K. and Milne, D. B. (1972). *Bioinorganic Chem.*, **1**, 331
214. Messer, H. H., Wong, K., Wegner, M., Singer, L. and Armstrong, W. D. (1972). *Nature New Biol.*, **240**, 218
215. Hagan, T. L., Pasternach, M. and Schaltz, C. C. (1954). *Publ. Hlth Rep. Washington*, **69**, 450
216. Heasman, M. A. and Martin, A. E. (1962). *Mon. Bull. Minist. Hlth.*, **21**, 150
217. World Health Organization (1970). *Fluorides and Human Health.* Chap. 6, 7 and 8.
218. Ericsson, Y. (1974). *Caries Res.*, **8**, (Suppl. 1), 16
219. Royal College of Physicians (1976). *Fluoride Teeth and Health.* (London: Pitman Medical)
220. Burk, D. and Yiamouyiannis, J. (1975). *Congress. Rec.*, **191**, H7172
221. Yiamouyiannis, J. and Burk, C. (1975). *Congress. Rec.* **191**, H12731
222. Doll, R. and Kinlen, L. (1977). *Lancet*, **1**, 1302
223. Oldham, P. D. and Newell, D. J. (1977). *Appl. Statist.*, **26**, 125
224. Yiamouyiannis, J. and Burk, D. (1977). *Fluoride*, **10**, 102
225. Longwell, J. (1957). *R. Soc. Hlth J.*, **77**, 361
226. Ramsey, A. C., Hardwick, J. L. and Tamacas, J. C. (1975). *Caries Res.*, **9**, 312
227. Rugg-Gunn, A. and Jenkins, G. N. (1978). *Caries Res.*, **12**, 109
228. Weidmann, S. M., Weatherell, J. A. and Jackson, D. (1963). *Proc. Nutr. Soc.*, **22**, 105
229. Singh, A. and Jolly, S. S. (1970). In *Fluorides and Human Health.* pp. 225 and 228. (World Health Organization)
230. Leone, N. C., Shimkin, M. B., Arnold, F. A., Stevenson, C. A., Zimmerman, E. R., Geiser, P. A. and Lieberman, S. E. (1954). *Publ. Hlth Rep. Washington*, **69**, 925
231. Zimmerman, E. R., Leone, N. C. and Armold, F. A. Jr. (1955). *J. Am. Dent. Assoc.*, **50**, 272
232. Leone, E., Stevenson, C. A., Hilbish, T. E. and Sosmen, M. C. (1953). *Am. J. Roentg. Radiv Ther. and Nucl. Med.*, **74**, 874
233. Agate, J. N. and other (1949). *Med. Res. Counc.*, No. 22. (London: HMSO)
234. Rall, T. W. and Sutherland, E. W. (1955). *J. Biol. Chem.*, **232**, 1065
235. Allman, D. W. and Benac, M. (1975). *J. Dent. Res.*, **54**, (Special Issue A), Abs. L32
236. Mornstad, H., Sundstrom, B. and Hedner, P. (1975). *J. Dent. Res.*, **54**, (Special Issue A), Abs. L39
237. Allman, D. W. and Benas, M. (1976). *J. Dent. Res.*, **55**, (Special Issue B), Abs. 523
238. Edgar, W. M., Jenkins, G. N. and Pru'dhoe, K. *J. Dent. Res.*, **58**, (Special Issue C), 1229
239. Waldbott, G. L. (1955). *Int. Arch. Allerg. Appl. Immunol.*, **7**, 70

240. Waldbott, G. L. (1956). *Acta Med. Scand.*, **156,** 157
241. Waldbott, G. L. (1959). *Acta Allerg.*, **13,** 456
242. Grimbergen, G. W. (1974). *Fluoride,* **7,** 146
243. Finn, R. and Cohen, H. M. (1978). *Lancet,* **1,** 426
244. Creighton, W. W., Savage, J. and Witter, D. M. (1964). *Publ. Hlth Rep. Washington,* **79,** 778
245. Yacavone, J. A. and Lisanti, F.(1960). *Arch. Oral Biol.,* **1,** 265
246. Horowitz, H. S. (1973). *Commun Dent. Oral Epidemiol.,* **1,** 104
247. Horowitz, H. S., Heifetz, S. B. and Law, F. E. (1972). *J. Am. Dent. Assoc.,* **84,** 832
248. Marthaler, T. M. and Schenardi, C. (1962). *Helv. Odontol. Acta,* **6,** 1
249. Toth, K. (1973). *J. Dent. Res.,* **52,** 533
250. Rusoff, L. L., Konikoff, B. S., Frye, J. B., Johnston, J. E. and Frye, W. W. (1962). *Am. J. Clin. Nutr.,* **11,** 94
251. Ziegler, E. (1964). *Helv. Paediatr. Acta,* **19,** 343
252. Personal Communication from Mr. E. W. Borrow, Director, Borrow Milk Foundation.
253. Marthaler, T. M. (1969). *Helv. Odontol. Acta,* **13,** 1
254. Stephen, K. W. and Campbell, D. (1978). *Br. Dent. J.,* **144,** 202
255. Horowitz, H. S. (1973). *J. Am. Dent. Assoc.,* **87,** 1013
256. Geddes, D. A. M., Jenkins, G. N. and Stephen, K. W. (1973). *Br. Dent. J.,* **134,** 426
257. Newbrun, E. (ed.) (1978). *Fluoride and Dental Caries.* 2nd edn. (Springfield: C. C. Thomas)
258. Duckworth, R. (1968). *Br. Dent. J.,* **124,** 505
258ᵃ Palmer, J. D. (1980). *Br. Dent. J.,* **149,** 48
259. Muhler, J. C., Boyd, T. M. and Van Huysen (1950). *J. Dent. Res.,* **29,** 182
260. Wei. S. H. Y. and Forbes, W. C. (1968). *Arch. Oral Biol.,* **13,** 407
261. Naylor, M. N. and Emslie, R. D. (1967). *Br. Dent. J.,* **123,** 17
262. Brudevold, F., Savory, A., Gardner, D. E., Spinnelli, M. and Spiers, R. (1963). *Arch. Oral Biol.,* **8,** 167
263. Wellock, W. D. and Brudevold, F. (1963). *Arch. Oral Biol.,* **8,** 179
264. Heifetz, S. B., Driscoll, W. S. and Creighton, W. E. (1973). *J. Am. Dent. Assoc.,* **87,** 364
265. Torell, P. and Ericsson, Y. (1965). *Acta Odontol. Scand.,* **23,** 287
266. Ericsson, Y. and Forsman, B. (1969). *Caries Res.,* **3,** 290
267. Hargreaves, J. A., Ingram, G. S. and Wagg, B. J. (1972). *Caries Res.,* **6,** 237
268   Kashket, S. and Rodriquez, V. M. (1976). *Arch. Oral Biol.,* **21,** 459.
269. Eisenberg, A. D. and Marquis, R. E. (1980). *J. Dent. Res.,* **59,** 1187
270. Kashket, S. and Bunick, F. J. (1978). *Arch. Oral Biol.,* **23,** 993
271. Hamilton. I. R. and Ellwood, D. C. (1978). *Infec. Immun.,* **19,** 434
272. Osis, D., Kramer, L., Wiatrowski, E. and Spencer, H. (1974). *J. Nutr.,* **104,** 1313
273. Taves, D. R. (1977). In Johansen, E., Taves, D. R. and Olsen, T. O. (eds.). A.A.A.S. Washington D.C. *Continuing Evaluation of the Use of Fluorides.* Chaps. 5, 6 (Washington D.C.: A.A.A.S.)
274. Whitford, G. M. and Pashley, D. H. (as 273). p. 188, 199
275. Whitford. G. M., Pashley. D. H. and Reynolds, K. E. (1977). *Am. J. Physiol..* **232,** F10
276. Wiseman, A. (1970). In Eichler, O., Farah, A., Herken, H. and Welch, A. D. (eds.). *Handbook of Experimental Pharmacology.* New Series, **20,** 48

Note: A useful source for recent references on fluoride and fluoridation is – Johansen, E., Taves, D. R. and Olsen, T. O. (eds.). *Continuing Evaluation of the Use of Fluorides* (Reference 273). A.A.A.S. Selected Symposium 11.

3
Nutritional status of North Americans

G. M. OWEN AND A. L. OWEN

INTRODUCTION

The nutritional status of a population group or of a community is evaluated by correlating results of dietary, clinical and biochemical studies. During the past 15 years, there have been a number of nutrition surveys in the United States, three or four of which can be considered national in scope[1]. Two major studies were initiated in the late 1960s and completed in the early 1970s. Another national study took place between 1971 and 1974 and a sequel to this study is currently in progress. In this limited review, major findings from three national surveys, which were completed, will be summarized and briefly discussed. Finally, data derived from smaller studies, undertaken since 1975, will be selectively examined to see what changes in nutritional status may be occurring.

MATERIALS AND METHODS
Objectives and sample designs

The data base to be described has been derived primarily from selected studies in which dietary, clinical, anthropometric and biochemical examinations were simultaneously performed within populations, some of which were better defined than others.

The Preschool Nutrition Survey (PNS) was conducted between November, 1968 and December, 1970[2]. The primary objective was to provide an overview of descriptive data on nutritional status of a cross-sectional sample of preschool children. Sampling was done by The University of Michigan Survey Research Center. Some 3400 children between 1 and 6 years of age were examined in 36 states and the District of Columbia.

The Ten State Nutrition Survey (TSNS) was undertaken almost simultaneously with the PNS but there was no overlap in sampling between the two studies[3-6]. The objective of this survey was to determine the prevalence of serious hunger, malnutrition and associated health problems that occur in low-income segments of the population. Sampling from the TSNS was designed in collaboration with the US Bureau of the Census, and was based on census tracts with the largest proportion of low-income families (Table 1).

The first National Health and Nutrition Examination Survey (N-HANES-I) was begun in 1971 and completed in 1974, some four years after the PNS and TSNS[7-12]. The immediate objective of N-HANES-I was to provide an initial overview of a cross-sectional sample of the entire US population. The longterm goal was to establish a continuing national nutrition surveillance system to measure nutritional status of the US population, and to monitor

Table 1 Characteristics of national surveys

	PNS	*TSNS*	*N-HANES-I*
Objectives:	Overview of nutritional status of preschool children	Incidence and location of malnutrition	Monitor change in nutritional status
Sample:	Cross-sectional Representative 1–6 years Individuals	Biased Low income 1–74 years Families	Cross-sectional Representative 1–74 years Individuals
Procedures:	One team One lab	Multiple teams Multiple labs	Two teams One lab

changes in this status over time. The US Bureau of Census co-operated with the National Center for Health Statistics in designing the sample and conducting interviews in selected households. Among 28 000 persons to be included in the original sample, there was some over-sampling of young children and other groups, especially among the poor, judged to be the most vulnerable segments of the population.

In two of these studies, the PNS and N-HANES-I, all individuals selected were to have clinical examinations, including various anthropometric measurements, estimates of dietary intakes and a battery of laboratory determinations (Table 2). In the TSNS, all subjects were to have clinical examinations and determinations of haemoglobin or packed cell volume (haematocrit), but only selected subjects were to have estimates of dietary intake and other laboratory determinations.

RESULTS

Sample

Both the PNS and N-HANES-I were designed to provide representative samples of the US population, preschool children in the former and all ages in the latter. Hence, the proportions of selected individuals who were Blacks, Whites or Hispanics were similar in these two surveys (Table 3). That Blacks comprised a slightly greater proportion of the N-HANES-I sample reflects the fact that there was some over-sampling among segments of the population

Table 2 Examinations performed in surveys

	PNS	TSNS	N-HANES-I
Dietary	All subjects 2-day record	Selected subjects 1-day recall	All subjects 1-day recall
Clinical	All	All	All
Hb/Hct	All	All	All
Other Lab	All	Selected	All

judged to be most vulnerable. Thus among 21 000 persons examined, some 4200 were Black, or nearly 20 % of the total. About one-third of the persons examined were under 17 years of age, one-third were young adults and one-third more than 45 years of age.

Within the predominantly low income census tracts sampled in the TSNS, Blacks and Whites each comprised about 40 % of the population and Hispanics some 17 %. More than half of the individuals examined in the TSNS were less than 17 years of age; two-thirds of the adults were between age 17 and 44 years and one-third more than 45 years. Some 3000 preschool children were represented in each of these national surveys (Table 4).

General findings

Income or socioeconomic status is a major determinant of nutritional status, but other factors – culture, geographic locale, level of education – play significant roles in the level of nutrition in the population. Signs of malnutrition based on clinical, anthropometric, dietary and biochemical findings were most common among Blacks, less common among Hispanics and least common among White persons.

Clinical examinations

Relatively few children had clinical signs suggestive of specific nutrition disorders (Table 5). Prevalence of clinical signs increased with age, findings that coincide with similar investigations in other industrialized nations. Many signs suggestive of nutritional deficiencies in older age groups are probably secondary to underlying medical disorders, e.g. alcoholism, and various degenerative diseases (Table 6). In the TSNS and N-HANES-I, Blacks manifested a somewhat greater prevalence of most signs than did Whites of the same age, sex and level of income.

Table 3 Survey samples by race or ethnic group

	PNS (%)	TSNS (%)	N-HANES-I (%)
Black	15	42	20
Hispanic	4	17	<1
White	80	40	79

Table 4 Survey samples by age

Age (yrs)	PNS (no.)	TSNS (no.)	N-HANES-I (mo)
1–5	3400	3700	3000
6–17	—	8000	4000
18–44	—	6000	7000
45 +	—	4700	6000

Table 5 Per cent of children with clinical findings

	<6 Years (%)	6–11 Years (%)	>11 Years (%)
Lips and Tongue	1	3–4	2–3
Gums	—	—	4
Skin	1	2	5
Bones	1	—	—

Table 6 Per cent of adults with clinical findings

	TSNS (%)	N-HANES-I (%)
Lips and Tongue	2–10	1.5
Gums	—	3–10
Skin	3–8	1–5
Bones	—	2–6
Thyroid	1–7	1–5
Nerves	—	1–10

Anthropometry

With increasing income or higher socioeconomic status, children in each of the three surveys were systematically heavier and taller, and advanced in skeletal maturity and dental development[2,3,5,6]. Some of these generalizations which hold within racial and ethnic groupings, are well demonstrated by height, weight and head circumference data for White children in the PNS (Table 7).

In all three surveys, Blacks tended to be smaller than Whites at birth, and until the age of 2 or 3 years. Thereafter, despite lower income levels, Blacks tended to grow more rapidly than Whites so that from the third year of life and through adolescence, Blacks were systematically taller and heavier than Whites and more advanced in skeletal and dental development, indicating that racial as well as nutritional factors affect growth and body size[5].

Subcutaneous fat thickness was measured in the three surveys by use of skinfold calipers. There were sufficient numbers of individuals in families in the TSNS to examine parent–child associations in relative fatness. Based on age- and sex-specific skinfold thickness percentiles, TSNS parents were classified as being lean (<15th P), medium (15th–85th P), or obese (>85th P) and

Table 7 Association between measurement of anthropometric variables and socioeconomic status of white children in PNS (Mean Z Scores)

Variable	I ($750)*	Warner ranks II ($1500)	III ($2125)	IV ($2827)
Height	−0.24	−0.04	0.05	0.16
Weight	−0.10	−0.02	0.00	0.14
Head circumference	−0.28	−0.04	0.06	0.15

* (median per capita income)

grouped into various combinations[6]. When lean–lean and obese–obese parent combinations were considered, there were clearcut parent–child similarities in relative fatness which increased with age of the children (Figure 1).

Depending upon age, between 10 and 30% of individuals examined in the three surveys could be considered to be obese by skinfold measurements

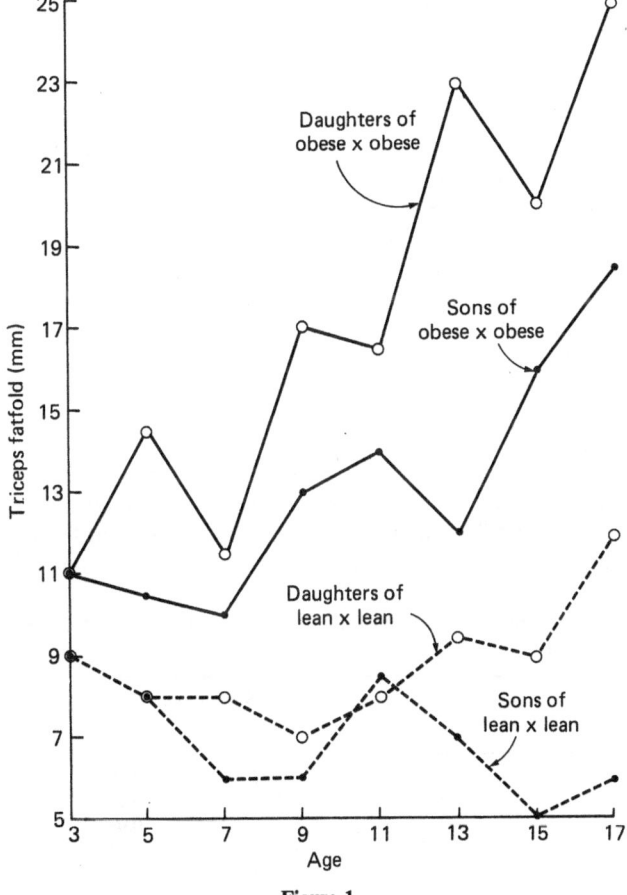

Figure 1

77

(Table 8). Obesity was most prevalent in adult women, particularly among low income Black women. In some groups, more than half the adult women were obese. Among adult males, obesity was substantially more prevalent among Whites than Blacks.

Table 8 Per cent of persons obese (triceps)

Age (yrs)	Males (%)	Females (%)
1–5	8	8
6–17	10	10
18–44	15	25
45+	15	30

Dietary and biochemical

Quantities of nutrients per 1000 kcal (4.18 MJ) showed little or no variation by race, ethnic group or socioeconomic status in the three surveys. This suggests that widely varying food preferences and food selections tend to yield diets which are comparable qualitatively.

In all three surveys, intakes of energy (calories) and of most nutrients reflected socioeconomic status. That is, when race, sex and age were held constant, intakes tended to increase with an increase in family income[2,4,11]. This association of nutrient intake with income was reflected in the association between laboratory variables and socioeconomic status which was most striking for vitamin C (Table 9).

In general, dietary intakes of protein were well above levels considered to be adequate. This was particularly true for children where average protein intakes were 50–100% greater than recommended dietary allowances for various age- and sex-groups. This was reflected in essentially normal levels of plasma albumin for all age groups studied. There were some pregnant women in the TSNS with somewhat low serum albumin levels but the significance of these is unknown.

Although nearly half the children in the PNS reported regular use of multivitamin supplements, there were differences in their use by age and socioeconomic status (Table 10). It is likely that comparable proportions of young children in N-HANES-I were taking vitamin supplements. While it was

Table 9 Association between laboratory variables and socioeconomic status of White children in PNS (mean Z-scores)

| Variable | Warner ranks | | | |
	I	II	III	IV
Haemoglobin	−0.14	−0.02	0.00	0.16
Vitamin C	−0.60	−0.14	0.15	0.41
Vitamin A	−0.36	−0.06	0.09	0.18
Iron	−0.17	−0.03	0.03	0.13
Cholesterol	−0.19	0.00	0.02	0.07

Table 10 Per cent of children in PNS using vitamin supplements

| Age (yrs) | Warner rank | | | |
	I	II	III	IV
1–2	36	51	70	84
2–3	31	46	65	69
3–4	32	47	54	64
4–5	29	47	61	55
5–6	22	41	57	56

estimated that approximately one-fourth of young children in the TSNS received vitamin supplement, specific figures are not actually available. Lacking this information makes it somewhat difficult to assess the significance of reported intakes of vitamins from food sources alone. For example, in all three surveys, Black children had consistently lower mean (or median) levels of retinol (vitamin A) in plasma than did White children of a comparable age. A major finding was that Hispanics living in southwestern states had lower levels of plasma vitamin A than did Black or White populations. Indeed, half the Hispanic children living in the southwest had plasma levels of vitamin A judged unacceptable, i.e. below 20 μg/dl.

Based on intake data and biochemical determinations (Table 11), there were some low income individuals who appeared to be in some jeopardy with respect to vitamin C nutriture. Adult males were more likely than females to have low levels of vitamin C in plasma.

A mean cholesterol value of 161 mg/dl (SD $\pm$ 35) was found for all children in the PSNS: 90% of plasma cholesterol values[2] were between 120 and 200 mg/dl. Similar values were found for TSNS preschool children[3]. In contrast, preschool children in N-HANES-I had slightly higher average values, approximately 170 mg/dl and 90% of values between 120 and 225 mg/dl suggesting a slight shift upward at the median and the upper end of the distribution curve[9]. Although little change in levels of total cholesterol was demonstrated during childhood and adolescence, irrespective of sex and race, a progressive increase in plasma cholesterol was demonstrable after age 17 years[10]. Mean levels between 240 and 250 mg/dl were reached by age 50–55 years in males and females, Blacks and Whites. Distributions had greater variability in adults than in children with standard deviations increasing from

Table 11 Per cent of individuals with abnormal laboratory test results

Blood or serum constituent	PNS (%)	TSNS (%)	N-HANES-I
Albumin	1–2	3–10	1–2
Vitamin A	1–2	2–20	1–10
Vitamin C	5–25	2–5	—
Haemoglobin	5–10	10–20	5–10
Transferrin sat.	20–35	—	10–15

approximately 35 mg/dl during childhood and adolescence to nearly 50 mg/dl after age 24 years.

In all three surveys, iron was the nutrient most often below standards with respect to intake. It is difficult to stipulate what constitutes a low intake, particularly in infants, young children, and adolescents because of marked variability in iron needs during the early months and adolescent years when rapid growth is occurring. Variability in needs in early life also reflects differences in body size at birth. In addition, there is considerable difference in the bioavailability of iron from various foods and mixed diets. Hence, at all ages, interpretation of the level of iron in the diet must take into account composition of the diet.

With respect to evidence of iron deficiency based on serum iron (transferrin saturation), findings in N-HANES-I supported those in the PNS; the greatest prevalence of iron deficiency occurred in young children (Table 11). Serum iron determinations in the TSNS were, for the most part, limited to individuals with anaemia; therefore, it was not possible to estimate prevalence of iron deficiency without anaemia in the TSNS population.

While there has been no unanimity in deciding what level of haemoglobin concentration shall be used to arbitrarily define anaemia in young children, most working groups have accepted levels between 10 and 11 g/dl. From data collected in the PNS, Black children were found to have haemoglobin levels which averaged about 0.5 g lower than those of White children of comparable age and socioeconomic status[13]. Other investigators confirmed the Black–White difference in haemoglobin concentrations for all age groups (Figure 2), and have raised the question whether there should be different criteria of screening for anaemia[14–18]. Using arbitrary definitions of anaemia

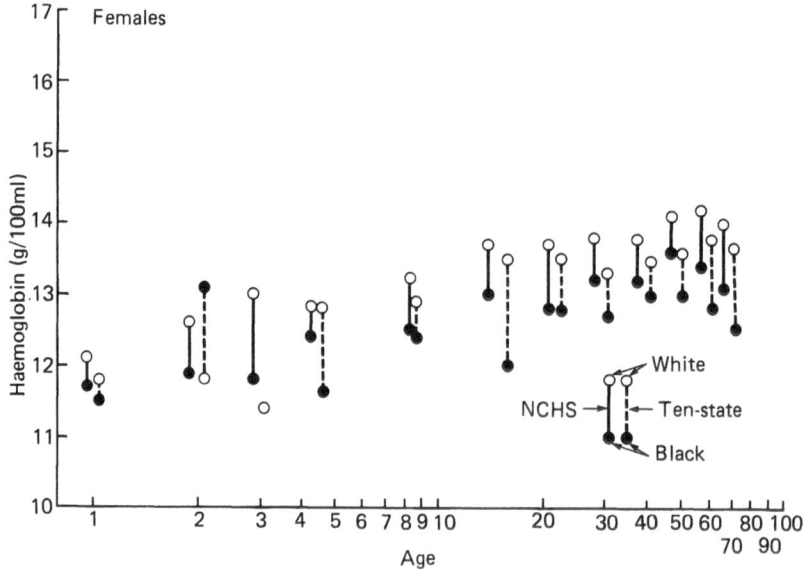

Figure 2

80

which take into account the Black–White differences in haemoglobin concentrations, the prevalence of anaemia in the three surveys differs by age and race (Table 12). Hispanics are included with other Whites. The greater prevalence of anaemia found in the TSNS reflects the significantly lower socioeconomic status of the population studied. Note the similar prevalence figures for anaemia among preschool children in PNS and N-HANES-I.

Table 12 Per cent of individuals with anaemia

Age (yrs)	PNS Black	White	TSNS Black	White	N-HANES-I Black	White
1–5	12	7	25	14	12	7
6–17	—	—	26	15	5	4
≥ 18	—	—	22	12	11	5

GENERAL COMMENTS

National surveys

Several observations may be made from these three major nutrition surveys undertaken in the US between 1968 and 1973.

1) There is a direct, positive correlation between level of intake of food (calories and most nutrients) and socioeconomic status within age-, sex- and race-specific groups.

2) Heights and weights of children within age-, sex- and race-specific groups correlate directly with socioeconomic status.

3) Iron deficiency, iron deficiency anaemia and obesity are the most prevalent nutrition-related disorders in the US.

4) Some segments of the population, predominantly low income groups, have low intakes of vitamin C and low levels of vitamin C in blood plasma. Similarly, some groups of Blacks, Hispanics and Native Americans have comparatively low levels of vitamin A in blood plasma.

Observations since N-HANES-I

While the PNS was in progress, a special study was undertaken with a population of Apache preschool children. Some 20% were anaemic and between 15 and 25% had low levels of vitamin A and C in plasma. In another cohort of preschool children on the same reservation studied some 7 years later (1976), the prevalence of anaemia was 10% and only 1 or 2% of children had low plasma levels of vitamin A and vitamin C[19]. Because both studies were undertaken by the same group of investigators using similar methods and procedures, it seems reasonable to conclude there had been a substantial improvement in the nutritional status of young children in this population.

The Center for Disease Control (CDC) initiated a nutrition surveillance system in 1973, with the continuing collection of selected indices of nutritional status including haemoglobin levels, haematocrits, heights and weights of children seen in a variety of health care situations. These data are summarized and distributed periodically and provide some insight into changes occurring among predominantly low income children. During the period between 1976 and 1979, it appears that between 12 and 15% of Black children and between 8 and 10% of White children had 'low' levels of haemoglobin. These figures suggest that during the past decade, intervention programmes have had some measurable impact on the problem of iron deficiency. Some care must be exercised in these data in view of the biased nature of populations being served in various public health care settings, and the basis for selection of individuals within these populations whose haemoglobin levels are determined.

In the mid-1970s, the nutritional status of a selected group of Kentucky teenagers was evaluated[20]. Included were 85 White and 33 Black adolescents with a mean age of approximately 15.2 years. Their nutrient intakes were very similar to those of adolescents in the TSNS and N-HANES-I except that Kentucky girls of both ethnic groups had lower average intakes of calories, iron and several of the B vitamins. Some 25% of females and 10% of males were classified as obese, on the basis of triceps skinfold thickness. Because a substantial number of individuals were on 'reducing' diets and restricted calorie intake, it was not surprising that some of the teenagers had significantly low intakes of iron, calcium and vitamin A. Between 15 and 50% of study participants had unacceptable levels of haemoglobin while between 10 and 25% had low levels of transferrin saturation. Folate nutriture was not evaluated. While mean serum cholesterol values of the Kentucky teenagers were in agreement with National data (N-HANES-I), approximately two-thirds of the Blacks had serum total cholesterol greater than 230 mg/dl. Levels of serum cholesterol and other lipid fractions correlated significantly with body weight among females but not among males. Questioning of teenagers indicated that about one-fourth of them irregularly took multivitamin supplements.

From a representative sample of adults in the State of Michigan, some 1100 White persons had measurements taken of height, weight and several skinfold thicknesses in 1978[21]. Michigan men and women in 1978 were on average 1.8 and 1.2 kg heavier, respectively, than their N-HANES-I counterparts, although average heights-for-age were the same. At all age groups with the exception of females at age 18–24 years, triceps and subscapular skinfolds were greater for Michigan adults (Figures 3 and 4). It will be of interest to see if these findings are confirmed by the N-HANES-I study, especially in view of the progressive decline in total serum cholesterol values among adults during the past decade.

In a study of nutritional status of elderly White persons in Missouri, it was reported that at least one-third consumed at least one vitamin and/or mineral supplement one or more times per week[22]. Among supplements reported were iron tablets, multivitamins, multivitamins plus minerals, Geritol®, calcium tablets and vitamin C. Although 20% of men and 10% of women had low levels of haemoglobin and serum iron, few individuals had low levels of vitamin

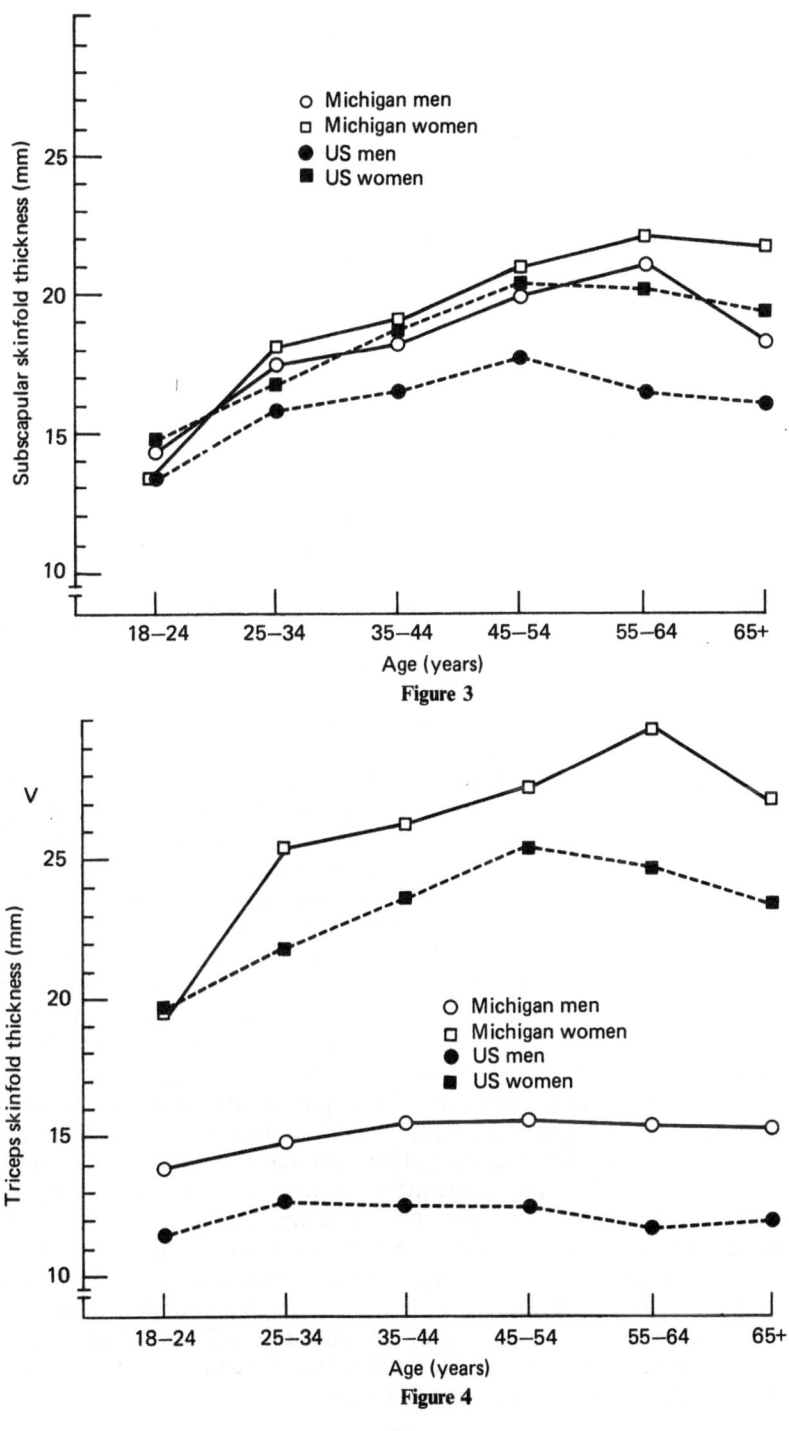

Figure 3

Figure 4

A, carotene, vitamin C, or riboflavin (erythrocyte glutathione reductase) in blood. Serum folacin was not measured. Although skinfolds were not measured in the Missouri study, the investigators concluded that more than half (59%) of the women and about one-fourth (22%) of men were obese, with body weights greater than 120% of desirable weight.

More recently, investigators in Florida reported that 14% of elderly Blacks living in the Dade county area were anaemic but not iron deficient[23]. At least one-fifth of these low income individuals were taking supplemental iron. Some 40% of the nearly 200 persons had low levels of serum folacin (< 6 ng/ml) and of these, some 60% were considered to be at 'high risk' because erythrocyte folacin levels were low (< 140 ng/ml). No information was given regarding use of supplemental vitamins.

CONCLUSIONS

Review of the medical literature since the mid-1970s indicates that a relatively small number of limited surveys or studies of nutritional status have been undertaken in the United States. N-HANES-II is in progress, and even preliminary findings are not available while the continuing CDC nutrition surveillance is somewhat restricted in its scope. Examination of some selected studies involving individuals of different ages living in different geographic locales indicates findings largely in keeping with those of major surveys conducted between 1968 and 1974. Anaemia is still a major problem and though iron deficiency is likely to be the major cause, there may be substantial numbers of adults with folacin deficiency.

While there are some problems of definition, obesity is probably the other most prevalent nutrition-related disorder in the United States. It is likely that a substantial proportion of the population from adolescence through later adult life is at any one point of time voluntarily restricting calorie intake to lose weight or control weight. This has some implications with respect to adequacy of intake of a number of micronutrients over extended periods of time even though it appears that some 25% or more of adolescents and adults are supplementing their diets with various vitamin and mineral preparations. Most major surveys and the majority of small scale or limited studies have concluded that protein intake was adequate. However, when calorie intake is low, some proportion of protein will be used as an energy source.

It is recognized that substance abuse, particularly alcohol and various illegal drugs may adversely affect the nutritional status of a significant number of individuals in the US. Similarly, there are many persons taking over-the-counter, as well as prescribed medicines which may interfere with ingestion, digestion, absorption, or metabolism of essential nutrients. One wonders to what extent restriction of calorie intake alone and in concert with other behaviours noted above including smoking, may contribute to less than optimal nutritional status. How much of the malnutrition, and risk of malnutrition, of persons admitted to hospitals reflects primary disease processes, how much reflects uncontrollable socioeconomic factors and how much reflects the individual's health behaviour[24,25]?

References

1. Owen, A. Y. (1978). Community nutrition in preventive health care services: a critical review of the literature. *DHEW Publ. No. (HRA)* **78–14017**
2. Owen, G. M., Kram, K. M., Garry, P. J., Lowe, J. E. and Lubin, A. H. (1974). A study of nutritional status of preschool children in the United States: 1968–1970. *Pediatrics*, **53**, 597
3. Ten State Nutrition Survey in the United States, 1968–1970 (1972). *DHEW Publ. No. (HSM)* **72–8130** to **72–8134**
4. Committee to Review Ten-State Nutrition: Reflections on dietary studies with children in Ten State Nutrition Survey of 1968–1970 (1975). *Pediatrics*, **56**, 320
5. Garn, S. M. and Clark, D. C. (1975). Nutrition, growth, development and maturation: Findings from Ten State Nutrition Survey of 1968–1970. *Pediatrics*, **56**, 306
6. Garn, S. M. and Clark, D. C. (1976). Trends in fatness and origins of obesity. Committee to Review the Ten State Nutrition Survey of 1968–1970. *Pediatrics*, **57**, 443
7. Preliminary Findings of the First Health and Nutrition Survey, United States, 1971–1972: Dietary and biochemical findings (1975). *DHEW Publ. No. (HRA)* **74–1219**
8. Preliminary Findings of the First Health and Nutrition Survey, (1975). *DHEW Publ. No. (HRA)* **75–1229**
9. Abraham, S. (1978). Total serum cholesterol levels of children 4–17 years, United States, 1971–1974. *Vital and Health Statistics: Series 11, Data from National Health Survey: No. 207. DHEW Publ. No. (PHS)* **78–1655**
10. Fulwood, R. (1980). Serum cholesterol levels of persons 4–74 years of age by socioeconomic characteristics, United States, 1971–1974. *Vital and Health Statistics: Series 11, Data from the National Health Survey; No. 217. DHEW Publ. No. (PHS)* **80–1667**
11. Caloric and selected nutrient values for persons 1–74 years of age, United States, 1971–1974 (1979). *Vital and Health Statistics: Series 11. Data from the National Health Survey: No. 209. DHEW Publ. No. (PHS)* **79–1659**
12. Johnson, C. L. and Abraham, S. (1979). Hemoglobin and selected iron-related findings of persons 1–74 years of age: United States, 1971–1974. *Advance Data No. 46, from Vital and Health Statistics, DHEW Publ. No. (PHS)* **79–1250**
13. Owen, G. M., Lubin, A. H. and Garry, P. J. (1973). Hemoglobin levels according to age, race and transferrin saturation in preschool children of comparable socioeconomic status. *J. Pediatr.*, **82**, 850
14. Garn, S. M., Smith, N. J. and Clark, D. C. (1975). Lifelong differences in hemoglobin levels between Blacks and Whites. *J. Natl. Med. Assoc.*, **67**, 91
15. Dallman, P. R., Barr, G. D., Allen, C. M. and Shinefield, H. R. (1978). Hemoglobin concentration in White, Black and Oriental children: Is there a need for separate criteria in screening for anemia. *Am. J. Clin. Nutr.*, **31**, 377
16. Meyers, L. D., Habicht, J. P. and Johnson, C. L. (1979). Components of the difference in hemoglobin concentrations in blood between Black and White women in the United States. *Am. J. Epidemiol.*, **109**, 539
17. Owen, G. M. and Owen, A. Y. (1977). Should there be a different definition of anemia in Black and White children? *Am. J. Publ. Hlth*, **67**, 865
18. Garn, S. M. and Clark, D. C. (1976). Problems in the nutritional assessment of Black individuals. *Am. J. Publ. Hlth*, **66**, 262
19. Owen, G. M., Garry, P. J., Seymoure, R. D., Harrison, G. G. and Acosta, P. B. (1981). Nutrition studies with White Mountain Apache preschool children in 1976 and 1969. *Am. J. Clin. Nutr.*, **31**, 266
20. Lee, C. J. (1978). Nutritional status of selected teenagers in Kentucky. *Am. J. Clin. Nutr.*, **31**, 1453
21. Moffatt, R. T., Sady, S. P. and Owen, G. M. (1980). Height, weight and skinfold thickness of Michigan adults. *Am. J. Publ. Hlth.*, **70**, 1290
22. Kohrs, M. D., O'Neal, R., Preston, A., Eklund, D. and Abrahams, O. (1978). Nutritional status of elderly residents in Missouri. *Am. J. Clin. Nutr.*, **31**, 2186
23. Barley, L. B., Wagner, P. A., Christakis, G. J., Araujo, P. E., Appledorf, H., Davis, C. G., Masteryanni, J. and Dinning, J. S. (1979). Folacin and iron status and hematological findings in predominantly Black elderly persons from urban low-income households. *Am. J. Clin. Nutr.*, **32**, 2346

24. Merritt, R. J. and Suskind, R. M. (1979). Nutritional survey of hospitalized pediatric patients. *Am. J. Clin. Nutr.*, **32,** 1320
25. Weinsier, R. L., Hunker, E. M., Krumdieck, C. L. and Butterworth, C. E. (1979). Hospital malnutrition: A prospective evaluation of general medical patients during the course of hospitalization. *Am. J. Clin. Nutr.*, **32,** 418

4
Nitrate, nitrite and *N*-nitroso compounds: biochemistry, metabolism, toxicity and carcinogenicity

L. C. GREEN, D. RALT AND S. R. TANNENBAUM

N-NITROSO COMPOUNDS
Definitions and toxicological significance

The addition of a nitroso group ($-N=O$) to a nitrogen atom is termed *N*-nitrosation: its product is an *N*-nitroso compound. These compounds include the nitrosamines $(RR'-N-N=O)$, nitrosamides $(R-\overset{\text{O}}{\underset{\|}{C}}-N-N=O)$, nitrosoureas $(R-\underset{\underset{\|}{\overset{\|}{O}}}{\overset{|}{N}}-\overset{\|}{C}-NH_2)$, and derivatives.

The simplest of *N*-nitroso compounds, and perhaps the most widespread, is *N*-nitrosodimethylamine (NDMA), or dimethylnitrosamine (DMN). The toxicity of DMN was apparently first studied by Freund in 1937[1]. Freund reported that two industrial chemists involved in the development and manufacture of DMN routinely developed headaches, weakness, anorexia and other signs of intoxication. One became acutely ill after cleaning up an accidental spill of DMN: this individual died following an exploratory laparotomy. Upon postmortem examination, an enlarged liver with signs of diffuse degeneration and intense regenerative proliferation was found. Freund showed that an experimental exposure of mice or dogs to DMN vapours for $\frac{1}{2}$ hour proved fatal; cirrhosis with ascites and other signs of hepatic damage were also evident in the animals postmortem. He concluded: 'Dimethylnitrosamine is a volatile toxic substance which upon inhalation exerts a destructive action on the liver. Its use should be considered as an industrial hazard.' A dozen years later, Hamilton and Hardy[2] noted that use of DMN in automobile factories had led to 'some illnesses'. These authors also reported that severe liver damage in dogs was experimentally induced by DMN.

In 1954, two cases of liver cirrhosis in laboratory workers employing DMN as a solvent were again reported[3]. The investigators, Barnes and Magee, showed by use of experimental animals that DMN was organ specific in its toxicity, i.e. that whether administered by mouth or by vein, severe damage in the liver would result. The authors considered, as had Freund, that DMN's toxicity might be the result of its reduction *in vivo* to the hydrazine. Their co-investigator Aldridge, however, dosed rabbits with 100 mg dimethylhydrazine/kg which, though lethal, did not induce liver damage. (The lethal dose for DMN in rabbits was 15 mg/kg). Barnes and Magee concluded that DMN was likely metabolized to another 'toxic breakdown product'. In the next 2 years, Magee and Barnes[4] showed that DMN was not only a toxin but also a carcinogen. It might be noted that by 1962, Magee and co-workers discovered that the 'toxic breakdown product' causing the damage and the cancer was in fact a methylating moiety[5-7].

Through the later 1950s, the field of nitrosamine investigations remained quite small, due no doubt to the belief that exposures to humans were only by inhalation and only in a few industrial settings. Things changed dramatically in the early 1960s. Outbreaks of toxic hepatosis with characteristic symptoms and lesions in sheep were reported[8,9]; a component of the feed – herring meal preserved with nitrite – was implicated[10]; the similarities between the hepatotoxic symptoms in the accidentally poisoned sheep and in experimentally poisoned animals strongly suggested the presence and action of DMN. Analysis revealed that toxic samples indeed contained the nitrosamine, at levels of 15–50 mg DMN/kg feed[11,12].

Since then, about 300 different *N*-nitroso compounds have been tested and found to be carcinogenic in animals. DMN itself has been shown to induce cancer in mice, rats, hamsters, guinea pigs, rabbits, ducks, fish, newts and frogs, causing benign and malignant tumours primarily of the liver, but also of the kidney, lung and nasal cavities. Dimethylnitrosamine appears to be carcinogenic whether inhaled or ingested and whether given by prenatal, single or multiple dosing. The potency of DMN is not insignificant: rats fed as little as 2 or 5 mg DMN/kg diet develop liver tumours[13]. Recent results suggest that doses as low as 0.1 mg DMN/l of drinking water are tumorigenic in rats[14]. The absorption and metabolic activation of DMN makes it more hazardous still: rats given DMN by gastric intubation or peritoneal injection show a dose-dependent alkylation of DNA from doses from 10 mg/kg body weight down to 1 μg/kg[15,16]. Finally, rat liver and human liver are similarly adept at metabolizing DMN to the active methylating species[7,17].

The scope of the problem is not small. The reader is referred to some of the excellent reviews on dimethylnitrosamine and other *N*-nitroso compounds[18-21]. This review makes mention of the *in vitro* and *in vivo* formation and occurrence of *N*-nitroso compounds, then focuses on the several aspects of nitrate and nitrite in microbial, animal and human metabolism and toxicity.

Formation and occurrence

Man may be exposed to *N*-nitroso compounds through a variety of circumstances:

(a) formation from precursors in the environment and exposure of man through food, water, or air,

(b) formation in the human body from precursors separately ingested in food, water, or air, and

(c) formation in the human body from precursors formed in the body.

Whether the formation of *N*-nitroso compounds is exogenous or endogenous, the chemical considerations are of a similar nature. Mirvish was the first to exploit the available knowledge on the chemical kinetics of nitrosation[22] and apply it to the problem of carcinogenesis[23]. He has more recently reviewed the entire field of nitrosation kinetics[20] and the reader is recommended to that article for details on rate equations and differences between classes of nitrogen compounds.

The chemistry of nitrite is complex. Some of the key equilibria for conversion of nitrite to a nitrosating agent are shown below (nitrosating agents are underlined:

$$H^+ + NO_2^- \rightleftharpoons HNO_2 \qquad pKa = 3.4$$

$$HNO_2 + H^+ \rightleftharpoons \underline{H_2NO_2^+}$$

$$2HNO_2 \rightleftharpoons \underline{N_2O_3} + H_2O$$

$$HNO_2 + HX \rightleftharpoons \underline{NOX} + H_2O \quad (X = halide \ or \ pseudohalide)$$

$$2NO_2 \cdot \rightleftharpoons \underline{N_2O_4}.$$

The field of nitrosamine chemistry is remarkable for its historical fictions. The most interesting of these is the belief that tertiary amines are unreactive to nitrosation, a comment commonly found in organic chemistry texts. Lijinsky and co-workers demonstrated the generality of tertiary amine nitrosation in 1972[24], and Lijinsky and Greenblatt[25] discovered what is most probably the most rapid known reaction leading to formation of DMN at ordinary temperatures – the nitrosation of aminopyrine. It is now recognized that any nitrogen compound, including quaternary ammonium compounds[26] and primary amines[27] may lead to the formation of *N*-nitroso compounds from starting materials as diverse as food constituents, drugs, agricultural chemicals, and industrial chemicals. The reader is referred to Scanlan[28] for details.

The environmental conditions which lead to formation of *N*-nitroso compounds depend upon the composition of the reaction medium. Aside from factors, such as high temperature, which normally accelerate chemical reactions, pH and ionic composition have significant effects. The halide ions and thiocyanate, for example, are among the most potent accelerators of nitrosation reactions. Their effect has been quantitatively described[29], and the extent of their effect is a complex function of pH and relative concentration of the reactants. The pH of the medium profoundly affects reaction rates[20], with maxima generally occurring at pH values of from 2 and 3.5 for secondary amines, increasing with increasing acidity for amides and ureas, and occurring at various pHs for tertiary amines.

Other factors can also play a role. Formaldehyde can promote nitrosation even in neutral or basic reaction media[30]: this effect also extends to other carbonyl compounds of selected structure[31]. Phenols and related compounds such as tannins have complex effects, which can be either inhibitory to amine nitrosation or can promote amine nitrosation[32,33]. These mixed effects have recently been shown to involve the process of transnitrosation, and may be explained by the structure of the particular phenol[34]. Nitrosation may also occur in basic solution under the influence of nitrogen oxides (NO_x)[35].

Important reactions compete with nitrosation in most environments. Primary amino acids, and secondary amines such as proline compete for nitrite, generally to form products that are either not nitrosamines or are not carcinogenic. Several other compounds compete for nitrite so effectively that amine nitrosation is blocked completely. The most effective of these compounds is ascorbic acid[36] which will inhibit nitrosation in many systems if it is present in twice the molar concentration of nitrite[37]. This effect has been exploited to impede nitrosation *in vivo*[38,39] and in foods that contain nitrite[40]. Other compounds which will compete for nitrite to form biologically inactive products include glutathione[41] and α-tocopherol[37,42]. The latter compound is lipophilic and therefore useful for blocking nitrosation in adipose tissue or in other multiphasic systems.

The entrance into the stomach of nitrite from food and saliva, followed by intragastric bacterial nitrate reduction under conditions of hypoacidity[43,44], may lead to the formation of N-nitroso compounds from nitrogenous constituents of foods, drugs, and agricultural chemicals. The concept of intragastric nitrosation as a process capable of generating carcinogenic N-nitroso compounds in man was originally proposed by Sander[45]. This view is supported by recent experiments which suggest the presence of nitrosamines in normal human blood[46,47]. The kinetics of intragastric nitrosation in animals and the quantative relations to carcinogenesis have been summarized by Mirvish[20]. It is important to note that experiments in rats and mice, however, may not reflect the condition in man. Diethylamine, for example, is not demonstrably nitrosated in the stomach of either rats or mice, but is nitrosated in the stomachs of both cats and rabbits[48]. This difference may be the result of differences in pH or in other ionic constituents of gastric juice.

Although foods may contain many secondary and tertiary amines[49], consideration must also be given to drugs and agricultural and industrial chemicals as sources of nitrosatable compounds. The chemistry of nitrosation of agricultural chemicals has been thoroughly explored[50,51]; in general these chemicals would be expected to be present in low concentrations in soils or as residues on agricultural products. In contrast, drugs and medicines may be taken in large doses by certain individuals, and several of these afford high yields of volatile and non-volatile N-nitroso compounds[52].

The nitrosation of food constituents may lead to N-nitroso compounds by complex and circuitous routes. Examples of this complexity are the formation of N-nitrososarcosine from creatine[53], the bacterial degradation of creatiné to methylguanidine followed by conversion to N-nitrosomethylcyanamide[54], the various reactions of nitrite with proteins[55], and the formation of N-nitrosodimethylamine from lecithin[56].

A situation of major concern has been the formation of N-nitrosopyrrolidine (Npyr) in fried bacon. The mechanism of formation of

Npyr has been the subject of several investigations[57–59]. Neither pyrrolidine (pyr) nor Npyr is present in uncooked bacon, but proline (pro) is present. A major question has been whether, during cooking, pro is first nitrosated to Npro and then decarboxylated to Npyr, or whether pro first decarboxylates to pyr and is then nitrosated to yield Npyr. Nitrosation does occur during cooking, since yields of Npyr are substantially reduced by the addition of the blocking agent ascorbyl palmitate to bacon prior to frying[60]. Npro in raw bacon is not a major source of Npyr in fried bacon[61]. ^{14}C-labelling experiments indicate that pyr is first formed and then nitrosated to yield Npyr[62].

A second source of exposure from food has been the formation of dimethylnitrosamine (DMN) in malted barley and its subsequent contamination of beer[63–65]. The nitrosamine is formed during the drying of the green malt when the drying gases contain NO_x as a result of direct flame heating. This problem has been solved through the use of sulphur burning, which produces SO_2 during drying and removes NO_x from the heated air, or by lowering flame temperature to reduce the rate of NO_x formation[66].

The most comprehensive survey of human exposure to nitrosamines from food has been conducted in the German market[66]. More than 3000 commercially available samples have been analysed, from which it has been estimated that there was an average daily intake of 1.1 μg DMN and of 0.1–0.15 μg Npyr *per capita* in 1978. Since almost 2/3 of the DMN was from beer, the 1980 exposure has been reduced considerably from the 1978 level.

Tobacco can also be a source of nitrosamines: pyrolysis products and naturally occurring alkaloids may form volatile and non-volatile *N*-nitroso compounds[67,68].

Nitrosamines can also form in the industrial environment. A major problem is the widespread use of nitrite salts as corrosion inhibitors in packaging materials[69] and in synthetic cutting fluids[70,71]. Quite high levels of *N*-nitroso compounds can form in these materials – in the order of hundreds of mg/l. *N*-nitrosodiethanolamine is the predominant product, and *N*-nitroso-morpholine is occasionally formed. Another source of industrial exposure is found in rubber factories, where the use of amines and diphenylnitrosamine, the presence of NO_x, and the possibility of transnitrosation, lead to serious air contamination, particularly from DMN and *N*-nitrosomorpholine[66,72]. Simulated atmospheric conditions have been studied with respect to the formation of nitrosamines and other derivatives of aliphatic amines[73].

It may be that man's exposure to nitrosamines through endogenous synthesis exceeds that from preformed compounds in the environment. An attempt has been made to estimate the order of magnitude of the flux of DMN, based upon blood concentrations and the assumption of a quasi steady state between formation and metabolism[74]. This analysis suggests that some individuals in the population may be exposed to very low rates of endogenous synthesis, while others may receive total body doses of up to 10 μg (kg body weight)$^{-1}$ d^{-1}. The total dose received by an individual from endogenous plus exogenous sources would be determined by his or her lifestyle exposure, occupation, and individual metabolism. The net result of these various factors is presently unknown.

OCCURRENCE OF NITRATE AND NITRITE

Nitrate occurrence is widespread. Its presence is the result of various processes that convert atmospheric N_2 into nitrogen oxides. These processes are of two general types:

(a) High temperature oxidation of nitrogen, resulting from the combustion of fuel, from lightning, volcanoes, etc.
(b) Biological nitrogen fixation and nitrification by micro-organisms.

As a result of these processes, nitrate can commonly be found in aerosols in the atmosphere[75,76], and in solution in water supplies, soils, and plants. Nitrate is often found in high concentrations in plant materials since it is the plants' primary source of nitrogen nutrition. Roots, tubers, leaves, and stems take up and store nitrate from soil and water: foods derived therefrom contain up to thousands of mg of nitrate/kg. These sources have been reviewed in a recent environmental assessment of nitrate[77].

The occurrence of nitrate in the food supply has been evaluated and the average intake estimated[78,79]. Table 1 summarizes the major vegetable sources of nitrate. The amount of nitrite in vegetables is variable, but low, although abnormally high levels may result from permissive conditions of storage (see p. 111). Prolonged storage of vegetables in the dark, for example, leads to reversible accumulation of nitrite, since nitrate reduction is uncoupled from photophosphorylation while nitrite reduction requires light. We have stored spinach in the refrigerator in the dark and measured nitrite concentrations as high as 700 ppm (unpublished data). Determining factors of nitrate content include plant variety, maturity, level and type of fertilization, rainfall, etc. Therefore, the values in Table 1 are to be taken only as estimates of average levels.

The known sources of exposure to nitrite were quantified by White in 1976[79] and are shown in Table 2. The various routes of nitrite exposure are discussed below.

Nitrite may be added to meat, cheese and poultry, according to a variety of regulations of the Food and Drug Administration and the Department of Agriculture in the USA and corresponding regulating agencies in other countries. The major use by far is in cured meat products, as a preservative against *Clostridium botulinum*. Currently allowed usage in the USA is 100–150 ppm (mg/kg) of sodium nitrite together with 550 ppm of ascorbic acid (or its erythro isomer). Under these conditions, the average residual nitrite content (ppm sodium nitrite × 0.67) at the earliest sampling time following manufacture was determined to be 24 ppm in 1977[80]. This may be compared to the value of 52.5 ppm nitrite used by White in his 1976 publication. When this lower residual nitrite value is substituted into the calculations in Table 2, the contribution from cured meat to overall nitrite exposure falls to 11%.

The fate of nitrite in cured meat products has been the subject of a great deal of investigation by Cassens *et al.*[81]. Using $^{15}NO_2^-$ they have demonstrated that most of the nitrite reacts with a variety of substrates, leading to binding or conversion to apparently innocuous products. A summary of these reactions is shown in Table 3.

Table 1 Source of nitrate and nitrite ingested from vegetables by the average US residence, 1972 (from White[78])

Item	Per capita consumption (lb/yr)	Per capita consumption (g/day)	Composition, ppm Nitrate	Composition, ppm Nitrite	Daily ingestion, µg Nitrate	Daily ingestion, µg Nitrite
Potatoes, white	96.0	119	119	0.4	14 200	47.6
Tomatoes and products	25.8	31.9	62	1.3	1980	41.5
Lettuce	17.9	22.2	850	0.4	18 900	8.9
Melons	17.4	21.6	433		9350	
Corn	13.8	17.1	45	2.0	770	34.2
Onions	9.60	11.9	134	0.7	1590	8.3
Beans, snap	8.23	10.2	253	0.9	2580	9.2
Pickles	7.70	9.5	59		560	
Carrots	7.02	8.70	119	0.8	1040	7.0
Cabbage	6.96	8.63	635	0.5	5480	4.3
Beans, dry	6.2	7.7	13		100	
Peas	5.70	7.07	28	0.7	198	4.9
Celery	5.52	6.84	2340	0.5	16 000	3.4
Potatoes, sweet	4.02	4.98	53		264	
Cucumbers	2.64	3.27	24	0.5	78	1.6
Peppers, sweet	2.16	2.68	125	0.7	335	1.9
Spinach	1.82	2.26	1860	2.7	4200	6.1
Beets	1.60	1.98	2760	6.0	5460	11.9
Sauerkraut	1.40	1.74	191	0.4	332	0.7
Broccoli	1.31	1.62	783	1.0	1270	1.6
Cauliflower	1.15	1.43	547	1.1	782	1.6
Asparagus	1.10	1.36	21	0.9	28	1.2
Beans, lima	0.99	1.23	54	1.1	66	1.3
Pumpkin/squash	0.74	0.92	413	0.7	380	0.6
Eggplant (Aubergine)	0.40	0.49	302	0.5	148	0.2
Total					86 mg	0.2 mg

Table 2 Estimated average daily ingestion of nitrate and nitrite for US resident

Source	Nitrate (mg)	Nitrate (%)	Nitrite (mg)	Nitrite (%)
Vegetables	86.1	86.3	0.20	1.8
Fruits, juices	1.4	1.4	0.00	0.0
Milk and products	0.2	0.2	0.00	0.0
Bread	2.0	2.0	0.02	0.2
Water	0.7	0.7	0.00	0.0
Cured meats	9.4	9.4	2.38	21.2
Saliva	30.0*	—	8.62	76.8
Total	99.8	100.0	11.22	100.0

* Not included in total.
From: White[79].

Since nitrate is naturally present in many vegetables and other foods, frequent opportunities exist for enzymatic reduction of nitrate to nitrite. This type of exposure to nitrite is highly variable, and dependent upon the methods of processing and storage of food. The occasional development of nitrite in this manner to levels toxic to infants is discussed in the Section on toxicity (p. 100).

A second source of inadvertent contamination involves certain types of dehydration processes, specifically those in which air is heated directly by flame or combustion. In these cases, the nitrogen oxides (NO_x) which are formed in the heated air may ultimately be deposited in the food product as nitrite. This has been documented for foods such as milk or soybean protein preparations which have been dried with direct-flame heated air. This source of exposure is also highly variable and therefore difficult to estimate. Concentrations of tens of parts per million of nitrite have been detected in divers dehydrated food products.

The existence of nitrite in saliva has been known for about 100 years[82]. Salivary nitrite arises from nitrate by bacterial reduction in the oral cavity, and while amounts of nitrite formed in saliva vary among people and among diets, this source is generally the largest single contribution to an individual's overall exposure to nitrite. Salivary nitrite is discussed further (p. 117). Exposure to nitrite may also include microbial nitrate reduction in the hypochlorhydric

Table 3 Fate of nitrite in cured meat

Substance	% of nitrite
Haem pigment	5–15
Non-haem protein	20–30
Bound to sulphydryl	5–15
Converted to nitrate	1–10
Bound to lipid	1–5
Converted to gaseous products	1–5
Residual nitrite	5–20

From: Cassens et al.[81].

stomach or the infected urinary tract. These contributions are considered later (p. 117).

Extensive use of nitrite as an industrial anti-corrosion agent may also be an important source of exposure[69]. Again, although this source is probably general, it is not possible at the present time to estimate the magnitude of its contribution.

Smoking of tobacco introduces a considerable amount of nitrogen oxides into the lungs[83]. Air pollution also increases exposure to NO_x; NO_2 is absorbed through the lungs and converted to nitrite and nitrate[84]. The contribution of this source to nitrite exposure is not known. It is of interest to note that mice gavaged with morpholine and exposed to NO_2 appear to synthesize nitrosomorpholine *in vivo*[85].

ENZYMOLOGY OF AMMONIA, AMINES AND NITRATE

Nitrogen oxidation

The oxidation of ammonia to nitrate is a continuous process in soils; it is part of the nitrogen cycle wherein atmospheric nitrogen is converted to the plant nutrient, nitrate. Until recently, this reaction was thought to occur exclusively in micro-organisms, but current evidence suggests that reduced nitrogen can be converted to nitrate in mammalian tissues (see p. 122). This section summarizes the known systems in micro-organisms, then postulates possible routes of nitrate metabolism in animals.

Most of the knowledge on microbial nitrogen oxidation derives from experiments with the autotrophic micro-organisms, *Nitrosomonas* and *Nitrobacter*[86]. *Nitrosomonas* catalyses the oxidation of ammonia and hydroxylamine to nitrite (Scheme 1), while *Nitrobacter* catalyses the oxidation of nitrite to nitrate.

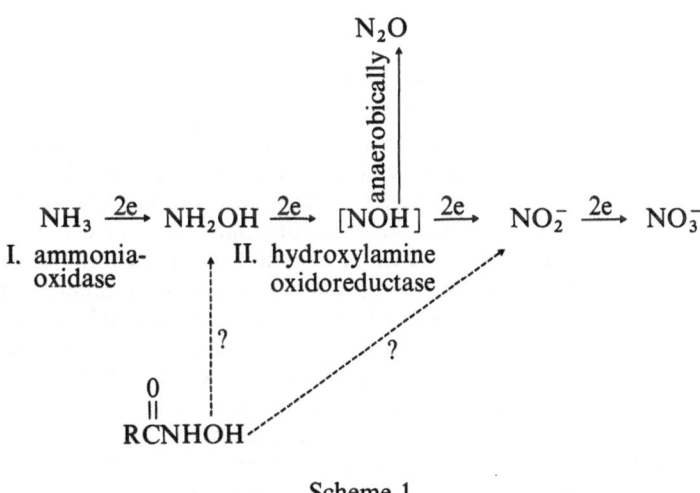

Scheme 1

Since *Nitrosomonas* catalyses the oxidation of ammonia as well as hydroxylamine to nitrite, it has been postulated that hydroxylamine is an intermediate in the oxidation of ammonia to nitrite. The intermediate between hydroxylamine and nitrite, however, remains unidentified. Apparently it is not hyponitrite, since cell-free extracts that oxidize hydroxylamine will not oxidize hyponitrite[87]. In the absence of oxygen, hydroxylamine will be oxidized to N_2O, and nitrite is not formed[88].

The first step of ammonia oxidation is probably catalysed by an oxygenase: it is unlikely that it is oxidized via the respiratory chain because of the high redox potential of the NH_4^+/NH_2OH couple $(+0.899 \, V)$[89].

Hydroxylamine oxidation, in contrast to ammonia oxidation, is catalysed via the respiratory chain[89] as described in Scheme 2:

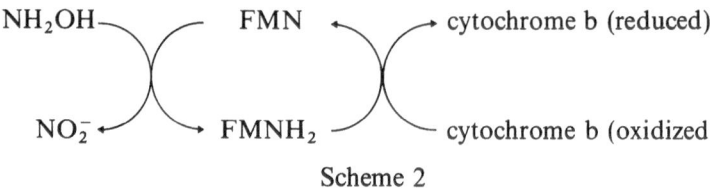

$$NH_2OH \qquad FMN \qquad cytochrome \; b \; (reduced)$$
$$NO_2^- \qquad FMNH_2 \qquad cytochrome \; b \; (oxidized)$$

Scheme 2

The enzyme hydroxylamine oxidoreductase has been purified, and its molecular weight measured to be about $200\,000$[90]. Hydroxylamine oxidation is probably closely coupled to the oxidation of ammonia, since there is always an induction period for ammonia oxidation which is eliminated following addition of trace amounts of hydroxylamine[87].

Nitrobacter catalyses the oxidation of nitrite to nitrate:

$$NO_2^- + \tfrac{1}{2}O_2 \rightarrow NO_3^- \qquad \Delta F = -17 \, \text{kcal/mol}$$

This oxidation involves a flavomolybdoprotein and cytochrome, which probably act sequentially. The activity is linked to the respiratory chain and is associated with the cell membrane[89]. The cytochrome concerned has been partially purified from *Nitrobacter* and some of its physical characteristics resemble those of mammalian cytochrome c[91].

A similar pathway has recently been demonstrated in heterotrophic bacteria[92]. Moreover, organic amine derivatives, such as acetohydroxamate or acetaldoxime, are also oxidized to nitrite by heterotrophic bacteria[93,94]. This pathway is suggested in Scheme 1. This portion of the scheme is only hypothetical, since this biochemistry in heterotrophic bacteria is not well-understood. It is not clear whether heterotrophic bacteria can utilize the energy dissipated from this oxidation, or whether the pathway is used for detoxification or other metabolic purposes (e.g. formation of siderophores)[94].

Although no one has demonstrated the oxidation of ammonia to hydroxylamine in mammalian tissues, it is well known that liver and other tissues catalyse the N-oxidation of numerous amines[95]. Heubner suggested as early as 1913 that methaemoglobin formation might be due to an N-hydroxy metabolite of certain aromatic amines (e.g. *p*-chloroaniline)[96]. Mammalian liver microsomes contain two distinct enzyme systems utilizing NADPH as a source of reducing equivalents for the subsequent oxidation of a variety of compounds. Two flavoproteins have been isolated from pig liver microsomes, one catalysing the reduction of the cytochrome P_{450} system, and the other catalysing the direct NADPH and oxygen dependent *N*-oxidation of amines[97]. During the last 5 years, interest has developed in metabolic *N*-oxidation of primary and secondary aliphatic amines[98], but the research has been focused on the immediate product (the hydroxylamine) and the possibility of second and third oxidation steps has been ignored.

The second postulated mammalian oxidation step is the oxidation of hydroxylamine to nitrite. Preliminary experiments from our work have shown that this reaction can occur even non-enzymatically using the Udenfriend system (ascorbic acid, Fe^{2+}, EDTA, O_2, pH 7), which mimics biological oxidation[99]. We have also demonstrated that the Udenfriend system oxidizes acetohydroxamate to nitrite to the same extent as hydroxylamine is oxidized[100].

The final oxidation step, the conversion of nitrite to nitrate, is a well known reaction that takes place in the red blood cell. Each mol of oxyhaemoglobin converted to methaemoglobin causes the oxidation of 1 mol of nitrite to nitrate[101].

One can hypothesize, then, a theoretical pathway for the formation of nitrate reduced nitrogen in mammals. This pathway could be a combination of various reactions originally functioning for other purposes, e.g. degradation, oxidation, or detoxification. Nitrate synthesis in mammalian tissues could be instead a new pathway for which the specific enzymes (and purposes) are yet to be discovered.

Alternatively, the observed formation of nitrate in mammals (see p. 122) could well be a result of non-enzymic oxidative processes, such as those involving superoxide or other reactive oxygen species.

Nitrogen reduction

The assimilatory reduction of nitrate to ammonia in plants and micro-organisms proceeds in two separate, well-defined, enzymatic steps:

(1) the reduction of nitrate to nitrite, catalysed by the flavomolybdoprotein, nitrate reductase;
(2) The reduction of nitrite to ammonia, catalysed by the iron-containing protein, nitrite reductase.

Nitrate reductase

Nitrate reductase, which catalyses the reduction of nitrate to nitrite, has been isolated from bacteria, fungi, algae and plants. The enzyme contains molybdenum (1 atom or less/mole), and has a molecular weight of $1.6–6 \times 10^5$ daltons; the K_m for nitrate varies from 0.015 to 1 mmol/l[102]. In bacteria, one or both of two nitrate reductases, 'A' and 'B', are found[103]. Enzyme 'A' reduces chlorate as well as nitrate, and is more sensitive to cyanide and azide than enzyme 'B'. Enzyme 'A' is particulate, inducible by nitrate, and repressed by O_2. Enzyme 'B' does not reduce chlorate, but is subject to chlorate inhibition, and has a higher activation energy than enzyme 'A'. The 'B' enzyme is soluble and, when constitutive, is unaffected by nitrate or oxygen.

Most enzymes utilize NADPH or NADH as primary electron donors: enzymes from higher plants more often utilize NADH[104]. Methyl and benzyl viologens can serve (with few exceptions) as electron donors[103].

Nitrate reductase has the following enzyme functions:

(a) nitrate reduction using NADPH as an electron donor,
(b) nitrate reduction using methyl viologen, benzyl viologen, $FMNH_2$, or $FADH_2$ as electron donors, and
(c) oxidation of NADPH using cytochrome c, ferricyanide, tetrazolium, etc. as electron acceptors.

The separate functions have been found through isolation of nitrate reductase-defective mutants[105]; and through selective enzyme denaturation experiments[106]. Loss of molybdenum through mutation or thermal denaturation, for example, leads to loss of ability to reduce nitrate, but cytochrome c reductase activity is retained[107]. Genetic evidence from *Aspergillus nidulans*[102] indicates that two 4.5 S flavin bearing cytochrome c reductase subunits are united into a 7.8 S wild type NADPH nitrate reductase via a cofactor subunit – cnx.

The cnx is a molybdenum binding protein of 10 000–20 000 daltons. It is thermolabile, stabilized by ionic molybdate, and dissociable, by treatment at pH 2–3, from plant and bacterial nitrate reductases, as well as from mammalian xanthine, aldehyde and sulphite oxidases[108].

The regulation of nitrate reductase is thought to be controlled by the dehydrogenase locus via one of the following mechanisms:

(a) A reversible inactivation by endogenous cyanide with a reductant, and reactivation by endogenous dehydrogenase oxidation[109], or
(b) Inactivation by reduction of the Mo in the enzyme from the oxidation state of V to state IV or III.

The redox state is controlled by the ratio of NAD(P)H to NAD(P)$^+$ [102,110].

Nitrite reductase

Nitrite reductase, which catalyses the reduction of nitrite to ammonia, has been isolated from bacteria, algae, fungi and plants. The enzyme contains iron, has a molecular weight of $0.6–1.2 \times 10^5$ daltons (*E. coli* and yeast enzymes are larger – $3.5–6.7 \times 10^5$ daltons), and a K_m for nitrite of 0.005–0.07 mmol/l[102].

Plant and algal enzymes are generally specific for single electron donors (ferredoxin, methyl viologen) and do not utilize NAD(P)H[111]. In yeast and bacteria, the enzyme is NAD(P)H specific and flavin dependent[112]. *Escherichia coli* has two nitrite reductases, one of which is specific for NADH and unable to reduce sulphite, and one which is specific for NADPH and can reduce sulphite. During anaerobic growth in the presence of nitrite, the NADPH-specific nitrite reductase is induced, together with a low potential c-type cytochrome (cytochrome c_{552}) that can be reoxidized by nitrite. The metabolic function of cyt c_{552} is as yet unclear[113]. Plant nitrite reductases do not reduce sulphite[114].

Most nitrite reductases reduce hydroxylamine[115], although the K_m for hydroxylamine is usually about 10 times higher than for nitrite. Furthermore, the reduction of hydroxylamine is inhibited by nitrite (but not vice versa). Pure preparations of nitrite reductase are unable to reduce hyponitrite or nitric oxide[111]. These data, and the fact that maximum yields of ammonia are produced from nitrite (by pure enzyme), suggest that once combined with nitrite, the enzyme may assume a configuration such that exchange between bound and free hydroxylamine does not occur. Regulation of the enzyme is controlled by the redox potential of the cell[116].

Nitrogen reduction in mammalian tissues

Complete reduction of nitrate to ammonia has not been described for mammalian systems, but partial reactions have been shown. For example, nitrate reductase activity has been demonstrated in a variety of rat tissues[117]. Although the enzyme has not been purified, its properties are similar to those of xanthine oxidase. Xanthine oxidase, as well as aldehyde oxidase (but not sulphite oxidase), can reduce nitrate to nitrite[118]. It is interesting to note that these enzymes share a common interchangeable factor, cnx (molybdenum-binding protein), with microbial nitrate reductase. Both xanthine oxidase and aldehyde oxidase have a molecular weight of 300 000 daltons. They consist of two equal subunits, each containing one atom of molybdenum, one molecule of flavin adenine dinucleotide and four nonhaem iron–sulphur groups[119].

Another system which is involved in reduction of nitrogenous compounds is the mixed function oxidase system, cytochrome P_{450}. Hepatic microsomal cytochrome P_{450} catalyses the reduction of tertiary amine oxides to their corresponding amines[120]. The reduction is NADPH and FMN dependent, and is strongly inhibited by carbon monoxide. It is worth noting that xanthine oxidase enhances N reduction in the presence of hypoxanthine, probably indirectly, through the reduction of FMN, which could then be reoxidized by the amine oxide. Another partial reduction reaction was discovered when hydroxylamine was incubated with rat liver mitochondria and NADPH: the hydroxylamine was reduced to ammonia[121].

It seems that the major systems for oxidation of a variety of carbon compounds are involved in the reduction of nitrogenous compounds. Most of the above studies, however, have been done with regard to specific drug metabolism. Thus, similar experiments with nitrite have not been carried out, and the possibility that nitrate and nitrite assimilation takes place in mammalian tissues has not been investigated since the early part of this century[122].

It is interesting to note that a dissimilatory mechanism has been suggested for nitrite reduction by bovine heart cytochrome c[123]. A scheme involving cyclic turnover of cytochrome c was suggested to yield NO from nitrite and an electron donor, which is similar to the *Pseudomonas aeruginosa* dissimilatory nitrite reductase. These mechanisms may be operative in muscle; nitric oxide has been identified as a product of the anaerobic incubation of fresh pig muscle with nitrite at pH 6.0[124].

Since nitrate and nitrite reductases are found both in nitrifying and denitrifying bacteria[103], one can postulate that mammalian tissues would carry out nitrite assimilation as well as dissimilation.

In conclusion, it appears that the enzyme units necessary for conversion of nitrate to ammonia are present in mammalian cells, although the complete reaction has not been observed.

TOXICITY OF NITRITE

Acute toxicity: methaemoglobinaemia

One of the most conspicuous actions of nitrite which has been recognized for a very long time is its reaction with haemoglobin to form methaemoglobin. This section begins by briefly describing haemoglobin and methaemoglobin, then outlines the mechanisms and results of their interconversion, describes the characteristics of, and proposed mechanisms for, the reaction of nitrite with haemoglobin, and ends by detailing the clinical consequences of nitrite induced methaemoglobinaemia.

Haemoglobin and methaemoglobin

Normal adult haemoglobin (HbA) is a tetramer composed of two pairs of subunits and so designated $\alpha_2\beta_2$. Each subunit consists of a haem group and a globin moiety: the structure of the globin portion determines the subunit type. Haem contains a central iron atom which is bonded with the four nitrogen atoms in the pyrrole residues that form a porphyrin ring. The globin moiety is a polypeptide chain that envelops the haem group: an imidazole nitrogen atom of the so-called proximal histidyl residue in the chain also bonds with the haem iron. The iron in deoxyhaemoglobin is ferrous, paramagnetic and therefore high spin, (all electrons in low spin ferrous iron are paired) and pentaco-ordinate[126-127]. In contrast, the iron in oxyhaemoglobin holds oxygen in a sixth co-ordination site. The nature of this iron–oxygen bond has been the matter of some controversy. Although it had been generally believed that the iron in oxyhaemoglobin was also in the ferrous form, in 1964 Weiss[126] proposed that the iron in oxyhaemoglobin was formally oxidized to the ferric state, having given up an electron to the oxygen ligand as shown:

$$\text{globin} \underset{N}{\overset{N}{-}} Fe^{2+} + O_2 \rightleftharpoons \text{globin} \underset{N}{\overset{N}{-}} Fe^{2+} \cdot O_2^-$$

deoxyhaemoglobin   oxyhaemoglobin

This model accounts for the observed diamagnetism[128] of oxyhaemoglobin. Thus although low spin ferric iron and free superoxide are both paramagnetic, having one unpaired electron each, in the sphere of a bound superoxide anion these electrons could spin-couple, giving rise to an overall diamagnetic molecule[127]. This description of oxyhaemoglobin as ferric haemoglobin-superoxide is further supported by the molecule's visible spectrum, its acid dissociation constant, and by molecular orbital calculations[129].

The globin chain of each α-subunit consists of 141 amino acid residues; the chain of each β-subunit has 146 amino acid residues. The tertiary structure of each subunit involves some helical and some nonhelical portions. The structure of each subunit surrounding the haem, and the effects of all four subunits acting in concert, determine the characteristics of haemoglobin as a respiratory transport molecule. Fetal haemoglobin (HbF), for example, is $\alpha_2\gamma_2$, and differs from HbA in several of its characteristics of oxygenation and oxidation.

The functional aspects of haemoglobin are often described by the use of an oxygen dissociation curve, shown below in Figure 1.

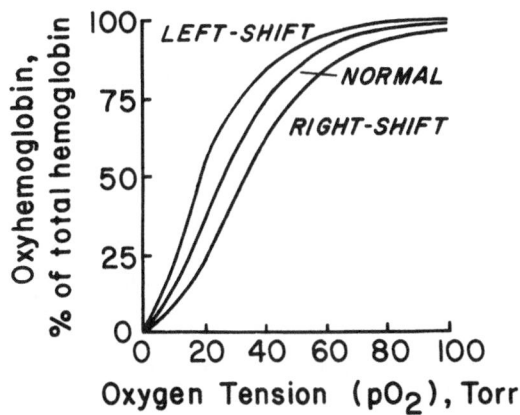

Figure 1   Oxygen dissociation curve of haemoglobin. The left shift is obtained when haemoglobin binds oxygen more tightly than usual and so releases less oxygen at tissue PO_2. The right shift has the opposite effect, and occurs under conditions of hypoxia and decreased pH[383]

The ability of haemoglobin to transport O_2 at physiologic oxygen tensions can be described as follows. The oxygen tension or partial pressure of oxygen (PO_2) in the capillaries at the lungs is normally 100 mmHg; at this pressure, haemoglobin is virtually 100% oxygenated. At the tissue oxygen tension of about 40 mmHg, haemoglobin has a much lower affinity for oxygen and so releases about 25% of its oxygen to the tissues. The oxy and deoxy forms of each monomeric subunit of haemoglobin are interconverted according to oxygen tension in a manner determined by the tetramer as a whole. The sigmoidal shape of the curve describes this four-fold co-operative reaction. The curve's shallow portion near the origin suggests that the oxygenation of the first or second Hb subunits is a relatively slow process; the steeply rising portion of the curve suggests that the second or third subunits react more quickly; the shallow portion from 75% to 100% oxygenation suggests that the fourth subunit is relatively limited in its reaction rate.

Perutz[130,131] envisions two states of haemoglobin structure as forming the basis of this co-operativity. Thus, the oxygenation of haemoglobin might proceed as follows. The four subunits of deoxyhaemoglobin start out in a 'tense' (T) configuration, with all haem groups relatively inaccessible to oxygen. As the partial pressure of oxygen increases, one and then two of the subunits become oxygenated, and the tetramer switches over to the 'relaxed' (R) configuration. The R state allows the remaining subunits to become oxygenated with relative ease. The curve flattens again as the fourth subunit is oxygenated, indicating the diminishing availability of deoxyhaem.

Many factors restrain this switching process, and thus determine the oxygen affinity of a particular type of haemoglobin. For example, 2,3-diphospho-glycerate (2,3-DPG) normally binds to the β-subunits of adult haemoglobin, tempering haemoglobin's oxygen affinity. Fetal haemoglobin $-\alpha_2\gamma_2-$ is considerably less restrained by 2,3-DPG, and so its overall oxygen affinity is higher than that of adult haemoglobin[132]. In graphical terms, the oxygen dissociation curve of HbF is shifted to the left.

Methaemoglobin (ferrihaemoglobin; hemiglobin) is haemoglobin with the haem iron in the oxidized ferric state and the ferric complex sextaco-ordinate, with water or hydroxide ion generally occupying the sixth co-ordination site. Several other ligands can bind there instead – some, like cyanide, with a considerably greater affinity – but oxygen cannot. Consequently, methaemo-globin does not transport oxygen. Methaemoglobin and oxyhaemoglobin are interconvertible, but not in the sense that oxyhaemoglobin and deoxyhaemo-globin are interconvertible. In the latter case, while deoxyhaemoglobin is both oxygenated and formally oxidized upon conversion to oxyhaemoglobin, the process is reversible by oxygen pressure such that the ligand generally returns the electron, leaves as free O_2, and regenerates the ferrous haem. In contrast, the formation of methaemoglobin, by the autoxidation of oxyhaemoglobin, for example, may be envisioned as the superoxide ligand *per se* dissociating itself from the haem iron without returning the borrowed electron[133].

Interconversion of haemoglobin and methaemoglobin

Neill[134] noted that the 'spontaneous' *in vitro* conversion of haemoglobin to methaemoglobin (metHb) had been observed beginning with the first descriptive work on metHb in the 1860s. The electronic mechanism remained conjectural until Conant's electrochemical studies of 1923[135] showed that one electron was transferred from oxyhaemoglobin in the formation of methaemoglobin. In 1925, Neill[134] demonstrated that spontaneous methaemoglobin formation was in fact the result of autoxidation by molecular or 'activated' oxygen. By 1931, Peters and Van Slyke had reviewed the work on the *in vitro* autoxidation of haemoglobin and concluded:

> The readiness with which methaemoglobin formation occurs indicates that methaemoglobin must be in the process of formation continually *in the circulation* and that a shifting equilibrium must occur between reduced, oxygenated and methaemoglobin, with the conditions such that normally only traces of methaemoglobin are present[136].

In 1944, Paul and Kemp[137] examined the blood of 120 individuals with no known exposure to methaemoglobin-forming xenobiotics. They detected metHb in all but one, in amounts ranging from 0.01 to 0.5 g/100 ml, and averaging 0.09 g/100 ml, or about 1.5 % of the total Hb. Subsequent work has corroborated the conclusion that circulating metHb levels in normal adults average from $<1\%$ to 3%[138-140].

Peters and Van Slyke were also correct in reasoning that normal physiologic processes must keep metHb levels in check. The investigations of Cox and Wendel in 1942[141] demonstrated that the *in vivo* reduction rate of metHb produced in dogs by a variety of compounds, including nitrite, was 11% of total Hb per hour. The authors concluded:

> There appears to be ample evidence that the maintenance of haemoglobin in a functionally active state is accomplished mainly if not entirely by enzyme systems contained within the circulating erythrocytes.[141]

Recognition of the occasional cases of chronically cyanotic people led to the description and isolation of the normal methaemoglobin reducing systems in man. François[142] in 1844 reported on an individual with normal heart and lung function who was nonetheless chronically cyanotic: no causal hypothesis was offered. Slosse and Wybauw[143] reported a similar case in 1912. These investigators confirmed the presence of metHb in the blood spectroscopically, and reduced it *in vitro*. They termed the case 'idiopathic' methaemoglobinaemia. Several other cases were reported during the 1930s and 1940s (reviewed by Sievers and Ryan[144]). Such cases 'in which the normal enzymic mechanisms for the removal of methaemoglobin is absent or has become suppressed'[145] were treated with ascorbic acid therapy[144-147].

Scott and Griffith[148] showed in 1959 that the enzyme normally responsible for *in vivo* metHb reduction utilized reduced diphosphopyridine nucleotide (DPNH; now termed NADH) and would reduce the substrates methaemoglobin, cytochrome c and 2,6-dichlorophenolidophenol (DCPIP), in increasing order of reaction rate. (Because of its very rapid reaction rate, the last substrate was typically used in *in vitro* assays: the 'diaphorase' activity of the preparation was measured by the decreased absorbance of the reduced dye at 600 nm). In 1960, Scott[149] showed that NADH-dependent diaphorase activity was very low in patients with congenital hereditary methaemoglobinaemia, and that parents of these individuals had about half of the normal enzyme activity. Jaffe[150] confirmed the marked attenuation of NADH-dependent diaphorase activity in erythrocytes from patients with congenital methaemoglobinaemia; other investigators showed that diaphorase activity and metHb reduction activity was somewhat lower in normal cord and infants' blood than in normal adults' blood[151-153]. Although Scott, Duncan and Ekstrand in 1965[154] had demonstrated that this NADH reductase was primarily responsible for metHb reduction, a few facts remained puzzling. The reaction rate of the enzyme with methaemoglobin as a substrate was really quite slow[154]. Furthermore, Kanazawa *et al.* in 1968[155] showed that the level of the enzyme in normal red blood cells *in vitro*, as measured by DCPIP reduction, did not correlate with the rate at which these cells reduced methaemoglobin.

The missing component proved to be cytochrome b_5. A generally overlooked report by Petragnani, Nogueira and Raw in 1959[156] showed that while hepatic NADH-cytochrome b_5 reductase did not itself catalyse reduction of methaemoglobin *in vitro*, a preparation of the enzyme with

NADH, metHb *and* cytochrome b_5 resulted in a very rapid reduction of methaemoglobin. The authors commented:

> It is interesting to note that the best preparation of erythrocyte methaemoglobin reductase reduced about 0.03 µmole/min/mgm of protein, whereas a rate of 200 µmole/min/mgm of protein is obtained with purified reduced diphosphopyridine nucleotide cytochrome b_5 reductase from pig liver[156].

A dozen years later, Hultquist and Passon[157,158] isolated and purified cytochrome b_5 and cytochrome b_5 reductase from human red blood cells, and showed that the slow reduction of metHb by the enzyme in the absence of cytochrome b_5 was markedly accelerated in its presence. Work by these and other investigators in the late 1970s[159,160] showed that erythrocyte NADH-cytochrome b_5 reductase and NADH-metHb reductase were identical entities, and that metHb reduction was accomplished by the enzymic reduction of the ferri- to the ferro-cytochrome, followed by this species' rapid, non-enzymic reduction of metHb to Hb[161]:

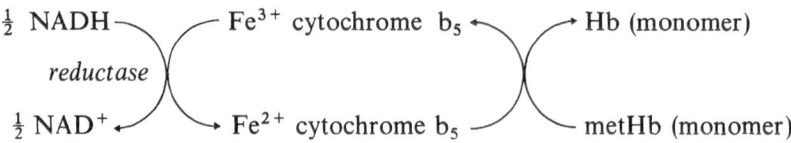

$$\tfrac{1}{2}\ \text{NADH} \qquad \text{Fe}^{3+}\ \text{cytochrome}\ b_5 \qquad \text{Hb (monomer)}$$
$$\textit{reductase}$$
$$\tfrac{1}{2}\ \text{NAD}^+ \qquad \text{Fe}^{2+}\ \text{cytochrome}\ b_5 \qquad \text{metHb (monomer)}$$

Another erythrocyte metHb reduction enzyme, this one utilizing NADPH as the electron donor, was investigated in the 1930s by Warburg and co-workers[162,163], in the 1940s by Kiese[164] and in the 1950s by Huennekens *et al.*[165,166]. This system seems to be little employed for the quotidian reduction of methaemoglobin due to autoxidation[133,167], but forms the basis for the clinical management of toxic rapidly induced methaemoglobin. The enzyme catalyses the reduction of the drug methylene blue to leucomethylene blue, which in turn effects the non-enzymic reduction of metHb[168]:

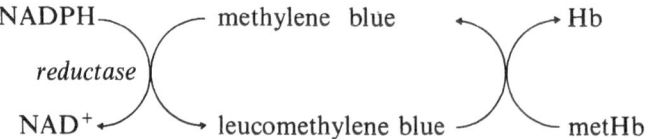

$$\text{NADPH} \qquad \text{methylene blue} \qquad \text{Hb}$$
$$\textit{reductase}$$
$$\text{NAD}^+ \qquad \text{leucomethylene blue} \qquad \text{metHb}$$

By 1978, more than 100 cases of chronic methaemoglobinaemia due to reductase deficiencies had been described[133]. Since the continuous autoxidation of oxyhaemoglobin is essentially unchecked in these people, they present with chronic marked cyanosis. Interestingly, no deaths have been ascribed to this genetic deficiency: the amount of methaemoglobin in untreated patients does not exceed 40 or 45% of total haemoglobin[133,169]. (This holds true only in the absence of methaemoglobin-producing agents, of course. Upon sufficient exposure of normal or of reductase-deficient people to such compounds, including nitrite, metHb levels of greater than 70% are reached: these are incompatible with life.) Since β subunits oxidize considerably more slowly, *in vitro*, than do α subunits[170], perhaps the rate at which the β chains autoxidize *in vivo* is sufficiently slow to be checked by patients' extant reducing systems. To lower the patients' methaemoglobin levels to the normal few per cent, ascorbic acid is still generally the drug of choice[133,171]. Riboflavin has also been used successfully[172], and menadione has some metHb reducing activity[173]. Physiologically available reductants such as ascorbic acid and glutathione may normally play a role in methaemoglobin reduction[154], but the reaction rates are too slow to be of use in the handling of acute toxic methaemoglobinaemia[173]. Conversely, it appears that the animal or person of marginal ascorbic acid status is not unusually susceptible to methaemoglobinaemia, given a normal enzyme status.

The hereditary absence or deficiency of glucose dehydrogenase, a much more common genetic trait than the absence of methaemoglobin reductase, prevents normal glycolysis and so does not provide for regeneration of NADPH[174,175]. Therefore, individuals with this deficiency cannot employ NADPH methaemoglobin reductase, but do not suffer from chronic methaemoglobinaemia, presumably due to their intact NADH reductase system. They are, however, more likely to succumb to acute toxic methaemoglobinaemia, since the administration of methylene blue is of no clinical use[150].

Brewer et al.[175] showed that glucose-6-P-dehydrogenase-deficient individuals were abnormally sensitive to nitrite-induced methaemoglobinaemia, but only after several consecutive days' administration of large amounts – from 1–4 g – of sodium nitrite.

Methaemoglobin is toxic both because it cannot deliver oxygen to the tissues and because it diminishes the ability of the remaining oxyhaemoglobin to do so. This effect is similar to that of carboxyhaemoglobin. In 1912, Douglas, Haldane and Haldane[176] showed that the deleterious effect of a combination of HbCO and HbO_2 was greater than that of the corresponding amounts of deoxyHb and HbO_2, by virtue of HbCO having shifted the oxygen dissociation curve of the remaining HbO_2 to the left. Darlington and Roughton[177] suspected that the simultaneous presence of metHb and O_2Hb might likewise result in O_2Hb having a higher affinity for oxygen and hence being less able to deliver O_2 to the tissues. The investigators found that increasing concentrations of metHb, from 0% to 77%, both increasingly shifted the oxygen dissociation curves of the remaining O_2Hb to the left and changed the curve shape from sigmoidal to hyperbolic. These results were obtained whether metHb was induced by autoxidation, by oxidation with ferricyanide, or by reaction with nitrite. The authors reasoned that these effects were the manifestations of Hb tetramers in which some of the subunits were in the methaem form and the remaining subunits in the oxyhaem form, and that consequently a mixture of wholly metHb tetramers and O_2Hb tetramers would not yield abnormal dissociation curves. Technical problems in their experiments, however, prohibited them from assessing this hypothesis. Thirty years later, Brewer[178] validated the proposition. Two groups of rats were transfused with different types of oxidized blood: the first group of rats received erythrocytes which had been uniformly oxidized in vitro to a methaemoglobin level of approximately 50%; the second group received blood in which equal parts of erythrocytes, which had been oxidized to 100%, were mixed with erythrocytes of 0 % methaemoglobin. The first group became hypoxic relative to the second group. Plotting the oxygen dissociation curves, Brewer found that the curve describing the second group of rats was normal, presumably because the oxyhaemoglobin tetramers were discreet from and not affected by the methaemoglobin tetramers. The oxygen dissociation curve of the first group of rats was shifted to the left, indicating that metHb subunits increase the oxygen affinity of O_2Hb subunits within the tetramer. Enoki, Tokui and Tyuma[179] note that $\frac{1}{3}-\frac{1}{2}$ of the hypoxic effect of toxic levels of metHb in human blood can be ascribed to its increasing the affinity of the remaining O_2Hb for oxygen.

Characteristics of the reaction of nitrite and haemoglobin

Nitrite, like a variety of other compounds[180-183], is toxic by virtue of its ability to form methaemoglobin more rapidly than methaemoglobin can be reduced. That nitrite reacts with haemoglobin to generate methaemoglobin has been appreciated for over 100 years[184,185]; the complete mechanism for this reaction, however, has remained elusive. The following outlines some of the salient characteristics of the reaction – its products, requirements, rate and stoichiometry – and attempts to reconcile the several suggested mechanisms. Finally, mention will be made of the special case of fetal haemoglobin in nitrite-induced methaemoglobinaemia.

The reaction of nitrite with oxyhaemoglobin *in vitro* yields nitrate in a stoichiometric amount[101]. The general statement that nitrite oxidizes haemoglobin in forming methaemoglobin is therefore incorrect; the reaction is instead a co-oxidation, in that both nitrite and haemoglobin are oxidized. Several earlier investigators reported that nitrate formed as a reaction product but do not indicate having actually measured it[186,187].

Hydrogen peroxide has been assumed to form in the reaction of nitrite with haemoglobin[188]: Cohen, Martinez and Hochstein[189] demonstrated the formation of H_2O_2 in an *in vitro* system with NO_2^- and Hb, but it is difficult to determine the actual amounts of H_2O_2 generated. These investigators suggested:

> Nitrite may act in part to destabilize the oxygen-hemoglobin complex and to promote oxidation of hemoglobin by oxygen; the H_2O_2 would then represent the reduced form of the oxidizing agent.[189]

A scheme might therefore be written following the general formulation of Castro, Wade and Belser[182] for the reaction of oxyhaemoglobin with proton donors:

$$Hb^{2+}O_2 + H^+NO_2^- \rightarrow Hb^{3+} + OOH^- + [NO_2\cdot]$$

Several investigators have measured the generation of gaseous O_2 following the reaction of NO_2^- with O_2Hb; and many different conclusions have been reached. Smith[190] measured less than 0.1 mol of O_2 evolved per mol of O_2Hb converted to metHb. Betke, Greinacher and Tietze[191] suggested that 0.5 mol of O_2 accompanied the formation of 1 mol of metHb; Greenberg, Lester and Haggard[186] measured 0.8 mol of O_2 evolved per mol of Hb oxidized. The most recent work using an oxygen electrode[101] revealed slightly less than 0.25 mol of O_2 evolved per mol of Hb converted. Meier[187] had suggested this stoichiometry in 1925.

The several schemes outlined above share the assumptions that oxy- rather than deoxyhaemoglobin is the species reactive to nitrite. Haldane, Makgill and Mavrogordata[185] stated that carboxyhaemoglobin would not react with nitrite. Kiese[180] noted that the reaction of nitrite with haemoglobin produced methaemoglobin more slowly under partially or fully anaerobic conditions than under normal aerobic conditions. Work by Kiese on metHb formation by aniline *N*-oxides[192], however, showed that these aniline derivatives reacted like nitrite in several respects, and that oxygen, i.e. oxyhaemoglobin, was an obligate reactant. Rodkey[193] reported that carboxyhaemoglobin would not react with nitrite to form metHb. The reaction was attempted at pH 8.1, however, and only monitored for 30 minutes: under these conditions, even O_2Hb would only partially have been oxidized. Mansouri[194] reported a very slow but measurable rate of nitrite-induced metHb formation under anaerobic conditions. Overall, it would appear that if deoxyHb can react with nitrite, it does so much less readily and probably by a different mechanism than does O_2Hb.

The reaction is further complicated by the fact that nitrite can act as a ligand for, and thereby alter the visible spectrum of, the methaemoglobin it produces[195–198]. The dissociation constant at pH 7.4 and 25°C for nitrosomethaemoglobin is $3 \, mM$[101,198–200]. This places NO_2^- in the following position in a list of increasing ligand strengths for methaemoglobin:

$$F^- < NO_2^- < N_3^- < HS^- < CN^- \quad \text{[197,198,201]}$$

Since *in vivo* concentrations of haemoglobin are about 8 mM, Smith noted that nitritomethaemoglobin was likely to form *in vivo* from toxic doses of nitrite[198].

Nitric oxide binds strongly to ferrous haemoglobin, forming the radical nitrosylhaemoglobin (HbNO)[202]. *In vivo* studies in the rat by Imaizumi *et al.*[203] showed that nitrite ingestion leads first to the formation of HbNO, detected by its electron resonance spectrum, and then to metHb: the maximum concentration of the former product is $\frac{1}{4}$ that of the latter. *In vitro*, hydrosulphite reduces NO_2^- in the presence of Hb to form HbNO[202]. The *in vitro* reaction of nitric oxide with methaemoglobin yields reduction of metHb, and also forms the HbNO complex[204]. It is unknown whether these reactions figure in the *in vivo* reactions of nitrite.

Several caveats should be noted concerning both the comparability among various *in vitro* studies on methaemoglobin formation, and the fidelity of *in vitro* results to *in vivo* situations. The interactions within the haemoglobin tetramer are profoundly affected by changes in ionic strength and phosphate concentration[205,206], but since this was not fully recognized until the late 1960s to mid 1970s, many studies have been performed in buffers chosen only with regard to pH. Oxygen tension is also a crucial reaction variable, since nitrite reacts quite differently with oxyHb than with deoxyHb. *In vivo*, Hb generally alternates between being fully saturated and half saturated with oxygen, but at the atmospheric oxygen pressures (140–150 Torr) of most *in vitro* experiments, Hb is fully saturated with oxygen. Furthermore, since nitrite both generates methaemoglobin and forms a complex with it, the absolute and relative concentrations of nitrite in reaction solutions are important. Finally, methaemoglobin formation *in vivo* is simultaneously countered by methaemoglobin reduction, while this reduction *in vitro* depends upon maintaining intact reductase systems, which depend upon maintenance of physiological levels of NADH, and in turn upon sufficient glucose concentrations.

The rates at which methaemoglobin is formed by nitrite *in vivo* and *in vitro* are somewhat unusual and characteristic for nitrite. Early work by Austin and Drabkin[195], demonstrated the presence of an initial lag phase, followed by a phase of rapid reaction. These authors considered the two phases to represent two types of reactions between NO_2^- and O_2Hb. Further study[186] suggested the existence of three phases – an induction period, a period of rapid reaction, and a slower final period: the data therefore describe a sigmoidal curve with methaemoglobin concentration plotted as a function of reaction time.

A variety of agents and conditions alter the overall reaction rate, generally by altering the length of the induction period. For example, the reaction rate depends heavily upon pH[195], such that the induction time for metHb formation *in vitro*, with excess NO_2^-, is quite prolonged above pH 8, is about 5 minutes at physiologic pH (7.4), and is considerably less than 1 minute at pH 6.4[193]. The overall reaction has been termed autocatalytic, since with the presence of small amounts of the product, methaemoglobin, in the starting mixture, the induction period is eliminated and the reaction kinetics are those of the rapid phase[193]. Conversely, the presence of CN^- in the starting mixture prohibits the reaction of NO_2^- and O_2Hb from accelerating beyond the slow rate of the induction period[193].

It seems likely that the curve describing the rate of nitrite-induced oxidation of haemoglobin is, like the Hb oxygenation curve, sharply sigmoidal because of co-operativity among the subunits of the Hb tetramer. Thus isolated β-subunits react with NO_2^- only slowly and follow a hyperbolic rather than sigmoidal rate curve[207]. Isolated $\alpha\beta$-dimers also react quite slowly, showing no autocatalytic phase and following a hyperbolic curve[193]. The presence of inositol hexaphosphate (IHP) significantly slows the *in vitro* reaction of NO_2^- with O_2Hb and abolishes the sigmoidal kinetics[208]. Since IHP, like 2,3-DPG, maintains haemoglobin in the T configuration, this result suggests that the normal sigmoidal rate depends upon the interconversion of the T and R configurations. Aquomethaemoglobin is predominantly in the R form in solution[206]. However, work by Mansouri[194] using haemoglobin in which the β-93 sulphydryl group had been iodoacetamide-blocked, suggested that conformational changes alone could not completely account for the reaction behaviour of Hb with NO_2^-.

The formation of nitritomethaemoglobin in reaction mixtures with sufficient nitrite concentrations may figure in the overall reaction rate. The rate profile of nitrite complexation with metHb is also sigmoidal[200]. Some investigators have suggested that nitritomethaemoglobin may donate nitrite for further methaemoglobin formation during the rapid reaction phase[193,198].

Of the several stoichiometries proposed to describe the reaction of oxyhaemoglobin with nitrite[186,187,191,193], the recent scheme by Kosaka *et al.*[101] is the most cogent. Having measured the amounts of nitrite, nitrate, oxygen and methaemoglobin in *in vitro* mixtures, they concluded that the reaction was described by the following equation:

$$4HbO_2 + 4NO_2^- + 4H^+ \rightarrow 4Hb^+ + 4NO_3^- + O_2 + 2H_2O,$$

where HbO_2 denotes an oxyhaemoglobin monomer and Hb^+, a methaemoglobin monomer. The stoichiometry of the Hb^+, NO_2^- and NO_3^- appears sound, but since the authors did not of course measure H_2O, and since their actual values of O_2:HbO_2 are closer to 0.85:4 than 1:4, it is conceivable that the simple accounting for O and H in the forms and ratios given may be inaccurate. The hydroxide ligand of the alkaline methaemoglobin is not included in the equation, although acknowledged in their report.

The kinetics of methaemoglobin formation *in vivo* involve a somewhat delayed and then sustained response for nitrite relative to several other methaemoglobinaemic agents[209]. Hydroxylamine is also a potent inducer of methaemoglobinaemia *in vivo*, but apparently nitrite and hydroxylamine react in different ways.

In the clinical section that follows, it will be noted that of the reported cases of nitrite-induced methaemoglobinaemia, the majority have occurred in infants. This susceptibility is likely due to the interactions of fetal haemoglobin with nitrite. Fetal haemoglobin is the predominant form of Hb at birth: it is increasingly replaced by HbA synthesis until HbF is only about 1 % of the total haemoglobin by the fifth or sixth month of life[132,211]. The progressive decline in circulating levels of metHb found in premature babies, full term babies and older children, in the absence of apparent exogenous oxidants[212], suggests that either metHb reduction is depressed in infants or that HbF is more readily oxidized than HbA. Several investigators have shown that NADH diaphorase activity is lowest in erythrocytes from premature babies, higher in those from full term and older babies, and highest in blood from adults[152,153]. The more important factor, however, is probably the greater susceptibility of HbF, relative to HbA, to autoxidation[170,213], to metHb formation by amino-phenols[183], and to metHb formation by nitrite[207]. Martin and Huisman[207] showed that HbF was converted by nitrite to metHb 2.5 times more rapidly than was HbA. Furthermore, infants may get a relatively larger proximate dose of nitrite from drinking nitrate-rich water, since they drink considerably more than do adults on a body weight basis, and since their relatively less acidic stomach invites colonization by nitrate-reducing flora.

Clinical consequences of nitrite-induced methaemoglobinaemia

The earliest reported cases of nitrate-related methaemoglobinaemia in humans were iatrogenic in nature, resulting from the use of the subnitrate salt of bismuth for obtaining X-ray images of the gut. In 1906, Bennecke and Hoffman[214] reported the death of a 3-week-old infant given a gastric gavage of 100 ml of a 3 % bismuth subnitrate solution to visualize a pyloric stenosis. Marked cyanosis led to death: methaemoglobinaemia was present postmortem. The next year, Boehme[215] reported the death of an 18-month-old child following the injection of a few grams of bismuth subnitrate into the rectum: metHb was again noted. Suspecting nitrite as the proximate cause of methaemoglobinaemia in this case, Boehme incubated human faeces with bismuth subnitrate and in fact observed the formation of nitrite. In 1909,

Beck[216] reviewed the reported cases of bismuth subnitrate poisoning, noted the similarities with acute nitrite poisoning, and concluded:

> The poisonous effects of bismuth subnitrate were not due to the absorption of the metallic bismuth, but to the absorption of nitrites, which caused methaemoglobin to precipitate in the blood... The intestine, and especially the sigmoid and the rectum, are the laboratories for the liberation of nitrites. The bacteria in this part of the intestinal tract evidently are the nitrite-splitting factors...

Beck suggested that radiographers switch from the nitrate to another salt of bismuth.

In 1929, Eusterman and Keith[217] reported the occurrence of transient cyanosis and methaemoglobinaemia in a 32-year-old man and a 47-year-old woman being treated with ammonium nitrate as a diuretic. Suspecting the nitrate as the cause, Keith injected dogs with comparable amounts of ammonium nitrate, but methaemoglobinaemia was not induced. The apparent resistance of the dogs, combined with the authors' 3 years of experience in giving ammonium nitrate 'in large doses to normal men and to a great number of patients with different types of dropsy' with no subsequent incidents of methaemoglobinaemia, led the authors to propose that the 'intestinal dysfunction' that both cases shared was necessary in this development of methaemoglobinaemia. They noted that previously reported cases of methaemoglobinaemia due to bismuth subnitrate were more severe when the agent was administered rectally, and speculated that reduction of NO_3^- to NO_2^- within the body was involved. Roe[218] reported the death from methaemoglobinaemia of a 1-month-old infant given bismuth subnitrate in the treatment of diarrhoea. Roe also stressed the involvement of intestinal bacteria in the nitrite poisoning arising from nitrate administration.

In the 1940s, another vehicle for nitrate exposure was discovered. Comly[219] reported a case of a 1-month-old infant presenting with diarrhoea. An allergy to her milk formula was suspected, so the patient was switched to a soy based formula to be reconstituted with boiled water. Within 2 days at home, the infant became markedly cyanotic and was taken back to the hospital. Treatment with methylene blue (still the agent of choice[171]) alleviated the cyanosis, which did not reappear during the patient's week-long hospital stay. Once at home, the infant again developed cyanosis, again was hospitalized, treated with methylene blue, and discharged. The cycle was repeated another two times. Comly remarked, 'it was realized that the only significant change in the infant's environment from hospital to farm home was in the water'. Analysis of the well water used at the patient's home revealed nitrate to be present at concentrations of 300–600 mg/l. The nitrite content of the water was below 1 mg/l. Comly noted that water samples from several other wells contained similarly high levels of nitrate, that several other paediatricians had reported cases of cyanosis among infants feeding on well water-diluted formulas, and that the underlying methaemoglobinaemia was similar to that occasionally induced by bismuth subnitrate. He concluded that intestinal bacterial conversion of nitrate to nitrite followed the ingestion of nitrate-rich water, and cautioned against the use of such water in the nourishment of babies.

Many reports of infantile methaemoglobinaemia from ingestion of well water followed that of Comly's. Lecks[220] noted that methaemoglobinaemia was a much more frequent occurrence in infants than in older children and adults. Cornblath and Hartmann[221] suggested that the characteristically higher gastric pH of newborns, especially those with diarrhoea, might allow the colonization of nitrite-producing bacteria in the stomach and thus allow a greater reduction of nitrate prior to absorption. Previous studies by Marriott, Hartmann and Senn[222] had shown that while the average pH of normal infants' stomachs was 3.7, the average gastric pH of a group of infants with diarrhoea was 5.7. Robertson and Riddell[223] added that other factors, such as an infant's total amount of haemoglobin and the efficacy of his enzyme systems responsible for methaemoglobin reduction, might figure in the infant's susceptibility to methaemoglobinaemia. These investigators tested 2000 samples of drinking water from wells in rural areas of Saskatchewan and Iowa, found 5–15% of the samples to contain greater than $300\,mg\;NO_3^-/l$, and identified ten cases of infantile methaemoglobinaemia associated with milk formulas made with nitrate-rich water.

Knotek and Schmidt[224] noted that the incidence of infantile methaemo-globinaemia in Czechoslovakia had risen with the use of dried milk formulas. The authors isolated spores of *Bacillus subtilis* from all of the dried milk products they tested, and showed that such milk reconstituted with nitrate-rich water led to considerable nitrite formation *in vitro* and methaemoglobin formation *in vivo*. Walton[225] reviewed the literature up to 1951 on infant methaemoglobinaemia due to nitrate in water. He noted a total of 287 reported cases with 14% fatality rate.

Simon *et al.*[226] published the results of a questionnaire on infant methaemoglobinaemia in Germany during the years 1956–1964. They reported 745 cases of infant methaemoglobinaemia due to nitrate contaminated water, 98% of which were associated with the use of private well water. Nitrate concentrations in water were not reported in many cases, but among those in which nitrate was measured, the concentration exceeded $100\,mg/l$ in 84% of cases. Nine per cent of cases were fatal. Shuval and Gruener[227] found that breast-fed or undiluted milk-fed infants did not have elevated methaemoglobin levels in areas where drinking water supplies contained from 50 to $90\,mg$ nitrate/l.

Interestingly, nitrates *per se* in vegetables have not been implicated in cases of methaemoglobinaemia, even though the nitrate content of some vegetables exceeds that of contaminated well waters by an order of magnitude. Methaemoglobinaemia has resulted from the ingestion of spinach or beets, for example, but in every reported case the food contained hundreds of mg of nitrite that had formed from the nitrate prior to ingestion[228].

The biochemistry of enzymic nitrate reduction in higher plants has been elucidated: nitrate reductase in spinach, for example, has been purified and characterized by Paneque *et al.*[229]. Schupan[230] demonstrated nitrite accumulation to several thousand mg per kg in fresh spinach stored for several days. Phillips[231–233] confirmed and extended this work, showing that tight packing of fresh spinach leaves might hasten nitrate conversion to nitrite by excluding oxygen, and that refrigerated storage generally slowed nitrate reduction but did not stop it as freezing would. Phillips also demonstrated that commercially canned foods made from vegetables originally high in nitrates did not show accumulation of nitrite, presumably because blanching inactivated plant and bacterial nitrate reductases, and also because pre-canning preparations leached out much of the nitrate. Heiser et al.[234] noted that conversion of nitrate to nitrite occurred much more readily in shredded, ground or juiced beets and spinach than in the intact vegetables.

Holscher and Natzscha[235] reported the development of methaemo-globinaemia in two infants, aged 2 and $3\frac{1}{2}$ months, caused by eating home prepared spinach. Analysis revealed a nitrite content of about 200 mg/kg spinach. Sinious and Wodsak[236] noted that 14 infants, ranging in age from 2 to 10 months, developed methaemoglobinaemia following ingestion of home pureed spinach.

Keating et al.[237] presented a case report of a 2-week-old infant who had become cyanotic after drinking 500 ml of home-prepared carrot juice. The patient's blood drawn in the Emergency Room contained 9 g methaemo-globin/100 ml, which was equivalent to 60% of the total haemoglobin. Methylene blue treatment of 1 mg/kg body weight reduced circulating methaemoglobin levels to 0.9 g/100 ml 1 hour later; complete recovery was noted by 12 hours. Fetal haemoglobin accounted for 33% of total haemoglobin. Analysis of the carrot juice revealed 500 mg nitrate and 800 mg nitrite per litre. Another bag of carrots similar to the suspect one was purchased at the same supermarket, processed into juice, assayed, and found also to contain several hundred mg nitrite and nitrate per litre. The high levels of nitrite in the carrots directly from the grocer's shelf suggested that mishandling at home was not to blame. Reduction of nitrate by plant enzymes rather than by those of contaminating bacteria was suspected.

Blatant misuse of sodium nitrite as a food additive has occasionally resulted in outbreaks of methaemoglobinaemia. Orgeron et al.[238] reported 10 cases of methaemoglobinaemia due to ingestion of wieners and bologna cured with illegally high amounts of nitrite. All of the persons affected were between $1\frac{1}{2}$ and 10 years old, and all recovered with methylene blue treatment. In another outbreak of nitrite poisoning, 48 people developed methaemo-globinaemia after dining on pigs' knuckles in tomato soup: the pork had been pickled mistakenly with pure sodium nitrite instead of the usual pickling medium[239].

Greenberg, Birnkrant and Schiftner[240,241] reported a bizarre outbreak of nitrite poisoning. Eleven elderly men had all breakfasted in the same cafeteria over the space of 3 hours, all turned cyanotic within 30 minutes of eating, all became acutely hypoxic, and one died. The common element of their breakfasts was oatmeal. The cook claimed that he had put a 'handful of salt' (approximately 100 g) into the 6 gallon batch of that morning's oatmeal. He typically kept his box of salt next to his box of saltpetre which he used for corning beef. The saltpetre box turned out not to contain $NaNO_3$ but rather $NaNO_2$, and it was into this box which the cook accidentally had reached. In addition, the salt shaker on the table where each subject had eaten accidentally contained $NaNO_2$ instead of NaCl. Each bowl of oatmeal probably contained about 1 g of nitrite. Not all the patrons who had eaten this oatmeal became frankly ill, but all eleven who salted their cereal at that table did, apparently adding a toxic extra bit.

Tepperman *et al.*[242] reported the hospital admission of two men on successive mornings, both of whom were deeply cyanotic and one of whom was also comatose. Both patients had eaten wheatcakes, butter and maple syrup at the same local diner hours before admission. Samples of the food were collected and aqueous extracts thereof fed to rats: the rats died within 35 minutes with marked methaemoglobinaemia. Separate testing of the pancake batter and the butter exonerated these components, while the putative maple syrup alone provoked methaemoglobinaemia. Interrogation at the diner revealed that a curing mixture, containing 8% nitrites, 4% nitrates and sucrose, had been mistakenly substituted for maple syrup. A retrospective diagnosis of moderate methaemoglobinaemia was made in five other individuals who had eaten similar breakfasts.

Bakshi, Fahey and Pierce[243] presented a case report of a man who had eaten about 1 pound of locally manufactured Polish blood sausage, became nauseated within 30 minutes, vomited, turned blue and collapsed. A blood sample revealed 4.1 g methaemoglobin/100 ml. The methaemoglobinaemia was successfully reduced upon treatment with methylene blue. This case was somewhat unusual, in that the patient had consumed comparable amounts of sausage on many occasions in the past, and in that analysis of the sausage revealed a nitrite content just under the legal limit. It seems likely that the nitrite analysis was in error.

In 1878, Hill[244] reported the death of a 2-year-old boy caused by his ingestion of 3–4 oz of the then common medicine Sweet Spirits of Nitre (4% ethyl nitrite in 70% ethyl alcohol). One hundred years later, Chilcote *et al.*[245] reported two poisonings, one of them fatal, due to the same over-the-counter drug. The patients were 4-month-old twins who had been given 1–2 teaspoons of the preparation for 'fussiness'. The twin who succumbed had 57% of his haemoglobin as fetal haemoglobin and methaemoglobin concentration of 80%. The surviving twin had 30% fetal haemoglobin and a methaemoglobin concentration of 38%, which was successfully lowered with treatment by methylene blue. The authors noted that ethyl nitrite was still a commonly used folk remedy and that the label contained no warning of toxicity along with its claim of usefulness as a 'mild diuretic'.

Accidental, homicidal and suicidal deaths have been reported from the ingestion of nitrite. Naidu and Venkatrao[246] reported the death of a 15-year-old boy who had apparently ingested pure potassium nitrite. These authors noted that nitrites were extensively used in making dyes in southern India: nitrite had been implicated in 19 cases of suicide and 9 homicides during the years 1935–1940 in India[247]. Greenberg, Birnkrant and Schiftner[240] noted that nitrite was also employed in the dye industry in the United States. The authors cited several incidents in which workers had brought home sodium nitrite from their manufacturing plants, mistaking it for sodium chloride, and had used the nitrite for cooking and seasoning: poisonings, often fatal, resulted[248–251]. More recent cases of methaemoglobinaemia include the poisonings of two men who had ingested sodium nitrite tablets, thinking them to be ordinary salt tablets[252,253]. Ironically, the nitrite tablets had been taken from first-aid cabinets. They are properly used as an antidote to cyanide, precisely because they can induce the formation of methaemoglobin which complexes cyanide and allows detoxification. Standefer *et al.*[254] report the suicide of an adult male following the ingestion of an estimated 50 g of nitrite. The postmortem blood contained 30 mg nitrate/litre, 0.55 mg nitrite/litre, and 90 % of the haemoglobin as methaemoglobin. The gastric contents contained 32 g nitrite/kg wet weight, while the liver contained no detectable nitrite or nitrate.

Death from methaemoglobinaemia resulted in one of three cases of workers who had been burned by molten nitrate salts during an industrial accident[255]. The *postmortem* blood sample revealed a methaemoglobin concentration of 65 % of total haemoglobin. The other two patients were successfully treated with methylene blue and exchange transfusions.

Henderson and Raskin[256] presented a case report of an adult male who had been experiencing headaches shortly after eating normal amounts of cured meats. The authors had seen several other such cases, and suspected nitrite as the cause of the 'hot-dog' headaches. To test this, they administered solutions containing either 10 mg sodium bicarbonate or 10 mg sodium nitrite to the patient. Nitrite induced headaches in eight of thirteen trials, while bicarbonate never did. 10 mg is not an inordinately large amount of nitrite, and it would have been interesting to determine whether the ingestion of celery juice or borscht, for example, would have provoked headaches in this patient. Although the authors do not substantiate a mechanism, the headaches may have been due to the individual's hypersensitivity to the vasodilatory action of nitrite[257].

Carcinogenicity

The major question concerning the chronic toxicity of nitrite is: Does nitrite cause cancer? Certainly nitrous acid – the protonated form of nitrite that predominates at pH's lower than 3.4 – causes mutations (reviewed by Zimmerman,[258]) in viruses[259], fungi[260,261] and bacteria[262,263], and causes chromosomal damage in animal cells in culture[264–266]. Nitrite does not, however, appear to genetically damage the germ cells of rats or mice fed up to 1 % dietary $NaNO_2$[267,268]. The results of several rodent feeding studies that have attempted to discern whether nitrite is a carcinogen are not all in agreement. These studies have either been designed to test whether nitrite *per se* is carcinogenic, or have simply included a group of animals fed nitrite as a control in studies designed to assess the simultaneous administration of nitrite and a nitrosatable precursor. Both types of studies are reviewed below.

Most chronic feeding studies have indicated that nitrite is not a carcinogen. In 1963, Druckrey *et al.*[269] reported that three successive generations of rats drinking 100 mg $NaNO_2$/kg daily did not suffer abnormal carcinogenic or teratogenic effects. The authors did note a moderately reduced life expectancy for the nitrite-treated animals. Van Logten *et al.*[270] fed, in restricted quantities, a diet of 40 % canned meat that had been treated with either 0.02 % or 0.5 % $NaNO_2$ to male and female specific pathogen free (SPF)-derived Wistar rats for up to 29 months. The nitrite treatment resulted in some slight decreases in animals' haematrocrits and in somewhat slower growth rates, but tumour incidence was not affected. Taylor and Lijinsky[271] found no major organ tumours in 27 male and 30 female Sprague-Dawley rats attributable to their having drunk limited quantities of 0.2% $NaNO_2$ in distilled water for 2 years. All nitrite-treated animals did develop benign endocrine tumours, but the authors noted that these types of tumours commonly arose in untreated control groups as well. Olsen and Meyer[272] fed a diet of 45% pork that had been treated with up to 0.4% $NaNO_2$ to two generations of Wistar SPF rats. No statistically significant differences were found between control groups and nitrite-treated groups with respect to the number of animals with tumours, or the number of benign or malignant tumours. In 1979, Inai, Aoki and Tokuoka[273] reported a study of 300 male and female ICR mice drinking solutions of 0.125%, 0.25% or 0.5% $NaNO_2$ for up to 109 weeks. A control group and the three test groups all showed high tumour incidences – 50 to 80% – but no differences in tumour induction time or overall incidence were ascribable to nitrite. The authors did note that the only four cases of myeloid cell proliferation occurred in the experimental groups.

Feeding nitrite alone proved to be an appropriate negative control in several *in vivo* nitrosation studies of amines, amides or ureas. Thus Sander[274] noted that 0.3% dietary $NaNO_2$ was not tumorigenic to any of three strains of female rats without the concurrent administration of dimethylurea in the drinking water. Greenblatt, Mirvish and So[275] reported that Swiss mice given 0.1% $NaNO_2$ alone in drinking water for 28 weeks did not differ from controls in the proportion of mice developing lung adenomas or in the number of adenomas per mouse. No other tumours arose within the nitrite-treated group during the 40 weeks of observation time (kept short to allow accurate scoring of the pulmonary adenomas in the other test groups) except for 1 malignant lymphoma: several of these developed within the control group, however. Scheunig, Horn and Mehnert[276] showed that while the concurrent administration of nitrite and aminopyrine by gastric intubation was extremely carcinogenic to male and female Wistar rats, the intubation of 0.1 mmol $NaNO_2$ alone, 3 times per week, for 29 months, was not carcinogenic for any major organ system.

Some feeding studies have indicated, however, that nitrite may be carcinogenic. In 1976, Shank and Newberne[277] reported on the effects of *in vivo* nitrosation of morpholine during a 2-year-long administration of various combinations of the amine and nitrite to Sprague-Dawley CD rats. Somewhat suprisingly, they found a 27% incidence of tumours in the lymphoreticular system for the group of rats receiving 0.1% dietary $NaNO_2$ with no added morpholine: this contrasted with a 6% incidence of lymphoreticular system tumours in the untreated control group. Furthermore, although the nitrite-treated group showed none of the increased incidences in hepatocellular carcinomas and angiosarcomas seen in the nitrite plus morpholine-dosed groups, the former did suffer an elevated incidence of glandular epithelium tumours and embryonal and mixed tissue tumours, as well as the aforementioned leukaemias and lymphomas. The next year, Matsukura *et al.*[278] reported that of the four male Wistar rats serving as nitrite-only controls in a nitrite plus methylguanidine feeding study, three developed liver tumours between 12 and 16 months of study, while none of the ten untreated controls bore tumours. Meanwhile, Newberne[279] was conducting a very much more extensive and systematic investigation of the effects on rats of nitrite in food or water. The 1979 report corroborated his earlier reported findings, suggesting that nitrite promotes the incidence of lymphoma in Sprague-Dawley CD rats. The overall combined incidence of lymphomas was 10.2% in the 1383 rats receiving 0.025%, 0.05%, 0.1% or 0.2% $NaNO_2$ in their food or drinking water, while the incidence in the 573 control animals was 5.4%. This increase was both statistically and politically significant. Although Newberne had noted that 'the data are only suggestive and the biological significance of nitrite associated lesions of the lymphoreticular system is unclear'[280], the US Food and Drug Administration considered the result sufficiently strong to merit a ban on nitrite as a food additive[281,282]. The proposed ban was accompanied by a not inconsiderable controversy[282–286]: a year later it was dropped[287]. Taylor and Morgenroth[288] reviewed several contrasting chronic nitrite feeding studies, but could not explain the variation in reti-culoendothelial pathologies observed.

Several investigators have focused on the effects of chronic nitrite exposure in pregnant rodents. Globus and Samuel[289] reported that the rather low dose of 0.5 mg $NaNO_2$ per pregnant CD-1 mouse per day stimulated fetal hepatic erythropoiesis, leading to transitorily increased percentages of polychromat-ophilic erythroblasts and mature erythrocytes in the offspring. No other signs of embryotoxicity were apparent at this dose. Other investigators employing much larger doses – 0.1–0.5% $NaNO_2$ in drinking water – have demonstrated reductions in the number, weight and survival of progeny from nitrite-treated pregnant mice, rats and guinea pigs[227,290–292]. Shuval and Gruener[227] also noted that rats chronically exposed to 0.01%, 0.1%, 0.2%, or 0.3% $NaNO_2$ in drinking water developed pathological cardiac and pulmonary changes with a frequency and severity that increased with increasing nitrite dose.

METABOLISM AND CORPORAL DISTRIBUTION OF NITRITE AND NITRATE

Nitrate and nitrite are both formed and destroyed *in vivo*. These processes may be the metabolic actions of microflora normally or abnormally resident in the animal host, or may result from the animal's own metabolism. For example, nitrate is reduced to nitrite by normal microflora in the mouth, by micro-organisms that colonize the abnormally hypochlorhydric or achlorhydric stomach, and by flora that inhabit the infected urinary tract or bladder. Nitrate may also be reduced by mammalian enzymes *in vitro*. Nitrate is formed both from nitrite via oxyhaemoglobin, and from more reduced nitrogen compounds by mammalian systems. This section discusses the metabolism, distribution and clearance of nitrate and nitrite in the animal and human body.

Reduction of nitrate to nitrite

People ingest from tens to several hundred mg of sodium nitrate per day from food and water[78, 293, 294]. As nitrate levels in saliva rise to reflect this ingestion, increased levels of salivary nitrite follow, due to the action of reductase systems of the oral microflora[295–301]. Both nitrate and nitrite levels in saliva peak from 2 to 4 hours after ingestion of nitrate-rich food or drink, reaching levels of up to several hundred mg/l depending on the ingested amount and concentration of nitrate[299–301]. The kinetics are governed by the absorption, distribution, and secretion of nitrate. Since the return to basal nitrite levels requires several hours, the contribution of nitrite by the saliva to the rest of the gastrointestinal system may be significant. Ishidate *et al.*[298] estimate that saliva might contribute 50–70 mg of nitrite following a nitrate-rich meal; Spiegelhalder, Eisenbrand and Preussmann[301] suggest 40 mg of nitrite could be formed within 5 hours after eating lettuce or other nitrate-rich vegetables or juices. Considerable variation in salivary nitrite production among individuals and among monkeys has been noted[302–304]. Lowenfels *et al.*[305] reported that oesophageal cancer patients as a group were no different from healthy controls in their ability to reduce nitrate to salivary nitrite. Fasting levels of salivary nitrite average 5–10 mg[301,306] and do not differ between smokers and nonsmokers[307].

Microbial reduction of nitrite is not confined to the oral cavity. The results of Klein *et al.*[308] suggest that microfloral production of nitrite continues in the oesophagus, and several investigators have shown that stomachs with reduced acidity and therefore favourable environments for microbial growth are likewise conducive to nitrite production. Thus Sander and Seif[309] showed that a fasting gastric pH of 4 or greater allowed nitrate reduction in patient's stomachs. Ruddell *et al.*[310] demonstrated the inverse relationship between nitrite and hydrogen ion concentration in the stomachs of normal individuals, ulcer patients, gastric cancer patients, and otherwise normal individuals with hypochlorhydria. Individuals with abnormally low, fasting, gastric acidity had average, gastric concentrations of 30–40 μmol NO_2^-/l (1–2 mg NO_2^-/l). These workers[311] also reported average nitrite concentrations of 120 μmol/l in the achlorhydric stomachs of pernicious anaemia patients. Normally acidic stomachs averaged 2–3 μmol NO_2^-/l. Tannenbaum and coworkers[43] also found considerably greater than normal concentrations of nitrite in the stomachs of individuals whose fasting gastric pH was 5 or higher. Jones, Davies and Savage[312] reported levels of 10–30 μmol NO_2^-/l in stomachs of post-partial-gastrectomy patients displaying dysplasia. Schlag *et al.*[313] also found elevated nitrite levels in Billroth II resected stomachs. It is generally hypothesized by the above cited authors that the increased gastric cancer risk of these patients with pernicious anaemia or resected stomachs might involve their increased levels of gastric nitrite.

In 1914, Cruickshank and Moyers[314] reported on the presence and significance of nitrite in urine. They assayed 600 urine samples for nitrite, and concluded that nitrite was not present in normal urine from healthy individuals, while in cases where nitrite was present, so were Gram-negative bacteria. Since then many investigators have tested the efficacy of diagnosing urinary tract infections using nitrite test strips[315–319]. It appears, however, that while false–positive results are very rare, the rather sizeable proportion of false–negatives (i.e. nitrite-free urines that belie infections) limits the usefulness of the screen. Several other investigators have studied urinary nitrite and urinary tract infections with respect to the *in situ* formation of nitrosamines[320-323].

In general, then, corporal sites containing both microflora and nitrate will generate nitrite. The small intestine and lower parts of the gastrointestinal tract are of course rife with micro-organisms, but nitrate and nitrite had generally not been found in the lower gut or in faeces[296,324]. Their apparent absence was presumed to be due to the rapid absorption of the bulk of dietary nitrate in the upper small intestine[325,326]. More recent work, however, has uncovered low levels of nitrate, nitrite, or both in the lower intestine and faeces of germfree and conventional rats[327,328] and in the faeces and ileostomy effluent of humans[329,330]. Witter, Balish and Gatley[331,332] suggested that either incomplete absorption, or re-introduction of absorbed nitrate into the intestinal lumen, could account for the presence of nitrate throughout the intestine.

Mammalian enzymes systems may also figure in *in vivo* nitrate reduction. (See p. 99 for details on enzymic nitrate reduction *in vitro*.) Fritsch, Saint-Blanquat and Derache[333] suggested that intestinal tissue was involved in nitrate reduction in the rat. It might be noted that several of the 19th century investigators in this field felt that mammalian enzymes might have the ability to reduce nitrate: Mitchell, Shonle and Grindley[122] reviewed the work in 1916 and concluded it 'probable that the tissues are able to reduce nitrates to nitrites and possibly to ammonia, though it is evident that under average conditions the nitrite stage must be transient ...'.

Distribution of nitrite

Pharmacodynamic studies on nitrite *per se* have been relatively few, due to the relative instability of the ion. Several investigators have shown that gastric loss of nitrite is rapid and substantial in laboratory animals gavaged with solutions of nitrite. The loss of sodium nitrite from the mouse stomach, for example, is very rapid, 85% of the ingested nitrite disappearing within 10 minutes of administration. The mechanisms by which nitrite is lost from the stomach include: direct absorption from the stomach to the blood, emptying to the duodenum with subsequent absorption in the intestine, decomposition within the stomach by oxidation or reduction, and/or utilization in chemical reactions with gastric contents. In the mouse, gastric absorption, probably of the anhydride N_2O_3, accounts for most of the nitrite loss, while oxidation of nitrite to nitrate is also an important pathway[334]. The stomach of the rat is also rapidly depleted of nitrite. Loss occurs via gastric absorption, emptying, and decomposition, although a diminishing remainder of nitrite persists for up to 5 hours, potentially available for intragastric nitrosation[335]. The concentration of nitrite in the stomach of the dog also decreases rapidly, with only 10% of the initial concentration remaining as detectable nitrite 30 minutes after gavage of a nitrite solution[336]. LaBar and Sander[337] fed either broth from boiled ham, or boiled ham itself, to fasted human volunteers. Their data, depicted in Figure 2, show that although the nitrite disappeared rather rapidly from the stomach, this disappearance was retarded when the food

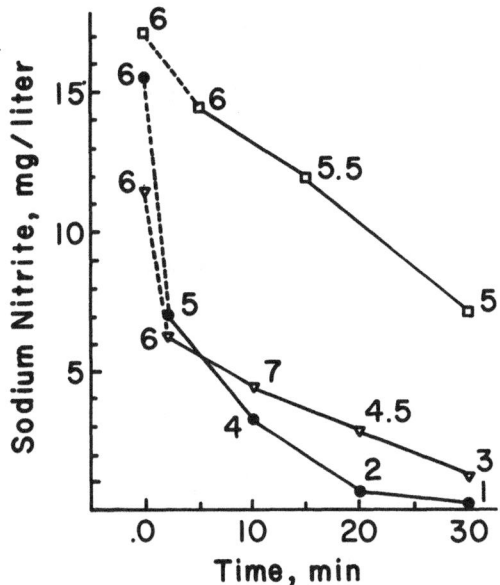

Figure 2 Decrease of nitrite concentration in 10 ml aliquots of the gastric contents after ingestion of a broth made by boiling 100 g boiled ham in 100 ml water (Experiment 1, △; Experiment 2, ●), and after ingestion of 100 g boiled ham (Experiment 3, □). Values at $t = 0$ represent the $NaNO_2$ in the broth, or in Experiment 3, the concentration in the meat (10 g) itself. The pH values are shown next to each nitrite value

rather than the aqueous extract was given. The repeated finding of intragastric nitrosation in laboratory animals and in humans (see p. 90) suggests that toxicologically significant levels of nitrite within the stomach are indeed obtained.

Upon absorption, nitrite is rapidly converted to nitrate via its reaction with oxyhaemoglobin[101]. Gruener *et al.*[338] showed, however, that in pregnant rats fed 30 mg $NaNO_2$/kg, nitrite was sufficiently stable to cross the placenta, resulting in elevated concentrations of both nitrite and the consequent methaemoglobin in the fetuses' blood. Nitrite did not appear to be transferred to suckling rats via the milk of nitrite-treated dams. Smith and Walters[339] showed that 12 minutes were required to halve a nitrite concentration of 60 mmol/l in whole pig blood at 37 °C *in vitro*.

Distribution and clearance of nitrate

Animals dosed with nitrate excrete the bulk of it into urine within a day[326,328,340,341]. For humans, the average elimination half-life of nitrate is 5 hours[342,343]. Nitrate excretion appears to follow first-order kinetics[343]. Although varying and dose-dependent recoveries of nitrate in urine have been reported, the amount of nitrate excreted generally reflects the amount of nitrate ingested[344-348] (see p. 122 on nitrate formation, however, for the very different case following low nitrate intakes). People on a variety of diets have urinary nitrate concentrations of about 1 mmol/l, and plasma nitrate levels of approximately 0.2 mmol/l[302], so a 5-fold concentration of nitrate typically is achieved by the kidney. In an experiment designed to mimic the effects of repeated nitrate ingestion with meals and water, Tannenbaum et al.[343] found diurnal patterns of nitrate excretion in urine and in nitrate and nitrite levels in saliva (Figure 3).

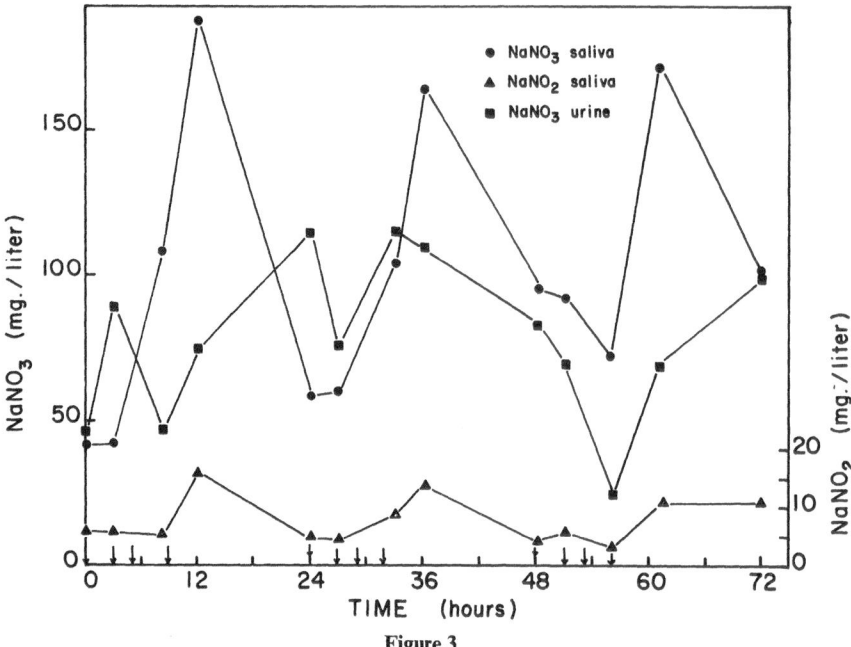

Figure 3

In sufficient quantities, nitrate causes diuresis. The effects of nitrate as a diuretic involve increased excretions of chloride, hydrogen and potassium into the urine. Circulating levels of chloride are progressively depleted, levels of bicarbonate, elevated, and an elevated blood pH, or alkalosis, established[341,349-353]. Nitrate acts by competing with chloride for active reabsorption, possibly Na-K-ATPase-mediated, in the ascending limb of the loop of Henle[353,354]. Since nitrate is less readily reabsorbed than chloride, large doses of nitrate–several grams per person–are required for effective competition and thus for diuretic effects. The considerably greater efficacy of a number of other diuretics ended the clinical use of nitrate for diuresis several decades ago[257].

While the kidney is responsible for most of the clearance of nitrate, a number of other glands also clear nitrate from blood, secreting it against a concentration gradient into other spaces or fluids. Thus the salivary, thyroid, mammary and gastric glands all appear to secrete nitrate into their lumina. Historically, nitrate uptake has been studied as a competitor of iodide uptake, the latter having been investigated both because of its importance in thyroid function and because of the availability and relative ease of studying the radioisotope ^{131}I. The thyroid, for example, normally concentrates iodide against a considerable gradient, generating thyroid to plasma concentration ratios of from 10 to more than 100 to 1[355]. Nitrate competes with this uptake of iodide, although since normal plasma concentrations of NO_3^- exceed those of I^- by four orders of magnitude, one would expect nitrate to be a very weak competitor under physiological conditions. Wyngaarden, Wright and Ways[356] studied the competitive effects of 100 μmol of each of several anions, injected intraperitoneally, on radio-iodide accumulation by the thyroid of the rat. They found no inhibitory effect on iodide from fluoride, chloride or bromide, a weakly inhibitory effect from nitrate, and strongly inhibitory effects from thiocyanate and perchlorate. A further study designed to determine the goiterogenic capabilities of selected anions showed that rats drinking 1% KNO_3 for 17 days showed thyroid glands with slightly greater than control levels of hypertrophy, and slightly decreased levels of iodine, while animals administered $KClO_4$ had thyroids with marked hyperplasia and very substantially decreased levels of iodine. Bloomfield et al.[357] confirmed that rats fed 0.5%, 1% or 2.5% dietary KNO_3 showed dose-dependent diminishment of thyroid uptake of $^{131}I^-$, and demonstrated that sheep fed 1.5% dietary NO_3^- also developed impaired thyroid function. Although these investigations suggest thyroidal uptake and secretion of nitrate at high doses, actual concentrations of nitrate in the thyroid under any conditions do not appear to have been measured.

As noted previously, salivary levels of nitrate and nitrite in man increase in response to nitrate doses. Plasma nitrate levels that normally average 0.2 mmol/l[302] were found to be rather insensitive to an aqueous dose of 4 mmol NO_3^-[342]. Since salivary nitrate would be expected to peak at several mmol/l 2–4 hours following such a dose[300, 301], the parotid gland probably achieves a considerable nitrate concentration against plasma. In the absence of nitrate dosing, however, it is not clear whether salivary nitrate levels generally exceed plasma nitrate levels. In contrast, normal salivary levels of I^- exceed normal plasma levels by 30-fold[358]. As noted above for the thyroid gland, $^{131}I^-$ uptake by the salivary gland is inhibited by a series of anions in the following decreasing order of efficacy[359, 360]:

$$ClO_4^- > SCN^- \geq {}^{127}I^- > NO_3^-$$

Iodide and nitrate uptake and secretion in saliva are due specifically, in a number of species, including man, to the action of the parotid gland[361]. In contrast to man, the rat does not concentrate iodide in its saliva[358, 362].

Humans, rabbits, guinea pigs, rats and mice[363, 364] also secrete and concentrate iodide via the mammary gland, achieving average milk to plasma concentration ratios of up to 30. Cows, goats and sheep, however, generate milk to plasma iodide concentration ratios of 2 or 3. As noted with other glands, the mammary gland's ability to concentrate iodide is markedly inhibited by perchlorate and thiocyanate, weakly by nitrate, and not at all by chloride or bromide[364]. This would seem to imply some concentration of nitrate within milk, although only one case is reported in the clinical literature in which a breast-fed infant appeared to develop methaemoglobinaemia when his mother drank nitrate-rich well water[365].

The rat, dog and human stomach secrete iodide, with gastric juice to plasma ratios of up to 40 at normal plasma iodide levels in man[358,363]. There is some indication that nitrate is also secreted by the human stomach[307,308], although gastric transport of nitrate against a concentration gradient has not been observed. In the rat, at low circulating levels of nitrate, the gastric juice to plasma ratio for nitrate is 20, and falls to unity when plasma nitrate concentrations reach 4.5–5 mmol/l[366]. These investigators also found that nitrate competed with $^{131}I^-$ for uptake and secretion by the rat gastric mucosa.

Nitrate appears to be concentrated by sections of the rat intestine[332]: the middle region of the small intestine in the rat also secretes iodide, and is competitively inhibited from so doing by perchlorate and thiocyanate[358].

In summary, NO_3^- appears to weakly compete with and mimic I^- in uptake, concentration and secretion by a number of glands. The results of the above cited references suggest this series of anionic strengths for competition with radio-iodide:

$$ClO_4^- > SCN^- \geq {}^{127}I^- > IO_3^- > NO_3^- > BrO_3^-;$$

F^-, Cl^-, Br^- are ineffective.

Formation of nitrate

Several investigators have found that laboratory animals and humans excrete more nitrate than they consume on diets low in nitrate. In 1916, Mitchell, Shonle and Grindley[122] reported on nutritional balance studies in which 12 human volunteers had eaten only low nitrate diets for 220 days. Although their average daily ingestion of nitrate was 0.25 mmol, their average daily excretion of nitrate in urine was 0.81 mmol. The authors noted considerable variability among days and among individuals, but found that nitrate excretion during low nitrate ingestion was continuously in excess of intake throughout the experiment. When nitrate was added to the diet (about 1 mmol consumed/day) urinary nitrate excretion increased, but less so than the nitrate ingestion had increased. Thus a deficit of urinary nitrate was obtained. This result was ascribed to a partial destruction of ingested nitrates. Although the current thinking was that urinary nitrates were derived solely from dietary nitrates, the investigators concluded, 'We believe, however, that the production of nitrates by animal tissues is a fact ...'. Investigations over the next several decades on nitrate in animal and human urine involved diets with moderate or high nitrate contents, and so found urinary nitrate deficits reflective of rather extensive corporal nitrate destruction[326,340,341,346,367]. In 1978, however, Tannenbaum *et al.*[330] confirmed the earlier observations that on low nitrate diets, nitrate appeared in the urine in a continuous excess. Balance studies by Kurzer and Calloway[368] also showed that humans ingesting 0.05 mmol NO_3^- daily excreted 3–4 times this amount in their urine. Radomski, Palmiri and Hearn[346] and Bartholomew *et al.*[347] found that people ingesting diets virtually free of nitrate excreted urine with a concentration of 0.3 mmol/l nitrate.

Several possibilities for the origin of the excess nitrate exist. Ingested nitrite would yield urinary nitrate[101], for example, but nitrite ingestion throughout these studies was most probably negligible. Nitrogen oxides in inspired air would be excreted and metabolized as nitrate[84], but these species would also not normally be present in sufficient amounts to substantially contribute to the excess urinary nitrate observed[369]. The emptying of a body pool of nitrate seemed unlikely, given the duration and magnitude of the excess, and was in fact excluded by stable isotope dilution studies. These studies, using ^{15}N-labelled nitrate in the rat[369] and in man[343], demonstrated that the body pool of nitrate was much too small and rapidly depleted to account for the phenomenon, and that *in vivo* nitrate synthesis was the most likely source of the excess urinary nitrate observed during restricted nitrate ingestion. The authors showed that endogenous nitrate synthesis is continuous and independent of dietary nitrate ingestion, but since it is smaller than the amount of ingested nitrate from moderate or high nitrate diets which is destroyed *in vivo*, in most studies it has not appeared as a net excess of excreted nitrate.

The sites and mechanisms for *in vivo* nitrate synthesis are currently unknown. Since many bacterial species oxidize ammonia and other reduced nitrogen substrates to nitrite and nitrate, nitrification by intestinal micro-organisms was a postulated source of synthesized nitrate[330]. Identical patterns of urinary nitrate excretion in germfree and in conventional rats, however, tended to disprove this hypothesis and to suggest that nitrate synthesis is a mammalian process[369].

EPIDEMIOLOGICAL ASSOCIATIONS OF NITRATE, NITRITE AND *N*-NITROSO COMPOUNDS WITH HUMAN CANCER

Several epidemiological studies have shown significant positive correlations between exposure to nitrate and cancer risk: nitrate in drinking water correlates with gastric cancer risk in Colombia[344] and in England[294]; exposure to nitrate-containing fertilizer also appears to be linked to gastric cancer mortality in Chile[370]. The situation, though, is complex. High risks for gastric cancer correlate not only with nitrate but also with several other dietary or environmental factors, and whether any of these associations actually involve causation is far from clear[371–375]. On the other hand, the operational insensitivity of the epidemiological method means that repeatedly finding a significant correlation between a putative carcinogen and a specific cancer may point to an agent of considerable public health significance.

Since many *N*-nitroso compounds elicit oesophageal neoplasms in laboratory animals[18], some investigators have looked for signs of nitrosamines in regions where people are at unusually high risks of developing oesophageal cancer. Bogovski *et al.*[376] noted that the high incidence of oesophageal cancer in northern France correlated with the local production and consumption of apple brandy (calvados). These workers collected and analysed 30 samples of farm-made calvados, and tentatively identified dimethylnitrosamine (DMN) at levels of 1–10 μg/kg in 14 samples. The two samples of commerical calvados showed no detectable DMN. Fong and

Newberne[377] found that oesophageal cancer patients had abnormally low tissue levels of zinc, and that some populations at abnormally high risks of oesophageal cancer were exposed to nitrosamines in their diets. These investigators then demonstrated that zinc deficiency and methylbenzyl-nitrosamine acted synergistically in inducing oesophageal cancer in rats. It is of interest to note that workers in the Chinese province of Henan, in Lin County, are employing a variety of methods to diminish the nitrate content of local crops, with the hope that reducing the population's exposure to nitrate will reduce its currently strikingly high incidence of oesophageal cancer[378].

Attempts have been made to identify the factors underlying the epidemiological associations between nitrate exposure and gastric cancer risk in Colombia[43, 344, 379, 380]. Correa et al.[381] found several differences between the stomachs of individuals from regions of low gastric cancer risk and those from regions of high gastric cancer risk, especially with respect to gastric nitrite concentrations (Tables 4 and 5). In vitro experiments, controlled for pH, nitrite concentration and precursor morpholine concentration, showed that nitrite both persisted longer and formed higher yields of nitrosomorpholine in samples of Colombian gastric juice than in samples of Bostonian (low risk) gastric juice[382]. The bases of these phenomena are unknown.

Table 4 Characteristics of individuals from low-risk and from high-risk regions of gastric cancer

	Low Risk	High Risk
Histology	Normal	Chronic Atrophic Gastritis
pH	<5	>5
Thiocyanate	present	present
Chloride	present	present
Nitrate	present	present
Nitrite	<0.5 ppm	>1 ppm
Bacteria	low to absent	abundant
Trace elements	present	present

Table 5 Nitrite concentration and histologic diagnosis

Type (no.)	pH	NO_2^- (ppm)	NO_3^- (ppm)
Normal + SG (5)	2.3	0.2	75
CAG (31)	5.2*	1.7*	86
pH <5 (18)	2.5	0.3	73
pH >5 (18)	7.0*	2.7*	95
No Necrosis (17)	5.0	1.7	76
Necrosis (19)	5.0	1.2	94
CAG (12)	4.8	2.0	40
CAG + IM (19)	5.4	1.5	115*

* $P < 0.001$

SG = superficial gastritis

CAG = chronic atrophic gastritis

IM = intestinal metaplasia

CONCLUDING REMARKS

It seems hardly necessary to state it: there is a lot unknown about nitrate, nitrite and *N*-nitroso compounds. These brief points suggest areas of current concern and current ignorance in the field.

(1) A low level of dimethylnitrosamine may be found in human blood and urine. If so, what is its source? Does it reflect endogenous nitrosation? If so, how and where in the body is the nitrosamine produced?

(2) Is nitrite *per se* an animal or human carcinogen? If so, what are the relative risks of nitrite from foods and nitrite from *in vivo* reduction of nitrate? Do higher than average environmental exposures to nitrate cause higher than average risks to cancer?

(3) Nitrate appears to be synthesized in the rat and in man. What is the site of endogenous nitrate production? Since the several species NO_3^-, NO_2^-, and $NO_2\cdot$ would all appear as NO_3^- upon absorption, which is actually the manufactured form? What is its toxicological significance?

ACKNOWLEDGEMENT

The authors gratefully acknowledge the support of the NIH Environmental Toxicology Training Grant No. 2-T32-ES07020 (LG) and NCI Grant No. 1-PO1-CA26731.

References

1. Freund, H. A. (1937). Clinical manifestations and studies in parenchymatous hepatitis. *Ann. Intern. Med.*, **10**, 1144
2. Hamilton, A. and Hardy, H. L. (1949). *Industrial Toxicology*. 2nd edn. p. 301. (New York: Paul B. Hoeber, Inc.)
3. Barnes, J. M. and Magee, P. N. (1954). Some toxic properties of dimethylnitrosamine. *Br. J. Ind. Med.*, **11**, 167
4. Magee, P. N. and Barnes, J. N. (1956). The production of malignant primary hepatic tumors in the rat by feeding dimethylnitrosamine. *Br. J. Cancer*, **10**, 114
5. Heath, D. F. (1962). The decomposition and toxicity of dialkylnitrosamines in rats. *Biochem. J.*, **85**, 72
6. Magee, P. N. and Hultin, T. (1962). Toxic liver injury and carcinogenesis. *Biochem. J.*, **83**, 106
7. Magee, P. N. and Farber, M. (1962). Toxic liver injury and carcinogenesis: methylation of rat liver nucleic acids by dimethylnitrosamine *in vivo*. *Biochem. J.*, **83**, 114
8. Hansen, M. A. (1964). An outbreak of toxic liver injury in ruminants. *Nord. Vet. Med.*, **16**, 323
9. Koppang, N. (1964). An outbreak of toxic liver injury in ruminants. *Nord. Vet. Med.*, **16**, 305
10. Ender, F., Havre, G., Helgebostad, A., Koppang, N., Madsen, R. and Cen, L. (1964). Isolation and identification of a hepatotoxic factor in herring meal produced from sodium nitrite preserved herring. *Naturwissenschaften*, **51**, 637
11. Sakshaug, J., Sognen, E., Hansen, M. A. and Koppang, N. (1965). Dimethylnitrosamine; its hepatotoxic effect in sheep and its occurrence in toxic batches of herring meal, *Nature (London)*, **206**, 1261

12. Ender, F., Havre, G., Madsen, R., Ceh, L. and Helgebostad, A. (1967). Studies on conditions under which N-nitrosodimethylamine is formed in herring meal produced from nitrite preserved herring. The risk of using nitrite uncritically as a preservative agent. *Tierphysiol. Tierernahr. Futtermittelk.*, **22**, 181

13. Terracini, B., Magee, P. N. and Barnes, J. M. (1967). Hepatic pathology in rats on low dietary levels of dimethylnitrosamine. *Br. J. Cancer*, **21**, 559

14. Crampton, R. F. (1980). Carcinogenic dose-related response to nitrosamines. *Oncology*, **37**, 251

15. Diaz Gomez, M. I., Swann, P. E. and Magee, P. N. (1977). The absorption and metabolism in rats of small oral doses of dimethylnitrosamine. *Biochem. J.*, **164**, 497

16. Pegg, A. E. and Hui, G. (1978). Formation and subsequent removal of O^6-methylguanine from deoxyribonucleic acid in rat liver and kidney after small doses of dimethylnitrosamine. *Biochem. J.*, **173**, 739

17. Montesano, R. and Magee, P. N. (1970). Metabolism of dimethylnitrosamine by human liver slices *in vitro*. *Nature (London)*, **228**, 173

18. Magee, P. N., Montesano, R. and Preussmann, R. (1976). N-Nitroso compounds and related carcinogens. In Searle, C. E. (ed.) *Chemical Carcinogens*, pp. 491–625. American Chemical Society Monograph 173, (Washington: American Chemical Society)

19. International Agency for Research on Cancer Working Group (1978). *Some N-Nitroso Compounds*. IARC Pub. No. 17 (Lyon: IARC)

20. Mirvish, S. S. (1975). Formation of N-nitroso compounds: chemistry, kinetics and *in vivo* occurrence. *Toxicol. Appl. Pharmacol.*, **31**, 325

21. Druckrey, H., Preussmann, R., Ivankovic, S. and Schmahl, D. (1967). Organotrope carcinogene Wirkungen bei 65 venschildenen N-nitroso-verbindungen an BD-ratten. *Z. Krebsforsch.*, **69**, 103

22. Ridd, J. H. (1961). Nitrosation, diazotisation and deamination. *Q. Rev. Chem. Soc., (London)*, **15**, 418

23. Mirvish, S. S. (1970). Kinetics of dimethylamine nitrosation in relation to nitrosamine carcinogenesis. *J. Natl. Cancer Inst.*, **44**, 633

24. Lijinsky, W., Keefer, L., Conrad, E. and Van de Bogart, R. (1972). Nitrosation of tertiary amines and some biologic implications. *J. Natl. Cancer Inst.*, **49**, 1239

25. Lijinsky, W. and Breenblatt, M. (1972). Carcinogen dimethylnitrosamine produced *in vivo* from nitrite and aminopyrine. *Nature New Biol..*, **236**, 177

26. Fiddler, W., Pensabene, J. W., Doerr, R. C. and Wasserman, A. E. (1972). Formation of N-nitrosodimethylamine from naturally occurring quaternary ammonium compounds and tertiary amines. *Nature (London)*, **236**, 307

27. Obiedzinski, M. W., Wishnok, J. S. and Tannenbaum, S. R. (1980). N-Nitroso compounds from reactions of nitrite with methylamine. *Food Cosmet. Toxicol.* (In press)

28. Scanlan, R. A. (1975). N-Nitrosamines in foods. *Crit. Rev. Food Technol.*, **5**, 357

29. Fan, T. Y. and Tannenbaum, S. R. (1973). Factors influencing the rate of formation of nitrosomorpholine from morpholine and nitrite: Acceleration by thiocyanate and other anions. *J. Agr. Food Chem.*, **21**, 237

30. Keefer, L. K. and Roller, P. P. (1973). N-Nitrosation by nitrite ion in neutral and basic medium. *Science*, **181**, 1245

31. Archer, M. C., Tannenbaum, S. R. and Wishnok, J. S. (1976). Nitrosamine formation in the presence of carbonyl compounds. In *Environmental N-Nitroso Compounds Analysis and Formation*. IARC Sci. Pub. No. 14, pp. 141–145. (Lyon: IARC)

32. Bogovski, P., Castegnaro, M., Pignatelli, B. and Walker, E. A. (1972). The inhibiting effect of tannins on the formation of nitrosamines. In Bogovski, P., Preussmann, R. and Walker, E. A. (eds.) *N-Nitroso Compounds: Analyses and Formation*. IARC Sci. Pub. No. 3, pp. 127–129. (Lyon: IARC)

33. Challis, B. C. (1973). Rapid nitrosation of phenols and its implications for health hazards from dietary nitrites. *Nature (London)*, **244**, 466

34. Davies, R. and McWeeny, D. J. (1977). Catalytic effect of nitrosophenols on N-nitrosamine formation. *Nature (London)*, **266**, 657

35. Challis, B. C. and Kyrtopoulos, S. A. (1979). Nitrosation of Amines by the Two Phase Interaction of Amines in Solution with Gaseous Oxides of Nitrogen. *J. Chem. Soc. Perkins Trans.* I, 299

36. Mirvish, S. S., Wallcave, L., Eagen, M. and Shubik, P. (1972). Ascorbate-nitrite reaction: Possible means of blocking the formation of carcinogenic *N*-nitroso compounds. *Science*, **177**, 65

37. Tannenbaum, S. R. and Mergens, W. (1980). Reaction of nitrite with vitamins C and E. Presented at *Conference on Micro-nutrient Interactions: Vitamins, Minerals and Hazardous Elements*, The New York Academy of Sciences, NY (In press)

38. Invankovic, S., Preussmann, R., Schmahl, D. and Zeller, J. (1974). Prevention by ascorbic acid of *in vivo* formation of *N*-nitroso compounds. In Bogovski, P., Walker, E. A. and Davis, W. (eds.) N-*Nitroso Compounds in the Environment*. IARC Sci. Pub. No. 9, pp. 101–102. (Lyon: IARC)

39. Mirvish, S. S., Cardesa, A., Wallcave, L. and Shubik, P. (1973). Effect of sodium ascorbate on lung adenoma induction by amines plus nitrite. *Proc. Am. Assoc. Cancer Res.*, **14**, 102

40. Fiddler, W., Pensabene, J. W., Piotrowski, E. G., Doerr, R. C. and Wasserman, A. E. (1973). Use of sodium ascorbate or erythorbate to inhibit formation of *N*-nitrosodimethylamine in frankfurters. *J. Food Sci.*, **38**, 1084

41. Sen, N. P. and Donaldson, B. (1974). The effect of ascorbic acid and glutathione on the formation of nitrosopiperazines from piperazine adipate and nitrite. In Bogovski, P., Walker, E. A. and Davis, W. (eds.) N-*Nitroso Compounds in the Environment*. IARC Sci. Pub. No. 9, pp. 103–106. (Lyon: IARC)

42. Kamm, J. J., Dashman, T., Kewmark, H. and Megens, W. J. (1977). Inhibition of amine-nitrite hepatotoxicity by α-Tocopherol. *Toxicol. Appl. Pharmacol.*, **41**, 575

43. Tannenbaum, S. R., Moran, D., Rand, W., Cuello, C. and Correa, P. (1979). Gastric cancer in Colombia. IV. Nitrite and other ions in gastric contents of residents from a high-risk region. *J. Natl. Cancer Inst.*, **62**, 9

44. Walters, C. L., Hill, M. J. and Ruddell, W. S. (1978). Gastric juice nitrite: its source and relationship to hydrogen ion concentration. In Walker, E. A., Castegnaro, M., Briciute, L. and Lyle, R. E. (eds.) *Environmental Aspects of N-Nitroso Compounds*. IARC Sci. Pub. No. 19, pp. 279–288. (Lyon: IARC)

45. Sander, J. (1967). Kann Nitrit in der menschlichen Nahrung Ursache einer Krebsenstenhung durch Nitrosaminbildung sein? *Arch. Hyg. Bakt.*, **151**, 22

46. Fine, D. H., Ross, R., Rounbehler, D. P., Silvergleid, A. and Song, L. (1977). Formation *in vivo* of volatile *N*-nitrosamines in man after ingestion of cooked bacon and spinach. *Nature (London)*, **265**, 753

47. Lakritz, L., Simenhoff, M. L., Dunn, S. R. and Fiddler, W. (1980). *N*-Nitrosodimethylamine in human blood. *Food Cosmet. Toxicol.*, **18**, 77

48. Sen, N. P., Smith, D. C. and Schwinghamer, L. (1969). Formation of *N*-nitrosamines from secondary amines and nitrite in human and animal gastric juice. *Food Cosmet. Toxicol.*, **7**, 301

49. Golovnya, R. V. (1976). Analysis of volatile amines contained in foodstuffs as possible precursors of *N*-nitroso compounds. In Walker, E. A. and Bogovski, P. (eds.) *Environmental N-Nitroso Compounds Analyses and Formation*. IARC Pub. No. 14, pp. 237–245. (Lyon: IARC)

50. Elespuru, R. K. and Lijinsky, W. (1973). Formation of carcinogenic nitroso compounds from nitrite and some types of agricultural chemicals. *Food Cosmet. Toxicol.*, **11**, 807

51. Eisenbrand, G., Unger, O. and Preussmann, R. (1974). Formation of *N*-nitroso compounds from agricultural chemicals and nitrite. In Bogovski, P., Walker, E. A. and Davis, W. (eds.) N-*Nitroso Compounds in the Environment*. IARC Sci. Pub. No. 9, pp. 71–74. (Lyon: IARC)

52. Lijinsky, W. (1974). Reaction of drugs with nitrous acid as a source of carcinogenic nitrosamines. *Cancer Res.*, **34**, 255

53. Archer, M. C., Clark, S. D., Thilly, J. E. and Tannenbaum, S. R. (1971). Environmental nitroso compounds: Reaction of nitrite with creatine and creatinine. *Science*, **174**, 1341

54. Endo, H., Takahashi, K. and Aoyagi, H. (1973). Identification and property of the mutagenic principle formed from a food component, methylguanidine, after nitrosation in simulated gastric juice. *Biochem. Biophys. Res. Commun.*, **54**, 1384

55. Knowles, M. E., McWeeney, D. J., Couchman, L. and Thorogood, M. (1974). Interaction of nitrite with proteins at gastric pH. *Nature (London)*, **247**, 288

56. Mohler, K. and Hallermayer, E. (1973). Buildung von Nitrosaminen aus Lecithin und Nitrit. *Z. Lebensmitteluntersuch. Forsch.*, **151**, 52

57. Bills, D. D., Hildrum, K. I., Scanlan, R. A. and Libbey, L. M. (1973). Potential precursors of N-nitrosopyrrolidine in bacon and other fried foods. *Agr. Food Chem.*, **21**(5), 876

58. Pensabene, J. W., Fiddler, W., Gates, R. A., Fagan, J. C. and Wasserman, A. E. (1974). Effect of frying and other cooking conditions on nitrosopyrrolidine formation in bacon. *J. Food Sci.*, **39**, 314

59. Fiddler, W., Pensabene, J. W., Fagan, J. C., Thorne, E. J., Piotrowski, E. G. and Wasserman, A. E. (1974). The role of lean and adipose tissue on the formation of nitrosopyrrolidine in fried bacon. *J. Food Sci.*, **39**, 1070

60. Sen, N. P., Seaman, S. and Miles, W. F. (1976). Dimethylnitrosamine and nitrosopyrrolidine in fumes produced during the frying of bacon. *Food Cosmet. Toxicol.*, **14**, 167

61. Hansen, T., Iwaoka, W., Green, L. and Tannenbaum, S. R. (1977). Analysis of N-nitrosoproline in raw bacon. Further evidence that nitrosoproline is not a major precursor of nitrosopyrrolidine. *J. Agric. Food Chem.*, **25**(6), 1423

62. Hwang, L. S. and Rosen, J. D. (1976). Nitrosopyrrolidine formation in fried bacon. *J. Agric. Food Chem.*, **24**, 1152

63. Spiegelhalder, B., Eisenbrand, G. and Preussmann, R. (1979). Contamination of beer with trace quantities of N-nitrosodimethylnitrosamine. *Food Cosmet. Toxicol.*, **17**, 29

64. Scanlan, R. A., Barbour, J. F., Hotchkiss, J. H. and Libbey, L. M. (1980). N-Nitrosodimethylamine in beer. *Food Cosmet. Toxicol.*, **18**, 27

65. Hotchkiss, J. H., Barbour, J. F. and Scanlan, R. A. (1980). Analysis of malted barley for N-nitrosodimethylamine. *J. Agr. Food Chem.*, **28**, 678

66. Preussman, R., Spiegelhalder, B. and Eisenbrand, G. (1980). Reduction of human exposure to environmental N-nitrosocarcinogens. Examples of possibilities for cancer prevention. *Carcinogenesis: Fundamental Mechanisms and Environmental Effects*, The 13th Jerusalem Symposium, Jerusalem, April 28–May 2, 1980 (In press)

67. Hoffmann, D., Rathkamp, C. and Liu, Y. Y. (1974). Chemical studies on tobacco smoke. XXVI. On the isolation and identification of volatile and nonvolatile N-nitrosamines and hydrazine in cigarette smoke. In Bogovski, P., Walker, E. A. and Davis, W. (eds.) N-*Nitroso Compounds in the Environment*. IARC Sci. Pub. No. 9, pp. 159–165. (Lyon: IARC)

68. Brunneman, K. D. and Hoffman, D. (1978). Chemical studies on tobacco smoke. LIX. Analysis of volatile nitrosamines in tobacco smoke and polluted indoor environments. In Walker, E. A., Castegnaro, M., Griciute, L. and Lyle, R. E. (eds.) *Environmental Aspects of N-nitroso Compounds*, IARC Sci. Pub. No. 19, pp. 343–356. (Lyon: IARC)

69. Archer, M. C. and Wishnok, J. S. (1976). Nitrosamine formation in corrosion-inhibiting compositions containing nitrite salts of secondary amines. *J. Environ. Sci. Hlth.*, **A11**(10 & 11), 583

70. Fan, T. Y., Morrison, J., Rounbehler, D. P., Ross, R. and Fine, D. H. (1977). N-nitrosodiethanolamine in synthetic cutting fluids: A part-per-hundred impurity. *Science*, **196**, 70

71. Rappe, C. and Zingmark, P.-A. (1978) Formation of N-nitrosamines in cutting fluids. In Walker, E. A., Castegnaro, M., Griciute, L. and Lyle, R. E. (eds.) *Environmental Aspects of N-Nitroso Compounds*, IARC Sci. Pub. No. 19, pp. 213–217. (Lyon: IARC)

72. Fajen, J. M., Carson, G. A., Rounbehler, D. P., Fan, T. Y., Vita, R., Goff, U. E., Wolf, M. H., Edwards, O. S., Fine, D. H., Reinhold, V. and Biemann, K. (1979). N-Nitrosamines in the rubber and tire industry. *Science*, **205**, 1262

73. Pitts, J. N., Grosjean, D., VanCauwenberghe, K., Schmid, J. P. and Fitz, D. R. (1978). Photooxidation of aliphatic amines under simulated atmospheric conditions: formation of nitrosamines, nitramines, amides, and photochemical oxidant. *Environ. Sci. Technol.*, **12**, 946

74. Tannenbaum, S. R. (1980). A model for estimation of human exposure to endogenous N-nitrosodimethylamine, *Oncology*, **37**, 232

75. Appel, B. R., Kothny, E. L., Hoffer, E. M., Hidy, G. M. and Wesolowsk, J. J. (1978). Sulfate and nitrate data from the California aerosol characterization experiment. *Environ. Sci. Technol.*, **12**, 418

76. Fishbein, L. (1976). Atmospheric mutagens. I. Sulfur oxides and nitrogen oxides. *Mutation Res.*, **32**, 309

77. National Research Council (1978). *Nitrates: An Environmental Assessment* (Washington, DC: National Academy of Sciences)

78. White, J. W. (1975). Relative significance of dietary sources of nitrate and nitrite. *J. Agric. Food Chem.*, **23**, 886
79. White, J. W. (1976). Relative significance of dietary sources of nitrate and nitrite: correction. *J. Agric. Food Chem.*, **24**, 202
80. American Meat Institute Survey. (Personal communication, Dr J. Birdsall)
81. Cassens, R. G., Greaser, M. L., Ito, T. and Lee, M. (1979). Reactions of nitrite in meat. *Food Technol.*, **33**, 42
82. Miller, W. D. (1980). *The Microorganisms of the Human Mouth*, p. 364. (Philadelphia: White)
83. Bokhoven, C. and Niessen, H. J. (1961). Amounts of oxides of nitrogen and carbon monoxide in cigarette smoke, with and without inhalation. *Nature (London)*, **192**, 458
84. Svorcova, S. and Kaut, V. (1971). Arteriovenous differences in the nitrite and nitrate ion concentrations in rabbits after inhalation of nitrogen oxides. *Cesk. Hyg.*, **16**, 71; (*Chem. Abstr. 75*, 33253 m)
85. Iqbal, Z. M., Dahl, K. and Epstein, S. S. (1980). Role of nitrogen dioxide in the biosynthesis of nitrosamines in mice. *Science.* **207**, 1475
86. Schmidt, E. L. (1978). Nitrifying microorganisms and their methodology. In Schlessinger, D. (ed.) *Microbiology.* pp. 288–291. (Washington, DC: American Society for Microbiology)
87. Hooper, A. B. (1978). Nitrogen oxidation and electron transport in ammonia oxidizing bacteria. In Schlessinger, D. (ed.) *Microbiology.* pp. 299–304. (Washington, DC: American Society for Microbiology)
88. Ritchie, G. A. F. and Nicholas, D. J. D. (1972). Identification of the sources of nitrous oxide produced by oxidative and reductive processes in *Nitrosomonas europaea. Biochem. J.*, **126**, 1181
89. Nicholas, D. J. D. (1978). Intermediary metabolism of nitrifying bacteria with particular reference to nitrogen, carbon and sulfur compounds. In Schlessinger, D. (ed.) *Microbiology.* pp. 305–309. (Washington, DC: American Society for Microbiology)
90. Rees, M. R. (1968). Studies of the hydroxylamine metabolism of *Nitrosomonas europaea. Biochemistry* **7**, 366
91. Butt, W. D. and Lees, H. (1958). Cytochromes of *Nitrobacter. Nature (London)*, **182**, 732
92. Focht, D. D. and Verstraete, W. (1977), Biochemical ecology of nitrification and denitrification. *Adv. Microbiol. Ecol.* **1**, 135
93. Obaton, M., Amarger, N. and Alexander, M. (1968). Heterotrophic nitrification of *Pseudomonas aeruginosa. Arch. Mikrobiol.*, **63**, 122
94. Verstraete, W. and Alexander, M. (1972). Heterotrophic nitrification by *Arthrobacter* sp. *J. Bacteriol.*, **110**, 955
95. Weisburger, J. H. and Weisburger, E. K. (1973). Biochemical formation and pharmacological, toxicological, and pathological properties of hydroxylamine and hydroxamic acids. *Pharmacol. Rev.*, **25**, 1
96. Heubner, W. (1913). Studien uber methamoglobinbildung. *Naunyn-Schmiedebergs Arch. Pharmakol. Exp. Pathol.*, **72**, 241
97. Masters, B. S. S. and Ziegler, D. M. (1971). The distinct nature and function of NADPH-Cytochrome c reductase and NADPH-dependent mixed function amine oxidase of porcine liver microsomes. *Arch. Biochem. Biophys.*, **145**, 358
98. Coutts, R. T. and Beckett, A. H. (1977). Metabolic N-oxidation of primary and secondary aliphatic medicinal amines. *Drug Metabol. Rev.*, **6**, 51
99. Udenfriend, S., Clark, C. T., Axelrod, J. and Brodie, B. B. (1954). Ascorbic acid in aromatic hydroxylation. *J. Biol. Chem.*, **208**, 731
100. Ralt, D. and Tannenbaum, S. R. (1980). Unpublished data.
101. Kosaka, H., Imaizumi, K., Imai, K. and Tyuma, I. (1979). Stoichiometry of the reaction of oxyhemoglobin with nitrite. *Biochim. Biophys. Acta*, **581**, 184
102. Hewitt, E. J. (1975). Assimilatory nitrate-nitrite reduction. *Ann. Rev. Plant Physiol.*, **26**, 73
103. Hewitt, E. J. (1974). Aspects of trace element requirements in plants and micro-organisms: The metallo enzymes of nitrate and nitrite reduction. *Plant Biochem.*, **11**, 199
104. Beevers, L., Schrader, L. E., Flesher, D. and Hageman, R. H. (1965). Aspects of trace element requirements in plants and micro-organisms: The metallo enzymes of nitrate and nitrite reduction. *Plant Physiol.*, **40**, 691
105. MacGregor, C. H. and Schnaitman, C. A. (1972). Restoration of reduced nicotinamide

adenine dinucleotide phosphate-nitrate reductase activity of a *Neurospora* mutant by extracts of various chlorate resistant mutants of *E. coli. J. Bact.*, **112**, 388

106. Villarreal-Moguel, E. I., Ibarra, V., Ruiz-Herrera, J. and Gitler, C. (1973). Resolution of the nitrate reductase complex from the membrane of *E. coli. J. Bact.*, **113**, 1264
107. Downey, R. J. (1972). Formation of NADPH nitrate reductase in *Aspergillus nidulans. Am. Soc. Microbiol. Ann. Meet.*, Abst. No. P236, p. 175
108. Johnson, J. L., Hainline, B. E. and Rajagopalan, K. V. (1980). Characterization of the molybdenum cofactor of sulfite oxidase, xanthine oxidase and nitrate reduction. *J. Biol. Chem.*, **255**, 1783
109. Solomonson, L. P. (1974). Regulation of nitrate reductase activity by NADH and cyanide. *Biochim. Biophys. Acta*, **334**, 297
110. Herrera, T., Paneque, A., Maldonado, T. M., Barea, J. L. and Losada, M. (1972). Regulation by ammonia of nitrate reductase synthesis and activity in *Chlamydomonas reinhardi. Biochem. Biophys. Res. Commun.*, **48**, 996
111. Hucklesby, D. P. and Hewitt, E. J. (1970). Nitrite and hydroxylamine reduction in higher plants. *Biochem. J.*, **119**, 615
112. Prabhakararao, K. and Nicholas, D. J. D. (1970). The reduction of sulphite, nitrite and hydroxylamine by an enzyme from Baker's yeast. *Biochim. Biophys. Acta*, **216**, 122
113. Abou-Jaoude, A., Pascal, M. C. and Chippaux, M. (1979). Formate–nitrite reduction in *E. coli* K12. *Eur. J. Biochem.*, **95**, 315
114. Zumft, W. G. (1972). Ferredoxin: nitrite reduction in *E. coli. Biochim. Biophys. Acta*, **276**, 363
115. Singh, J. (1973). Cytochrome oxidase from *Pseudomonas aeruginosa*. III. Reduction of hydroxylamine. *Biochim. Biophys. Acta*, **333**, 28
116. Losada, M. (1973). Interconversion of nitrate and nitrite reductase of the assimilatory type. *3rd Int. Symp. Metab. Interconversion of Enzymes.* pp. 257–270. Seattle, Washington
117. Cohen, B. S. and Weinhouse, S. (1971). Reduction of nitrate to nitrite in tissues of the rat. Abstract No. 179 *162nd American Chemical Society Natl. Meeting*, Washington, DC
118. Rajagopalan, K. V., Fridovich, I. and Handler, P. (1962). Hepatic aldehyde oxidase. I. Purification and properties. *J. Biochem. Chem.*, **237**, 922
119. Krenitsky, T. A. (1978). Aldehyde oxidase and xanthine oxidase: functional and evolutionary relationships. *Biochem. Pharmacol.*, **27**, 2763
120. Kato, R., Iwasaki, K. and Noguchi, H. (1978). Reduction of tertiary amine *N*-oxides by cytochrome R-450. *Molec. Pharmacol.*, **14**, 654
121. Bernheim, M. L. C. and Hochstein, P. (1968). Reduction of hydroxylamine by rat liver mitochondria. *Arch. Biochem. Biophys.*, **124**, 436
122. Mitchell, H. H., Shonle, H. A. and Grindley, H. S. (1916). The origin of the nitrates in the urine. *J. Biol. Chem.*, **24**, 461
123. Orii, Y. and Shimada, H. (1978). Nitrite metabolism by muscle *in vitro. J. Biochem.*, **84**, 1543
124. Walters, C. L. and Taylor, A. M. (1963). Nitrite metabolism by muscle *in vitro. Biochim. Biophys. Acta*, **86**, 448
125. Nobbs, C. L., Watson, H. C. and Kendrew, J. C. (1966). Structure of deoxymyoglobin: A crystallographic study. *Nature (London)*, **209**, 339
126. Weiss, J. J. (1964). Nature of the iron–oxygen bond in oxyhaemoglobin. *Nature (London)*, **202**, 83
127. Wittenberg, J. B., Wittenberg, B. A., Peisach, J. and Blumber, W. E. (1970). On the state of the iron and the nature of the ligand in oxyhemoglobin. *Proc. Natl. Acad. Sci.*, **67**, 1846
128. Pauling, L. and Coryell, C. D. (1936). The magnetic properties and structure of hemoglobin, oxyhemoglobin and carbon-monoxyhemoglobin. *Proc. Natl. Acad. Sci.*, **22**, 210
129. Viale, R. O., Maggiora, G. M. and Ingraham, L. L. (1964). Molecular orbital evidence for Weiss's oxyhaemoglobin structure (Letter). *Nature (London)*, **203**, 183
130. Perutz, M. F. (1970). Stereochemistry of cooperative effects in haemoglobin. *Nature (London)*, **228**, 726
131. Perutz, M. F. (1978). Hemoglobin structure and respiratory transport. *Sci. Am.*, **239**(6), 92
132. Bard, H. and Teasdale, F. (1979). Red cell oxygen affinity, hemoglobin type, 2,3-diphosphoglycerate, and pH as a function of fetal development. *Pediatrics*, **64**, 483
133. Schwartz, J. M. and Jaffe, E. R. (1978). Hereditary methemoglobinemia with deficiency of NADH dehydrogenase. In Stanburg, J. *et al.* (eds.) *The Metabolic Basis of Inherited Disease*, pp. 1452–1464.

134. Neill, J. M. (1925). Studies on the oxidation-reduction of hemoglobin and methemoglobin. *J. Exp. Med.*, **41**, 561

135. Conant, J. B. (1923). An electrochemical study of hemoglobin. *J. Biol. Chem.*, 401

136. Peters, J. P. and Van Slyke, D. D. (1931). *Quantitative Clinical Chemistry, Interpretation.* pp. 631–632. (London: Baillière, Tindall and Cox)

137. Paul, W. D. and Kemp, C. R. (1944). Methemoglobin: a normal constituent of blood. *Proc. Soc. Exp. Biol. Med.*, **56**, 55

138. VanSlyke, D. D., Hiller, A., Weisiger, J. R. and Cruz, W. O. (1946). Determination of carbon monoxide in blood and of total and active hemoglobin by carbon monoxide capacity: Inactive hemoglobin and methemoglobin contents of normal blood. *J. Biochem.*, **166**, 121

139. Scott, E. M. (1968). Congenital methemoglobinemia due to DPNH-diaphorase deficiency. In Beutler, E. (ed.) *Hereditary Disorders of Erythrocyte Metabolism.* (New York: Grüne and Stratton)

140. Goldsmith, J. H., Rokaw, S. N. and Shearer, L. A. (1975). Distributions of percentage methaemoglobin in several population groups in California. *Int., J. Epidemiol.*, **4**, 207

141. Cox, W. W. and Wendel, W. G. (1942). The normal rate of reduction of methemoglobin in dogs. *J. Biol. Chem.*, **143**, 331

142. Francois (1844–1845) Cas de cyanose congeniale sans cause apparente. *Bull. Acad. R. M. Belg.*, **4**, 698

143. Slosse, A. and Wybauw, R. (1912). Un cas de methemoglobinemie idiopathique. *Ann. Bull. Soc. R. Sci. Med. Nat. Bruxelles*, **70**, 206

144. Sievers, R. F. and Ryan, J. B. (1945). Congenital idiopathic methemoglobinemia: favorable response to ascorbic acid therapy. *Arch. Intern. Med.*, **76**, 299

145. Gibson, Q. H. (1943). The reduction of methaemoglobin by ascorbic acid. *Biochem. J.*, **37**, 615

146. Deeny, J., Murdock, E. T. and Rogan, J. J. (1943). Familial idiopathic methaemoglobinaemia with a note on the treatment of two cases with ascorbic acid. *Br. Med. J.*, **1**, 721

147. King, E. J., Gikhrest, M. and White, J. C. (1944). A case of methemoglobinemia. *Biochem. J.*, **38**

148. Scott, E. M. and Griffith, I. V. (1959). The enzymic defect of hereditary methemoglobinemia: Diaphorase. *Biochim. Biophys. Acta*, **34**, 584

149. Scott, E. M. (1960). The relation of diaphorase of human erythrocytes to inheritance of methemoglobinemia. *J. Clin. Invest.*, **39**, 1176

150. Jaffe, E. R. (1963). The reduction of methemoglobin in erythrocytes of a patient with congenital methemoglobinemia, subjects with erythrocyte glucose-6-phosphate dehydrogenase deficiency and normal individuals. *Blood*, **21**, 561

151. Ross, J. D. and Desforges, J. F. (1959). Reduction of methemoglobin by erythrocytes from cord blood. *Pediatrics*, **23**, 718

152. Ross, J. D. (1963). Deficient activity of DPNH dependent methemoglobin diaphorase in cord blood erythrocytes. *Blood*, **21**, 51

153. Bartos, H. R. and Desforges, J. F. (1966). Erythrocyte DPNH dependent diaphorase levels in infants. *Pediatrics*, **37**, 991

154. Scott, E. M., Duncan, I. W. and Ekstrand, V. (1965). The reduced pyridine nucleotide dehydrogenases of human erythrocytes. *J. Biol. Chem.*, **240**, 481

155. Kanazawa, Y., Hattori, M., Kosaka, K. and Nakao, K. (1968). The relationship of NADH-dependent diaphorase activity and methoglobin reduction in human erythrocytes. *Clin. Chim. Acta*, **19**, 524

156. Petragnani, N., Nogueira, O. C. and Raw, I. (1959). Methaemoglobin reduction through cytochrome b5. *Nature (London)*, **184**, 1651

157. Hultquist, D. E. and Passon, P. G. (1971). Catalysis of methaemoglobin reduction by erythrocyte cytochrome b5 and cytochrome b5 reductase. *Nature New Biol.*, **229**, 252

158. Hultquist, D. E. (1978). Erythrocyte cytochrome b5; structure, role in methemoglobin reduction, and solubilization from endoplasmic reticulum. *Prog. Clin. Biol. Res.*, **21**, 199

159. Leroux, A., Torlinski, L. and Kaplan, J. C. (1977). Soluble and microsomal forms of NADH-cytochrome b5 reductase from human placenta: similarity with NADH-methemoglobin reductase from human erythrocytes. *Biochim. Biophys. Acta*, **481**, 50

160. Abe, K. and Sugita, Y. (1979). Properties of cytochrome b5 and methemoglobin reduction in human erythrocytes. *Eur. J. Biochem.*, **101**, 423

161. Hultquist, D. E. (1978). Methemoglobin reduction system of erythrocytes. *Methods Enzymol.*, **52**, 463

162. Warburg, O. and Christian, W. (1931). Uber Aktivierung der Robisonschen Hexose-monophosphorsaure in roten Blutzellen und die Gewinnung aktivierender Fermentlosungen. *Biochem. Z.*, **242**, 206

163. Warburg, O. and Griese, A. (1935). Wasserstoffubertragendes Co ferment, seine Zusammensetzung und Wirkungsweise. *Biochem. Z.*, **282**, 157

164. Kiese, M. (1944). Die Reduktion des Hamoglobins. *Biochem. Z.*, **316**, 264

165. Huennekens, F. M., Caffrey, R. W., Basford, R. E. and Gabrio, B. W. (1957). Erythrocyte metabolism. IV. Isolation and properties of methemoglobin reductase. *J. Biol. Chem.*, **227**, 261

166. Huennekens, F. M., Lin, L., Myers, H. A. P. and Gabrio, B. W. (1957). Erythrocyte metabolism. III. Oxidation of glucose. *J. Biol. Chem.*, **227**, 253

167. Sass, M. D., Caruso, C. J. and Farhangi, M. (1967). TPNH-methamoglobin reductase deficiency: A new red-cell enzyme defect. *J. Lab. Clin. Med.*, **70**, 760

168. Sass, M. D., Caruso, C. J. and Axelrod, D. R. (1969). Mechanism of the TPNH-linked reduction of methemoglobin by methylene blue. *Clin. Chim. Acta*, **24**, 77

169. Tomoda, A., Takeshita, M. and Yoneyama, Y. (1978). Analysis of met-form hemoglobin in glucose-deleted human red cells. *FEBS Lett.*, **88**, 247

170. Mansouri, A. and Winterhalter, K. H. (1973). Nonequivalence of chains in hemoglobin oxidation. *Biochemistry*, **12**, 4946

171. Isselbacher, K. J., Adams, R. D., Braunwald, E., Petersdorf, R. G. and Wilson, J. D. (1980). *Harrison's Principles of Internal Medicine*, 9th ed., p. 1552. (New York: McGraw-Hill)

172. Kaplan, J. C. and Chirouze, M. (1979). Therapy of recessive congenital methaemoglobinaemia by oral riboflavin. (letter). *Lancet*, **2**, 1043

173. Jaffe, E. R. and Neumann, G. (1964). A comparison of the effect of menadione, methylene blue and ascorbic acid on the reduction of methaemoglobin *in vivo*. *Nature (London)*, **202**, 607

174. Tarlov, A. R., Brewer, G. J., Carson, P. E. and Alving, A. S. (1962). Primaquine sensitivity. Glucose-6-phosphate dehydrogenase deficiency: an inborn error of metabolism of medical and biological significance. *Arch. Intern. Med.*, **109**, 209

175. Brewer, G. J., Tarlov, A. R., Kellermeyer, R. W. and Alving, A. S. (1962). The hemolytic effect of primaquine. XV. Role of methemoglobin. *J. Lab. Clin. Med.*, **59**, 905

176. Douglas, C. G., Haldane, J. S. and Haldane, J. B. S. (1912). The laws of combination of haemoglobin with carbon monoxide and oxygen. *J. Physiol.* **44**, 275

177. Darling, R. C. and Roughton, F. J. W. (1942). The effect of methemoglobin on the equilibrium between oxygen and hemoglobin. *Am. J. Physiol.*, **137**, 56

178. Brewer, G. J. (1971). Clinical implications of variation in erythrocyte oxygen affinity: A. Blood storage and B. Arteriosclerosis. In Astrup, P. and Rorth, M. (eds.) *Oxygen Affinity of Hemoglobin and Red Cell Acid Base Status*. pp. 629–645. (New York: Academic Press)

179. Enoki, Y., Tokui, H. and Tyuma, I. (1969). Oxygen equilibria of partially oxidized hemoglobin. *Respir. Physiol.*, **7**, 300

180. Kiese, M. (1966). The biochemical production of ferrihemoglobin forming derivatives from aromatic amines, and mechanisms of ferrihemoglobin formation. *Pharmacol. Rev.*, **18**, 1091

181. Smith, R. P. and Olson, M. V. (1973). Drug-induced methemoglobinemia. *Semin. Hematol.*, **10**, 253

182. Castro, C. E., Wade, R. S. and Belser, N. O. (1978). Conversion of oxyhemoglobin to methemoglobin by organic and inorganic reductants. *Biochemistry*, **17**, 225

183. Wind, M. and Stern, A. (1977). Comparison of human adult and fetal hemoglobin: Aminophenol-induced methemoglobin formation. *Experientia*, **33**, 1500

184. Gamgee, A. (1880). *A Text-book of the Physiological Chemistry of the Animal Body.* pp. 109–112. (London: Macmillan and Co.)

185. Haldane, J., Makgill, R. H. and Mavrogordato, A. E. (1897). The action as poisons of nitrites and other physiologically related substances. *J. Physiol.*, **21**, 160

186. Greenberg, L. A., Lester, D. and Haggard, H. W. (1943). The reaction of hemoglobin with nitrite. *J. Biol. Chem.*, **151**, 665

187. Meier, R. (1925). Studien uber Methamolgobinbildung. VII. Nitrit. *Arch. Exp. Pathol. Pharmakol.*, **110**, 241

188. Harvey, J. W. and Kaneko, J. J. (1976). Oxidation of human and animal haemoglobins with ascorbate, acetylphenylhydrazine, nitrite, and hydrogen peroxide. *Br. J. Haematol.*, **32**, 193

189. Cohen, G., Martinez, M. and Hochstein, P. (1964). Generation of hydrogen peroxide during the reaction of nitrite with oxyhemoglobin. *Biochemistry*, **3**, 901

190. Smith, R. P. (1970). Some features of the reaction between cobalt, nitrite and hemoglobin. *Toxicol. Appl. Pharmacol.*, **17**, 634

191. Betke, K., Greinacher, I. and Tietze, O. (1956). Oxidation menschlicher und tierischer oxyhamoglobin durch natrium nitrit. *Arch. Exp. Pathol. Pharmakol.*, **229**, 220

192. Kiese, M. (1967), Reactions of *N,N*-dimethylamine-*N*-oxide with hemoglobin. *Molec. Pharmacol.*, **3**, 9

193. Rodkey, F. L. (1976). A mechanism for the conversion of oxyhemoglobin to methemoglobin by nitrite. *Clin. Chem.*, **72**, 1986

194. Mansouri, A. (1979). Oxidation of human hemoglobin by sodium nitrite – effect of beta-93 thiol groups. *Biochem. Biophys. Res. Commun.*, **89**, 441

195. Austin, J. H. and Drabkin, D. L. (1935). Spectrophotometric studies. III. Methemoglobin. *J. Biol. Chem.*, **112**, 67

196. Jung, F. and Remmer, H. (1949). Uber die Umsetzung zwischen Nitrit und Hamoglobin. *Arch. Exp. Pathol. Pharmakol.*, **206**, 459

197. Assendelft, O. W. V. and Ziljstra, W. G. (1965). The formation of hemiglobin using nitrites. *Clin. Chim. Acta*, **11**, 571

198. Smith, R. P. (1967). The nitrite methemoglobin complex – its significance in methemoglobin analysis and its possible role in methemoglobinemia. *Biochem. Pharmacol.*, **16**, 1655

199. Gibson, Q. H., Parkhurst, L. G. and Gevaci, G. (1969). The reaction of methemoglobin with some ligands. *J. Biol. Chem.*, **244**, 4668

200. Uchida, H. and Klapper, M. H. (1970). Evidence for an irreversible reaction between nitrite and human methemoglobin. *Biochim. Biophys. Acta*, **221**, 640

201. Smith, R. P. and Gosselin, R. E. (1966). On the mechanism of sulfide inactivation by methemoglobin. *Toxicol. Appl. Pharmacol.*, **8**, 159

202. Coryell, C. D., Pauling, L. and Dodson, R. W. (1939). The magnetic properties of intermediates in the reactions of hemoglobin. *J. Phys. Chem.*, **43**, 825

203. Imaizumi, K., Tyuma, I., Imai, K., Kosaka, H. and Ueda, Y. (1980). *In vivo* studies on methemoglobin formation by sodium nitrite. *Int. Arch. Occup. Environ. Hlth*, **45**, 97

204. Chien, J. C. W. (1969). Reactions of nitric oxide with methemoglobin. *J. Am. Chem. Soc.*, **91**, 2156

205. Benesch, R., Benesch, R. E. and Yu, C. I. (1968). Reciprocal binding of oxygen and diphosphoglycerate by human hemoglobin. *Proc. Natl. Acad. Sci.*, **59**, 526

206. Perutz, M. F., Ferscht, A. R., Simon, S. R. and Roberts, G. C. K. (1974). Influence of globin structure on the state of heme. II. Allosteric transitions in methemoglobin. *Biochemistry*, **13**, 2174

207. Martin, H. and Huisman, T. H. J. (1963). Formation of ferri-haemoglobin of isolated haemoglobin types by sodium nitrite. *Nature (London)*, **200**, 898.

208. Tomoda, A., Matsukawa, S., Takeshita, M. and Yoneyama, Y. (1977). Effect of inositol hexaphosphate on hemoglobin oxidation by nitrite and ferricyanide. *Biochem. Biophys. Res. Commun.*, **74**, 1469

209. Smith, R. P., Alkaitis, A. A. and Shafer, P. R. (1967). Chemically induced methemoglobinemias in the mouse. *Biochem. Pharmacol.*, **16**, 317

210. Smith, R. P. and Layne, W. R. (1969). A comparison of the lethal effects of nitrite and hydroxylamine in the mouse. *J. Pharmacol. Exp. Therap.*, **165**, 30

211. Bunn, H. F., Forget, B. G. and Ranney, H. M. (1977). *Human Hemoglobins* (Philadelphia: W. B. Saunders)

212. Kravitz, H., Elegant, L. D., Kaiser, E. and Kagan, B. M. (1956). Methemoglobin values in premature and mature infants and children. *Am. J. Dis. Child.*, **91**, 1

213. Kunzer, W., Schuzz, A. and Schutz, E. (1956). Vergleichende Untersuchung der Spontanoxydation edes Blutfarbstoffes in Nabelschnur- und Erwachsenen-erythrocyten nach Glykolysehemmung. *Acta Haematol.*, **16**, 137

214. Bennecke and Hoffman (1906). First fatal case of bismuth subnitrate poisoning reported in the literature. *Muench. Med. Wochenschr.*

215. Boehme (1907). Report of fatal case of Bismuth Subnitrate poisoning. *Arch. Exp. Pathol. Pharmakol.*

216. Beck, E. G. (1909). Toxic effects from bismuth subnitrate. *J. Am. Med. Assoc.*, **52**, 14
217. Eusterman, G. B. and Keith, N. M. (1929). Transient methemoglobinemia following administration of ammonium nitrate. *Med. Clin. North Am.*, **12**, 1489
218. Roe, H. E. (1933). Methemoglobinemia following the administration of bismuth subnitrate: report of a fatal case. *J. Am. Med. Assoc.*, **101**, 352
219. Comly, H. H. (1945). Cyanosis in infants caused by nitrates in well water. *J. Am. Med. Assoc.*, **129**, 112
220. Lecks, H. L. (1950). Methemoglobinemia in infancy. *Am. J. Dis. Child.*, **79**, 117
221. Cornblath, M. and Hartmann, A. F. (1948). Methemoglobinemia in young infants. *J. Pediatr.*, **33**, 421
222. Marriott, M. W., Hartmann, A. F. and Senn, M. J. E. (1933). Observations on the nature and treatment of diarrhoea and the associated systemic disturbances. *J. Pediatr.*, **3**, 181
223. Robertson, H. E. and Riddell, W. A. (1949). Cyanosis of infants produced by high nitrate concentration in rural waters of Saskatchewan. *Canad. J. Pub. Hlth*, **40**, 72
224. Knotek, Z. and Schmidt, P. (1964). Pathogenesis, incidence and possibilities of preventing alimentary nitrate methemoglobinemia in infants. *Pediatrics*, **34**, 78
225. Walton, G. (1951). Survey of literature relating to infant methemoglobinemia due to nitrate-contaminated water. *Am. J. Pub. Hlth*, **41**, 986
226. Simon, C., Manzke, H., Kay, H. and Mrowetz, G. (1964). Über Vorkommen, Pathogenese und Moglichkeiten zur Prophylaxe der durch Nitrit verursachten Methamoglobinamie. *Z. Kinderheilkd.*, **91**, 124
227. Shuval, H. I. and Gruener, N. (1972). Epidemiological and toxicological aspects of nitrates and nitrites in the environment. *Am. J. Pub. Hlth*, **62**, 1045
228. Simon, C. (1966). Nitrite poisoning from spinach (letter). *Lancet*, **1**, 872
229. Paneque, A., DelCampo, F. F., Ramirez, J. M. and Losada, M. (1965). Flavin nucleotide nitrate reductase from spinach. *Biochim. Biophys. Acta*, **109**, 79
230. Schuphan, W. (1965). Der Nitrategehalt von Spinat (*Spinacia oleraces L.*) in Beziehung zur Methamoglobinanamie. *Z. Ernaehrungswiss.*, **5**, 207
231. Phillips, W. E. J. (1968). Changes in the nitrate and nitrite contents of fresh and processed spinach during storage. *J. Agr. Food Chem.*, **16**, 88
232. Phillips, W. E. J. (1969). Lack of nitrite accumulation in partially consumed jars of baby food. *Canad. Inst. Food Tech. J.*, **2**, 160
233. Phillips, W. E. J. (1971). Naturally occurring nitrate and nitrite in foods in relation to infant methaemoglobinaemia. *Food Cosmet. Toxicol.*, **9**, 219
234. Heisler, E. G., Siciliano, J., Krulick, S., Feinberg, J. and Schwartz, J. H. (1974). Changes in nitrate and nitrite content, and search for nitrosamines in storage-abused spinach and beets. *Agric. Food Chem.*, **22**, 1029
235. Holscher, P. M. and Natzschka, J. (1964). Methamoglobinanamie bei jungen Sauglingen durch nitrithaltigen Spinat. *Dtsch. Med. Wochenschr.*, **89**, 1751
236. Sinious, A. and Wodsak, W. (1965). Die spinatvergiftung des Sauglings. *Dtsch. Med. Wochenschr.*, **90**, 1856
237. Keating, J. P., Lell, M. E., Stauss, A. W., Zarkowsky, H. and Smith, G. E. (1973). Infantile methemoglobinemia caused by carrot juice. *N. Engl. J. Med.*, **288**, 824
238. Orgeron, J. D., Martin, J. D., Caraway, C. T., Martine, R. M. and Hanser, G. H. (1957). Methemoglobinemia from eating meat with high nitrite content. *Pub. Hlth Rep.*, **72**, 189
239. Golba, J., Klecha, I., Kurowski, M. and Waluszkiewicz, H. (1977). Mass food poisoning with sodium nitrite. *Pol. Tyg. Lek.*, **32**, 1275
240. Greenberg, M., Birnkrant, W. G. and Schiftner, J. J. (1945). Outbreak of sodium nitrite poisoning. *Am. J. Pub. Hlth*, **35**, 1217
241. Roueche, B. (1954). *Eleven blue men and other narratives of Medical Detection.* (Boston: Little Brown)
242. Tepperman, J., Marquardt, R., Reifenstein, G. and Lozner, E. (1951). Methemoglobinemic cyanosis – report of an epidemic due to corning extract substituted for maple syrup. *J. Am. Med. Assoc.*, **146**, 923
243. Bakshi, S. P., Fahey, J. L. and Pierce, L. E. (1967). Sausage cyanosis – acquired methemoglobinemic nitrite poisoning. *N. Engl. J. Med.*, **277**, 1072
244. Hill, T. W. (1878). Poisoning from an overdose of sweet spirits of nitre, resembling a case of acute alcoholic poisoning. *Lancet*, **2**, 766

245. Chilcote, R. R., Williams, B., Wolf, L. J. and Baenher, R. L. (1977). Sudden death in an infant from methemoglobinemia after administration of 'sweet spirits of nitre'. *Pediatrics*, **59**, 280

246. Naidu, S. R. and Venkatrao, P. (1936). Case of nitrite poisoning. *Br. Med. J.*, **1**, 1300

247. Naidu, S. R. and Venkatrao, P. (1945). The toxicology of nitrites. *Calcutta Med. J.*, **42**, 79

248. Huziter-Kramer, H. (1936). Sodium nitrite poisoning. *Samml. Vergiftungsfaellen*, **7**, 15

249. McQuiston, T. A. C. (1936). Fatal poisoning by sodium nitrite. *Lancet*, **2**, 1153

250. Padberg, L. E. and Martin, T. (1939). Three fatal cases of poisonings. *J. Am. Med. Assoc.*, **113**, 1733

251. Ruegg, H. (1935). Nitrite poisoning. *Schweiz. Med. Wochenchschr.*, **16**, 809

252. Wilson, L. G. (1976). Accidental sodium nitrite ingestion. *Med. J. Aust.*, **1**, 505

253. Sevier, J. N. and Berbatis, G. G. (1976). Accidental sodium nitrite ingestion. *Med. J. Aust.*, **1**, 847

254. Standefer, J. C., Jones, A. M., Street, E. and Inserra, R. (1979). Death associated with nitrite ingestion: report of a case. *J. Forensic Sci.*, **24**, 768

255. Harris, J. C., Rumack, B. H., Peterson, R. G. and McGuire, B. M. (1979). Methemoglobinemia resulting from absorption of nitrates. *J. Am. Med. Assoc.*, **242**, 2869

256. Henderson, W. R. and Raskin, N. H. (1972). 'Hot-dog' headache: individual susceptibility to nitrite. *Lancet*, **2**, 1162

257. Sollman, T. (1957). *A Manual of Pharmacology*. 8th edn. (Philadelphia: W. B. Saunders)

258. Zimmermann, F. E. (1977). Genetic effects of nitrous acid. *Mutat. Res.*, **39**, 127

259. Wittmann-Liebold, B. and Wittman, H. G. (1965). Localization of amino acid exchanges of nitrite mutants of tobacco mosaic virus. *Z. Vererbungsl.*, **97**, 305

260. Barnet, W. E. and DeBusk, A. G. (1960). Nitrous acid induced reverse mutation in *Neurospora crassa*. *Genetics*, **45**, 973

261. Gutz, H. (1961). Nitrous acid induced mutations in the genetic fine structure of the *ad*-7 locus of *Schizosaccharomyces pombe*. *Nature (London)*, **191**, 1125

262. Kaudewitz, F. (1958). Production of bacterial mutants with nitrous acid. *Nature (London)*, **183**, 1829

263. Zahmenhof, S. (1958). Induction of mutations by deamination. *Microb. Genet. Bull.*, **16**, 33

264. Ishidate, M. and Odashima, S. (1977). Chromosome Tests with 134 compounds on Chinese hamster cells *in vitro* – a screening for chemical carcinogens. *Mutat. Res.*, **48**, 337

265. Kodama, F., Umeda, M. and Tsutsui, T. (1976). Mutagenic effect of sodium nitrite on cultured mouse cells. *Mutat. Res.*, **40**, 119

266. Utakoji, T. (1974). Chromosomal aberrations caused by sodium nitrite ($NaNO_2$) in PHA cultures of human peripheral blood lymphocytes (meeting abstract). *Gann Proceedings of the Japanese Cancer Assoc.*, 33rd Annual Meeting, p. 27, Sendai, Japan

267. Sauro, F., Friedman, L. and Green, S. (1973). Biochemical, mutagenic and pathological effects of nitrosamines in rats (meeting abstract). *Toxicol. Appl. Pharmacol.*, **25**, 449

268. Knudsen, I. and Meyer, O. A. (1977). Mutagenicity studies on rats and mice given canned, heated nitrite-treated pork. *Mutat. Res.*, **56**, 177

269. Druckrey, H., Steinhoff, D., Beuthner, H., Schneider, H. and Klarner, P. (1963). Prufung von Nitrit auf chronisch toxische Wirkung an Ratten. *Arzneim. Forsch.*, **13**, 320

270. Van Logten, M. J., Den Tonkelaar, E. M., Kroes, R., Berkvens, J. M. and Van Esch, G. J. (1972). Long-term experiment with canned meat treated with sodium nitrite and glucono-ω-lactone in rats. *Food Cosmet. Toxicol.*, **10**, 475

271. Taylor, H. H. W. and Lijinsky, W. (1975). Tumor induction in rats by feeding heptamethyleneimine and nitrite in water. *Cancer Res.*, **35**, 812

272. Olsen, P. and Meyer, O. (1976). Carcinogenicity study on rats fed on canned heated nitrite-treated meat: preliminary communication. *Proc. 2nd Intl. Symp. Nitrite Meat Prod.*, pp. 275–278.

273. Inai, K., Aoki, Y. and Tokuoka, S. (1979). Chronic toxicity of sodium nitrite in mice, with reference to its tumorigenicity. *Gann*, **70**, 203

274. Sander, J. (1970). Induction of malignant tumors in rats by oral administration of *N,N'*-Dimethylurea and sodium nitrite. *Arzneim. Forsch.*, **20**, 418

275. Greenblatt, M., Mirvish, S. and So, B. (1971). Nitrosamine studies: Induction of lung adenomas by concurrent administration of sodium nitrite and secondary amines in Swiss mice. *J. Natl. Cancer Inst.*, **46**, 1029

276. Scheunig, G., Horn, K. H. and Mehnert, W. H. (1979). Induction of tumors in Wistar-rats after oral application of amino pyrine and nitrite. *Arch. Geschwulstforsch.*, **49**, 220

277. Shank, R. C. and Newberne, P. M. (1976). Dose-response study of the carcinogenicity of dietary sodium nitrite and morpholine in rats and hamsters. *Food Cosmet. Toxicol.*, **14**, 1

278. Matsukura, N., Kawachi, T., Sasajima, K., Sano, T., Sugimura, T. and Ho, N. (1977). Induction of liver tumors in rats by sodium nitrite and methylguanidine. *Z. Krebsforsch.*, **90**, 87

279. Newberne, P. M. (1979). Nitrite promotes lymphoma incidence in rats. *Science*, **204**, 1079

280. Lachance, P. A. (1978). Nitrites: The Newberne Report (letter). *Science*, **202**, 576

281. Food and Drug Administration and U.S. Department of Agriculture. (1978). *FDA's and USDA's Action Regarding Nitrite*, August, 1978

282. Hartman, S. L. (1979). Case history of FDA actions on M.I.T. nitrite study. *Congressional Record*, September 12, 1979, p. H7787–7792

283. Expert Panel on Nitrites and Nitrates. (1978). *Final Report on Nitrites and Nitrosamines.* Report to the Secretary of the US Department of Agriculture, February, 1978

284. Council for Agricultural Science and Technology. (1978). Nitrite in meat curing: risks and benefits. *Congressional Record*, **124**, 95th Congress, 2nd Session

285. Committee on Government Operations. (1972). Nineteenth Report. Regulation of food additives–nitrites and nitrates. *Union Calendar No. 701, 92nd Congress, 2nd Session*, House Report No. 92-1338 (Washington, DC: US Govt. Printing Office)

286. Culliton, B. J. (1978). Nitrites – to ban or not to ban? *Br. Med. J.*, **2**, 1613

287. Anonymous (1980). Plan to ban nitrites in foods dropped for now. *Chem. Eng. News*, p. 11. August 25, 1980

288. Taylor, J. M. and Morgenroth, V. H. (1979). Comparison of studies on saccharin and sodium nitrite. *J. Assoc. Off. Anal. Chem.*, **62**, 883

289. Globus, M. and Samuel, D. (1978). Effect of maternally administered sodium nitrite on hepatic erythropoiesis in fetal CD-1 mice. *Teratology*, **18**, 367

290. Sleight, S. D. and Atallah, O. A. (1968). Reproduction in the guinea pig as affected by chronic administration of potassium nitrate and potassium nitrite. *Tox. Appl. Pharmacol.*, **12**, 179

291. Sinha, D. P. and Sleight, S. D. (1971). Pathogenesis of abortion in acute nitrite toxicosis in guinea pigs. *Toxicol. Appl. Pharmacol.*, **18**, 340

292. Anderson, L. M., Giner-Sorolla, A., Ebeling, D. and Budinger, J. M. (1978). Effects of imipramine, nitrite and dimethylnitrosamine of reproduction in mice. *Res. Commun. Pathol. Pharmacol.*, **19**, 311

293. Kawabata, T., Oshima, H., Uibu, J., Nakamura, M., Matsui, M. and Hamano, M. (1979). Occurrence, formation and precursors of *N*-nitroso compounds in Japanese diet. In Miller, E. C. *et al.* (eds.) *Naturally Occurring Carcinogens-Mutagens and Modulators of Carcinogenesis.* pp. 195–209. (Baltimore: University Park Press)

294. Hill, M. J., Hawksworth, G. and Tattersall, G. (1973). Bacteria, nitrosamines and cancer of the stomach. *Br. J. Cancer*, **28**, 562

295. Ville, J. and Mestrezat, W. (1907). Origine des nitrites contenus dans la salive; leur formation par reduction microbrenne des Nitrates elimines par ce liquide. *C. R. Soc. Biol.*, **73**, 231

296. Keith, N. M., Whelan, M. and Bannick, E. G. (1930). The action and excretion of nitrates. *Arch. Intern. Med.*, **46**, 797

297. Goaz, P. W. and Biswell, H. A. (1961). Nitrate reduction in whole saliva. *J. Dent. Res.*, **40**, 355

298. Ishidate, M., Harada, M., Ishiwata, H., Nakamura, Y. and Tanimura, A. (1975). Studies on *in vivo* formation of nitrite. *Proc. Japan Cancer Assoc.*, p. 66. *33rd Annual Meeting*, October, 1974

299. Harada, M., Ishiwata, H., Nakamura, Y., Tanimura, A. and Ishidate, M. (1975). Studies on *in vivo* formation of nitroso compounds. I. Changes of nitrite and nitrate concentration in human saliva after ingestion of salted Chinese cabbage. *J. Food Hyg. Soc.*, **16**, 11

300. Tannenbaum, S. R., Weisman, M. and Fett, D. (1976). The effect of nitrate intake on nitrite formation in human saliva. *Food Cosmet. Toxicol.*, **14**, 549

301. Spiegelhalder, B., Eisenbrand, G. and Preussmann, R. (1976). Influence of dietary nitrate on nitrite content of human saliva: possible relevance *in vivo* formation of *N*-nitroso compounds. *Food Cosmet. Toxicol.*, **14**, 545

302. Fett, D. R. (1977). The effect of diet on nitrate metabolism in man. (*Masters Thesis.* Massachusetts Institute of Technology)

303. Okabe, S. (1973). Fundamental studies on nitrite contents in human saliva. *Hikone-Ronso*, **162**, 165

304. Hayashi, N., Watanabe, K., Ishiwata, H., Mizushiro, H., Tanimura, A. and Kurata, H. (1978). Fate of nitrate and nitrite in saliva and blood of monkey administered orally sodium nitrate solution, and microflora of oral cavity of the monkey. *J. Food Hyg. Soc., Japan*, **19**, 391

305. Lowenfels, A. B., Tuyns, A. J., Walker, E. A. and Roussel, A. (1978). Nitrite studies in oesophageal cancer. *Gut*, **19**, 199

306. Tannenbaum, S. R., Sinskey, A. J., Weisman, M. and Bishop, W. (1974). Nitrite in human saliva. Its possible relationship to nitrosamine formation. *J. Natl. Cancer Inst.*, **53**, 79

307. Ruddell, W. S. J., Blendis, L. M. and Walters, C. L. (1977). Nitrite and thiocyanate in the fasting and secreting stomach and in saliva. *Gut*, **18**, 73

308. Klein, D., Gaconnet, N., Poullain, B. and Derby, G. (1978). Effet d'une charge en nitrate sur le nitrite salivaire et gastrique chez l'homme. *Food Cosmet. Toxicol.*, **16**, 111

309. Sander, J. and Seif, F. (1969). Bacterial reduction of nitrate in the human stomach as a cause for nitrosamine formation. *Arzneim. Forsch.*, **19**, 1091

310. Ruddell, W. S. J., Bone, E. S., Hill, M. J., Blendis, L. M. and Walters, C. L. (1976). Gastric-juice nitrite: A risk factor for cancer in the hypochlorhydric stomach? *Lancet*, **1**, 1037

311. Ruddell, W. S. J., Bone, E. S., Hill, M. J. and Walters, C. L. (1978). Pathogenesis of gastric cancer in pernicious anaemia. *Lancet*, **1**, 521

312. Jones, S. M., Davies, P. W. and Savage, A. (1978). Gastric-juice nitrite and gastric cancer [letter]. *Lancet*, **1**, 1355

313. Schlag, P., Ulrich, H., Merkle, P., Bockler, R., Peter, M. and Herfarth, C. (1980). Are nitrite and N-nitroso compounds in gastric juice risk factors for carcinoma in the operated stomach? *Lancet*, **1**, 727

314. Cruickshank, J. and Moyers, J. M. (1914). The presence and significance of nitrite in urine. *Br. Med. J.*, **2**, 712

315. Guignard, J. P. and Torrado, A. (1978). Nitrite indicator test strips for bacteria (letter). *Lancet*, **1**, 47

316. Jogart, G. (1978). Screening for bacteriuria of school children by the nitrite reaction. *Int. Urol. Nephrol.*, **10**, 33

317. Kunin, C. M. and DeGroot, J. E. (1977). Sensitivity of a nitrite indicator strip method in detecting bacteriuria in preschool girls. *Pediatrics*, **60**, 244

318. Scheifele, D. W. and Smith, A. L. (1978). Home-testing for recurrent bacteriuria using nitrite strips. *Am. J. Dis. Child.*, **132**, 46

319. Sinaniotis, C. A. (1978). Nitrite indicator strip test for bacteriuria [letter]. *Lancet*, **1**, 776

320. Hill, M. J. and Hawksworth, G. (1972). Bacterial production of nitrosamines *in vitro* and *in vivo*. In Bogovski, P., Preussmann, R. and Walker, E. A. (eds.), N-*Nitroso Compounds Analysis and Formation*, IARC Scientific Publication No. 3, pp. 116–121. (Lyon: IARC)

321. Brooks, J. B., Cherry, W. B., Thacker, L. and Alley, C. C. (1972). Analysis of gas-chromatography of amines and nitrosamines produced *in vivo* and *in vitro* by *Proteus mirabilis*. *J. Infect. Dis.*, **126**, 143

322. Hicks, R. M., Walters, C. L., Elsebai, I., El-Aasser, A. B., El-Merzabani, M. and Gough, T. A. (1977). Demonstration of nitrosamines in human urine: Preliminary observations on a possible etiology for bladder cancer in association with chronic urinary tract infections. *Proc. R. Soc. Med.*, **70**, 413

323. El-Merzabani, M. M., El-Aasser, A. A. and Zakhary, N. I. (1979). A study on the aetiological factors of Bilharzial bladder cancer in Egypt. 1. Nitrosamines and their precursors in urine. *Eur. J. Cancer*, **15**, 287

324. Hill, M. J. and Hawksworth, G. (1974). Some studies on the production of nitrosamines in the urinary bladder and their subsequent effects. In Bogovski, P., Walker, E. A. and Davis, W. (eds.). N-*Nitroso Compounds in the Environment*, Int. Agency Res. Cancer Sci. Publ. 9, pp. 220–222. (Lyon: IARC)

325. Burns, H. S. and Visscher, M. B. (1934). The influence of various anions of the lyotropic series upon the sodium and chloride content of fluid in the intestine. *Am. J. Physiol.*, **110**, 490

326. Hawksworth, G. M. and Hill, M. J. (1971). Bacteria and the N-nitrosation of secondary amines. *Br. J. Cancer*, **25**, 520

327. Witter, J. P. and Balish, E. (1979). Distribution and metabolism of ingested NO_3^- and NO_2^- in germfree and conventional-flora rats. *Appl. Environ. Microbiol.*, **38**, 861

328. Wang, C. F., Cassens, R. G. and Hoekstra, W. G. Metabolic fate of ingested 1,5-N-labeled nitrate and nitrite in the rat. *J. Food Sci.* (In press)

329. Saul, R. L., Kabir, S. H., Cohen, Z., Bruce, W. R. and Archer, M. C. A re-evaluation of nitrate and nitrite levels in the human intestine. (In preparation)

330. Tannenbaum, S. R., Fett, D., Young, V. R., Land, P. D. and Bruce, W. R. (1978). Nitrite and nitrate are formed by endogenous synthesis in the human intestine. *Science*, **200**, 1487

331. Witter, J. P., Gatley, S. J. and Balish, E. (1979). Distribution of Nitrogen-13 from labeled nitrate ($^{13}NO_3^-$) in humans and rats. *Science*, **204**, 411

332. Witter, J. P., Balish, E. and Gatley, S. J. (1979). Distribution of nitrogen-13 from labeled nitrate and nitrite in germfree and conventional-flora rats. *Appl. Environ. Microbiol.*, **38**, 870

333. Fritsch, P. and DeSaint-Blanquat, G. (1976). Formation of nitrite from nitrates in the digestive tract. *Ann. Nutr. Aliment.*, **30**, 793

334. Friedman, M. A., Greene, E. J. and Epstein, S. S. (1972). Rapid gastric absorption of sodium nitrite in mice. *J. Pharm. Sci.*, **61**, 1492

335. Mirvish, S. S., Patil, K., Ghadirian, P. and Kommineni, V. R. C. (1975). Disappearance of nitrite from the rat stomach: contribution of emptying and other factors. *J. Natl. Cancer Inst.*, **54**, 869

336. Mysliwy, T. S., Wick, E. L., Archer, M. C., Shank, R. C. and Newberne, P. M. (1974). Formation of N-nitrosopyrrolidine in a dog's stomach. *Br. J. Cancer*, **30**, 279

337. LeBar, J. and Sander, J. (1975). Carcinogenic N-Nitrosodimethylamine from the reaction of the analgesic amido pyrine and nitrite extracted from foodstuffs. *Z. Krebsforsch.*, **84**, 299

338. Gruener, N., Shuval, H. I., Behroozi, K., Cohen, S. and Shechter, H. (1973). Methemoglobinemia induced by transplacental passage of nitrites in rats. *Bull. Environ. Contamin. Toxicol.*, **9**, 44

339. Smith, P. L. R. and Walters, C. L. (1978). The transport of nitrite in the blood [proceedings]. *Biochem. Soc. Trans.*, **6**, 665

340. Kilgore, L., Almon, L. and Gieger, M. (1959). The effects of dietary nitrate on rabbits and rats. *J. Nutr.*, **69**, 39

341. Greene, I. and Hiatt, E. P. (1954). Behavior of the nitrate ion in the dog. *Am. J. Physiol.*, **176**, 463

342. Ruiz de Luzuriaga, K. F. (1980). Human nitrate metabolism: effect of dietary variables. (*Masters Thesis*. Massachusetts Institute of Technology)

343. Tannenbaum, S. R., Green, L. C., Ruiz de Luzuriaga, K., Gordillo, G., Ullman, L. and Young, V. R. Endogenous carcinogenesis: nitrate, nitrite and N-nitroso compounds. In *Carcinogenesis: Fundamental Mechanisms and Environmental Effects*, Thirteenth Jerusalem Symposium, Jerusalem, April 28 – May 2, 1980. (In press)

344. Cuello, C., Correa, P., Haenszel, W., Gordillo, G., Brown, C., Archer, M. and Tannenbaum, S. (1976). Gastric cancer in Colombia. I. Cancer risk and suspect environmental agents. *J. Natl. Cancer Inst.*, **57**, 1015

345. Ishiwata, H., Mizushiro, H., Tanimura, A. and Murata, T. (1978). Metabolic fate of precursors of N-nitroso compounds (III). Urinary excretion of nitrate in man. *J. Food Hyg. Soc., Japan*, **19**, 318

346. Radomski, J. L., Palmiri, C. and Hearn, W. L. (1978). Concentrations of nitrate in normal human urine and the effect of nitrate ingestion. *Tox. Appl. Pharmacol.*, **45**, 63

347. Bartholomew, B., Caygill, C., Darbar, R. and Hill, M. J. (1979). Possible use of urinary nitrate as a measure of total nitrate intake. *Proc. Nutr. Soc.* (Engl.)

348. Maruyama, S., Shimizu, S. and Muramatsu, K. (1979). Dietary intake of nitrate and urinary excretion of nitrate in the population of several areas in Nagano prefecture. *J. Food Hyg. Soc. Japan*, **20**, 276

349. Cahn, A. (1886). Die Magenverdauung im Chlorhunger. *Z. Physiol. Chem.*, **10**, 522

350. Hiatt, E. P. (1940). Extreme hypochloremia in dogs induced by nitrate administration. *Am. J, Physiol.*, **129**, 597

351. Greene, I. and Hiatt, E. P. (1955). Renal excretion of nitrate and its effect on excretion of sodium and chloride. *Am. J. Physiol.*, **180**, 179

352. Berkman, P. M., deStrihou, C. Y., Needle, M. A., Gulyassy, P. F. and Schwartz, W. B. (1967). Factors which determine whether infusion of the sodium salt of an anion will induce metabolic alkalosis in dogs. *Clin. Sci.*, **33**, 517

353. Kahn, T., Bosch, J., Levitt, M. F. and Goldstein, M. H. (1975). Effect of sodium nitrate

loading on electrolyte transport in the renal tubule. *Am. J. Physiol.*, **229**, 746

354. Weiner, M. W. (1978). Effects of chloride, nitrate and sulfate on ATPase of renal cortex and medulla. *Proc. Soc. Exp. Biol. Med.*, **158**, 370

355. Ganong, W. F. (1975). *Review of Medical Physiology* (Los Altos, California: Lange Medical Publications)

356. Wyngaarden, J. B., Wright, B. M. and Ways, P. (1952). The effect of certain anions upon the accumulation and retention of iodide by the thyroid gland. *Endocrinology*, **50**, 537

357. Bloomfield, R. A., Weisch, C. W., Garner, G. B. and Muhrer, M. E. (1961). Effect of dietary nitrate on thyroid function. *Science*, **134**, 1690

358. Brown-Grant, K. (1961). Extrathyroidal concentrating mechanisms. *Physiol. Rev.*, **41**, 189

359. Edwards, D. A., Fletcher, K. and Rowlands, E. N. (1954). Antagonism between perchlorate, iodide, thiocyanate and nitrate for secretion in human salvia. *Lancet*, **1**, 498

360. Fletcher, K., Honour, A. J. and Rowlands, E. N. (1956). Studies on the concentration of radioiodide and thiocyanate in slices of the salivary gland. *Biochem. J.*, **63**, 194

361. Burgen, A. S. V. and Emmelin, N. E. (1961). *Physiology of the Salivary Glands*. (Baltimore: Williams and Wilkins)

362. Cohen, B. and Myant, N. B. (1959). Concentration of salivary iodide: A comparative study. *J. Physiol.*, **145**, 595

363. Honour, A. J., Myant, N. B. and Rowlands, E. N. (1952). Secretion of radioiodine in digestive juices and milk in man. *Clin. Sci.*, **11**, 447

364. Brown-Grant, K. (1957). The iodide concentrating mechanism of the mammary gland. *J. Physiol.*, **135**, 644

365. Donahoe, W. E. (1949). Cyanosis in infants with nitrates in drinking water as cause. *Pediatrics*, **3**, 308

366. Bloomfield, R. A., Hersey, J. R., Welsch, C. W., Garner, G. B. and Muhrer, M. E. (1962). Gastric concentration of nitrate in rats. (Meeting Abstract) *J. Animal Sci.*, **21**, 1019

367. Whelan, M. (1935). The nitrate content of animal tissues, and the fate of ingested nitrate. *Biochem. J.*, **29**, 782

368. Kurzer, M. and Calloway, D. H. (1979). Endogenous nitrate production in humans (Meeting Abstract). *Fed. Proc.*, **38**, 607

369. Green, L. C., Tannenbaum, S. R. and Goldman, P. (1981). Nitrate synthesis in the germfree and conventional rat. *Science*, **212**, 56

370. Zaldivar, R. and Robinson, H. (1973). Epidemiological investigation on stomach cancer mortality in Chileans: association with nitrate fertilizer. *Z. Krebsforsch.*, **80**, 289

371. Doll, R. (1956). Environmental factors in the aetiology of cancer of the stomach. *Gastroenterologia*, **86**, 320

372. Boyd, J., Langman, M. and Doll, R. (1964). The epidemiology of gastrointestinal cancer with special reference to causation. *Gut*, **5**, 196

373. Dungal, N. (1961). The special problem of stomach cancer in Iceland. *J. Am. Med. Assoc.*, **178**, 789

374. Haenszel, W., Kurihara, M., Locke, F. B., Shimuzu, K. and Mitsuo, S. (1976). Stomach cancer in Japan. *J. Natl. Cancer Inst.*, **56**, 265

375. Tempia, E., Health effects of water quality: a case study (personal communication)

376. Bogovski, P., Walker, E. A., Castegnaro, M. and Pignatelli, B. (1975). Some evidence of the presence of traces of nitrosamines in cider distillates. In N-*Nitroso Compounds in the Environment*, IARC Sci. Pub. No. 9, pp. 192–196. (Lyon: IARC)

377. Fong, L. Y. Y. and Newberne, P. M. (1978). Nitrosobenzylmethylamine, zinc deficiency and oesophageal cancer. In *Environmental Aspects of N-Nitroso Compounds*, IARC Sci. Pub. No. 19, pp. 503–513. (Lyon, France: IARC)

378. Song, Puju (1980). Personal communication

379. Haenszel, W., Correa, P., Cuello, C., Guzman, N., Burbano, L. C., Lores, H. and Munoz, J. (1976). Gastric cancer in Colombia. II. Case-control epidemiologic study of precursor lesions. *J. Natl. Cancer Inst.*, **57**, 1021

380. Correa, P., Cuello, C., Duque, E., Burbano, L. C., Garcia, F. T., Oscar, B., Brown, C. and Haenszel, W. (1976). Gastric cancer in Colombia. III. Natural history of precursor lesions. *J. Natl. Cancer Inst.*, **57**, 1027

381. Correa, P., Cuello, C., Gordillo, G., Zarama, G., Lopez, J., Haenszel, W. and Tannenbaum, S. The gastric microenvironment in populations at high gastric cancer risk. *JNCI Monographs on Cancer*, in press

382. Tannenbaum, S. R. and Moran, D. (1980). Epidemiological studies of nitrate, nitrite and gastric cancer. In *Proc. of Conference on Safety Evaluation of Nitrosatable Drugs and Chemicals*, January 24/25, London. (In press)
383. Rifkind, R. A., Bank, A., Marks, P. A. and Nossel, H. L. (1976). *Fundamentals of Hematology*. (Chicago: Year Book Medical Publishers)

5
Vitamin D

H. F. DELUCA

INTRODUCTION

In the past few years the view of vitamin D has greatly changed, primarily as the result of intensive investigation into the metabolic alterations to which the vitamin is subjected before it can function. It must be recognized that vitamin D would not be required in the diet of man and domestic animals should they subject themselves to sufficient amounts of ultraviolet light. We now know that vitamin D can be produced in the skin by the photolysis of 7-dehydrocholesterol, a sterol which is biosynthesized in abundant quantities in skin and elsewhere in the body. A requirement for vitamin D can, therefore, only be demonstrated under conditions where this photolysis reaction is prevented. In man this is primarily because he chooses to live inside structures protecting him from ultraviolet light, and also because he wears clothing over much of his body so even exposure to ultraviolet light is not as effective in producing vitamin D as it would be otherwise. Finally, the pollution of the atmosphere with industrial wastes and by-products of our population density also reduces the incidence of ultraviolet light, again diminishing the chances of biosynthetic sources of vitamin D. Fortunately, animals and man can absorb vitamin D from their intestinal tract as will be discussed in a subsequent section of this chapter. Therefore, as a result of the living habits to which man has subjected himself, vitamin D has become a dietary requirement; and thus vitamin D is a vitamin only because of the manner in which man chooses to live or raise his domestic animals. Consistent with this is the fact that vitamin D is not widely distributed in nature and is found in very few sources throughout the plant and animal kingdom. Recent work has also demonstrated that vitamin D is the precursor of at least one hormone which functions in calcium and phosphorus metabolism. Again, this is unique among the family of vitamins in which a vitamin serves as a precursor to a hormone. By following the above reasoning, namely that vitamin D is not required in the diet under conditions of adequate ultraviolet irradiation of skin and that it is the precursor of a hormone, it is likely that the vitamin is not truly a vitamin but must be regarded as a prohormone. These arguments, however, are only semantic; the fact remains that vitamin D *is* taken in the diet and it is an extremely potent substance which prevents a deficiency disease.

This chapter will focus on the recent developments in the understanding of vitamin D metabolism and function, but will also draw on some important facts which are necessary to understand vitamin D as a nutrient as well.

HISTORICAL PERSPECTIVE

A deficiency of vitamin D results in the disease rickets in the young and osteomalacia in the adult. Although rickets became much more prominent following the industrial revolution, descriptions of the rachitic symptoms occur even in ancient literature. The first clear and accurate description of the disease is attributed to Whistler[1] in 1645. However, the cause of the disease was not clear until placed on an experimental basis by Sir Edward Mellanby[2]. He produced the disease in dogs by dietary means and prevented or cured it with cod liver oil[3]. Inasmuch as McCollum et al.[4] had discovered the 'fat-soluble vitamine A' in cod liver oil, Sir Edward Mellanby attributed the ability of the cod liver oil to cure rickets to the vitamin A. McCollum et al.[5] demonstrated that heating and oxygenation of the cod liver oil destroyed the vitamin A activity, but the ability to cure rickets remained. He, therefore, concluded that the antirachitic activity resulted from another fat-soluble substance which he called vitamin D. However, at the time of Mellanby's brilliant work, Huldshinsky found that rachitic children could be cured by ultraviolet light[6]. This dichotomy was resolved when Steenbock and Black, and somewhat later Hess and co-workers, demonstrated that ultraviolet light converts a fat soluble substance present in skin and food to the antirachitic vitamin[7,8]. This discovery provided the basis for elimination of rickets as a major medical problem by the irradiation of food, and also for the isolation of the D vitamins. In 1931 Askew and co-workers[9] and somewhat later Windaus and his colleagues[10] isolated and identified vitamin D_2. Vitamin D_3 was subsequently isolated and identified in 1936[11], essentially drawing to a close the era of vitamin D discovery and isolation.

A new era was subsequently opened in 1966[12] with the discovery that vitamin D is converted in the body to active forms before it functions. This recent advance will be highlighted in the ensuing chapter.

DEFICIENCY DISEASES

A deficiency of vitamin D results in a variety of pathological states, the most well recognized being rickets, the deficiency disease generally encountered in young growing animals and children[13]. Simply put, this disease results from a failure to mineralize the newly laid down organic matrix of both epiphyseal chondroblasts and osteoblasts. Two types of bone growth are recognized; endochondral mediated long bone growth and intramembraneous growth. In the former the resting chondroblasts proliferate and hypertrophy in the epiphyseal plate. The hypertrophic chondroblasts elaborate collagen matrix plus mucopolysaccharide. At maturity this matrix calcifies with amorphous calcium phosphate and crystalline hydroxyapatite with death of the chondroblasts. Both matrix and mineral are resorbed by invading osteoblasts and blood vessels. The osteoblasts lay down new bone collagen and mucopolysaccharides, which calcify first as amorphous calcium phosphate and then as hydroxyapatite. In the case of membraneous bone or periosteal bone growth, osteoblasts elaborate the collagen matrix which then calcifies as just described.

In rickets both processes occur except that the collagen matrix of all types fails to calcify, giving wide epiphyseal plates and large areas of uncalcified bone, termed osteoid. Because the soft and pliable rope collagen structures (organic matrix) fail to calcify, they cannot carry out the structural functions of bone. It is the mineral component that imparts rigidity to the collagen fibrils and thus to the skeleton. Without this, the ends of long bones especially become twisted and bent giving rachitic symptoms as shown in Figure 1. Thus the epiphyseal plate may become damaged with displacement, the ribs show a rosary appearance, the legs become bowed, and the cranium soft and misshapen.

In adults the epiphyseal plate is closed and no long bone growth occurs. However, bone is continually being remodelled in the usual sequence in which cells are activated to resorb bone followed by new osteoblastic mediated bone growth replacement[14]. It is this new bone that fails to calcify, resulting in large osteoid seams or uncalcified bone. This disease is called osteomalacia.

The failure to calcify in both rickets and osteomalacia can be attributed primarily to insufficient supply of calcium and phosphorus to the calcification sites. Although there may be a direct role of some form of vitamin D at the calcification site, evidence to support this belief is lacking.

Another deficiency disease which is even more critical than rickets or osteomalacia is hypocalcaemic tetany. At low ionized calcium levels of the plasma the neuromuscular junction fails to operate satisfactorily, and a continuous and uncontrolled convulsion ensues (tetany); this disease is quickly fatal unless corrected. Both vitamin D and parathyroid hormone are necessary to prevent the disease by the elevation of plasma calcium concentration. Both humoral agents are necessary at physiologic concentrations.

Vitamin D is necessary for normal absorption of calcium, and permits the intestine to adapt its efficiency of calcium absorption to satisfy the body's needs[15, 16]. Inadequate vitamin D levels reduce this function which leads to a reliance on the skeleton for support of serum calcium levels. A continual drain on the skeletal calcium stores for a long period of time gives rise to reduced bone mass or osteoporosis. Thus adequate vitamin D intake is also needed to help prevent osteoporosis.

Finally, vitamin D stimulates muscle strength and tone[17, 18]. Exactly how this function occurs is unknown but nevertheless this phenomenon represents an important function requiring investigation.

It is important to realize that these functions of vitamin D take place throughout life. Thus vitamin D is required throughout life and claims that adults do not require vitamin D are incorrect. The daily requirement for vitamin D is between 200 and 400 units/day ($5-10\,\mu g$ of vitamin D_3)[19].

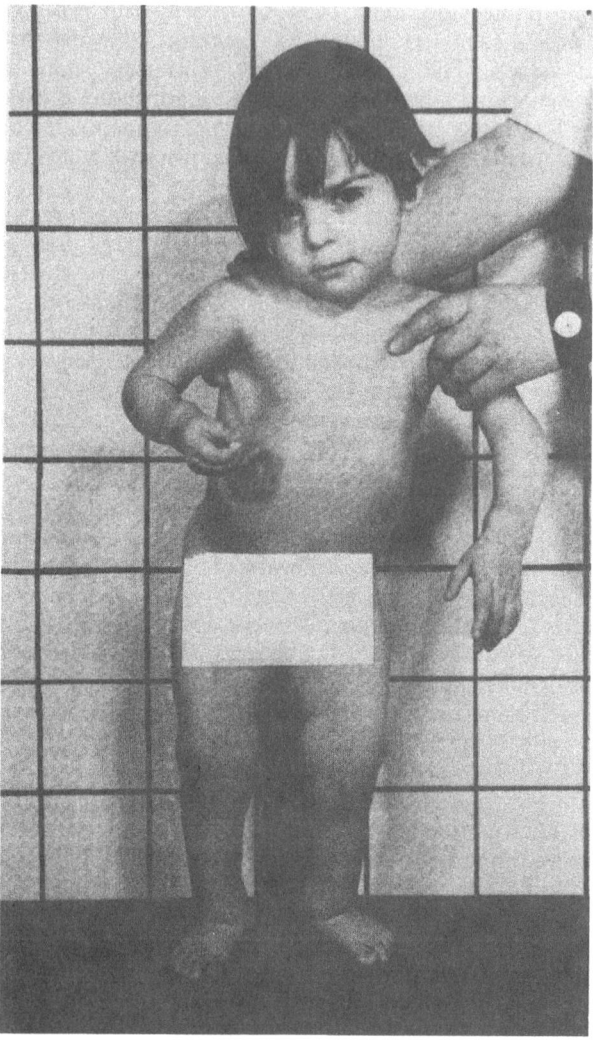

Figure 1 Photograph of a child suffering from vitamin D-deficiency rickets (courtesy of Dr Sonia Balsan, Paris)

THE D VITAMINS AND THEIR PRECURSORS

Figure 2 illustrates the known nutritional forms of vitamin D of any significance. The D vitamin of greatest importance is vitamin D_3, which has in the past been called cholecalciferol and whose systematic chemical name is 9,10-seco-5,7,10(19)-cholestatrien-3β-ol. It is this form of vitamin D which is made in skin under the influence of ultraviolet light, and thus can be regarded as the natural form of the vitamin. Vitamin D_3 has an ultraviolet absorption

144

maximum at 265 nm with an absorption minimum at 228 nm. Its molar extinction coefficient is 18 200 which results from the cisoid triene structure of the 9,10, 5,6 and 7,8 double bonds. X-ray crystallography has been completed on the vitamin D_3 compound, and its detailed chemical structure is fully understood as well as spacial arrangement of all of the carbon and hydrogen atoms[20, 21]. Vitamin D_3 crystallizes in two forms in which the A ring can assume one of two conformations[21]. It is unlikely that this conformational option plays any biological role. The physical properties of vitamin D and many of its analogues are well known and interested readers are referred to other chemically oriented publications for this information[22 – 25].

Vitamin D_2 is the form of vitamin D which is made from the irradiation of ergosterol. Although this form of vitamin D is found in nature, it is probably

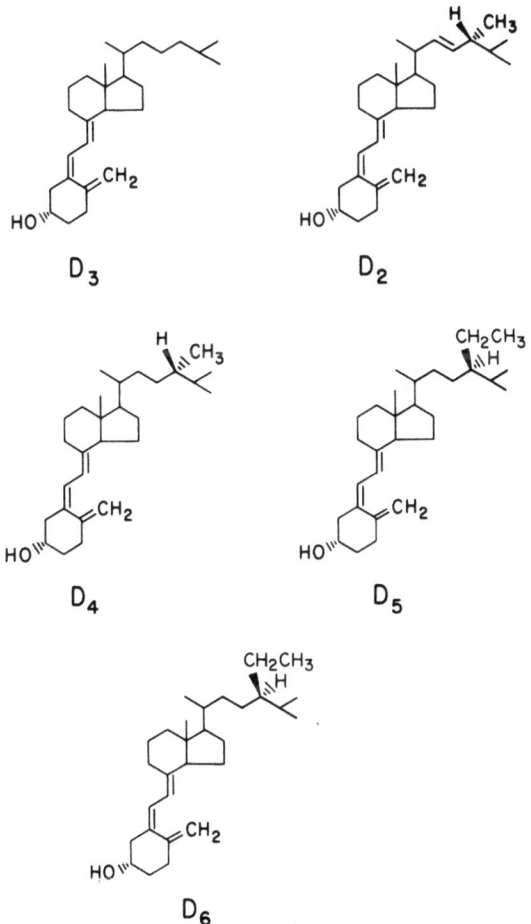

Figure 2 Structures of the known vitamin D compounds. Vitamin D_2 and vitamin D_3 are considered the only practically significant forms

present in only small amounts but represents the major synthetic form of vitamin D used during the past 40 years. It, like vitamin D_3, has the same absorption characteristics, and a similar extinction coefficient as vitamin D_3, but has somewhat different chemical properties because of the 22,23 double bond and because of the added methyl group on carbon 24 in the R configuration. The systematic chemical name for this compound is 9,10-seco-5,7,10(19),22-ergostatetraen-3β-ol.

Vitamin D_4 is a chemical curiosity which was originally synthesized by Windaus and Trautman[26] and later by DeLuca et al.[27]. The synthesis is involved the reduction of the 22,23 double bond prior to photolysis of the 5,7 diene structure of ergosterol, yielding vitamin D_4 or 22,23-dihydrovitamin D_2.

Other minor forms of vitamin D include the 24-methyl vitamin D_3 (vitamin D_5) and the 28-methyl vitamin D_2 (vitamin D_6). Little is known concerning their biological activity and they appear to be of minor significance in terms of their appearance in foods following irradiation.

The precursor of vitamin D_3 is 7-dehydrocholesterol whose structure is shown in Figure 3 along with the precursors of the other forms of vitamin D discussed above. 7-Dehydrocholesterol has a complex absorption spectrum with absorption maxima at 293, 281 and 271 with a shoulder at 265. The molar extinction coefficient is 11 900 at 281 nm. The complex absorption spectrum is the result of the 5,7-diene system contained in a restrained cyclic system. The

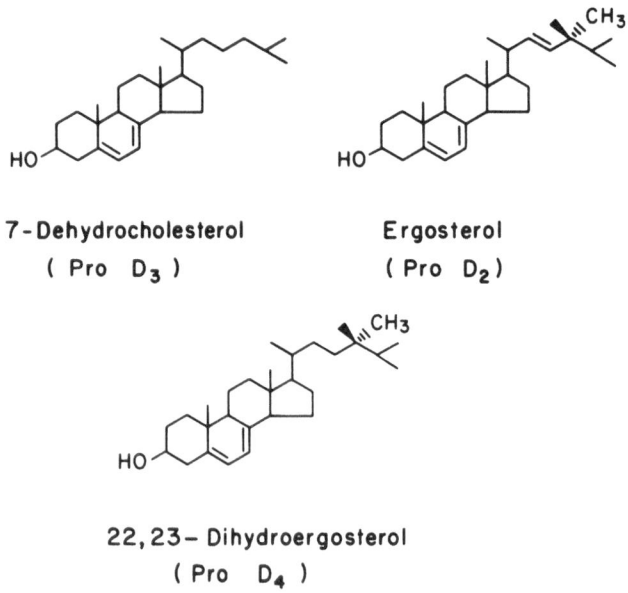

7-Dehydrocholesterol
(Pro D_3)

Ergosterol
(Pro D_2)

22,23- Dihydroergosterol
(Pro D_4)

Figure 3 The precursors of the major forms of vitamin D

other precursor sterols are well known especially ergosterol which has a wide distribution in nature, being found both in plants and in micro-organisms. It is commercially produced from yeast and from ergot mould, accounting for as much as 2% of their weight when grown in appropriate conditions. The physical properties of ergosterol are well known and interested readers are referred to other more chemically oriented texts for that information[22-25]. The 5,7-diene sterol precursors of the other forms of vitamin D indicated above are also known and interested readers are referred elsewhere for that information[22-25].

The 5,7-diene sterols are converted to vitamin D_3 by exposure to ultraviolet light of 270–300 nm. The exact nature of the photolysis is not fully understood although Figure 4 represents the current concept regarding the activation of vitamin D by ultraviolet light when the precursors are dissolved in organic solvents such as ethanol or diethylether. Commercially, photolysis is carried out in organic solvents and the unconverted 5,7-diene is often crystallized out of solution and recycled through another irradiation sequence. By irradiating the remaining 5,7-diene and some of the photolysis side reaction products such as tachysterol, it is possible to achieve up to 60–80% conversion of the corresponding sterol to the D vitamin. Both vitamin D_2 and vitamin D_3 are used as food supplements and as sources of vitamin D for fortification of dairy products and for supplementation of the diets of domestic animals.

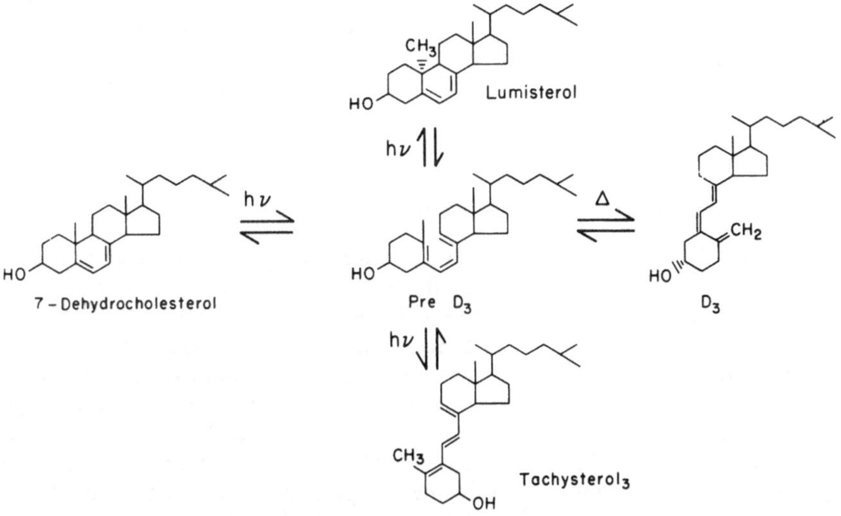

Figure 4 The structural modification of 7-dehydrocholesterol by ultraviolet irradiation during the production of vitamin D. Note that the reaction of previtamin D to vitamin D_3 is thermally accelerated

METABOLISM OF VITAMIN D

Absorption and transport

It is not yet clear where in the intestinal tract vitamin D is absorbed. When absorption of vitamin D from an alcoholic solution is examined, the most active site is the upper part of the small intestine[28]. When absorption from oily solutions is examined, absorption is from the ileum along with other fats[29, 30]. Bile is required for optimal absorption, as might be suspected[28, 31]. The absorbed vitamin D is incorporated into chylomicrons[32] which are cleared by the liver[33]. Vitamin D may also be transported on a vitamin D transport protein which appears in the α-globulin fraction on electrophoresis. Some of it is also associated with β-lipoprotein but it is not carried on albumin[33-35].

The plasma protein which transports vitamin D_3 and its major polar metabolite has been isolated in pure form from human plasma[36-38] and from rat plasma[39]. It has a molecular weight of about 52 000, is an α-globulin and is identical with the group specific protein previously isolated[40]. The plasma binding protein is used to assay the 25-hydroxyvitamin D_3 (25-OH-D_3) and other vitamin D metabolites[41-44].

Excretion of vitamin D

The primary route of excretion appears to be in the faeces, accounting for virtually all the vitamin D given[29, 30, 45]. Only 2–4 % appears to be excreted in the urine[32, 46]. The bile undoubtedly accounts for much of the faecal excretion, with as much as 30 % of a physiological dose appearing in this fluid in the first 48 h after dose. The nature of these excretory products has not been determined, although there is some evidence that glucuronides[29, 32, 47] and sulphate esters[48] are present. Two major biliary metabolites have recently been identified: 25-hydroxyvitamin D_2-25-glucuronide[49] and 24,25,26,27-tetranorvitamin D carboxylic acid[50, 51].

Production of vitamin D_3 in skin

Following the work of Huldshinsky[6] it is well accepted that the exposure of man or of animals to ultraviolet light results in elimination of rickets and of osteomalacia. Although the biochemical basis of this was not understood, the work of Steenbock and Black[7] and Hess et al.[8] demonstrated that this was due to the conversion of a sterol precursor to the antirachitic substance induced by ultraviolet light. It is now well known that the epidermis contains large amounts of the sterol 7-dehydrocholesterol[52, 53] which was shown to be a precursor of vitamin D_3 by Windaus et al.[54] In addition, there is considerable evidence that ultraviolet light incident upon skin can penetrate to the epidermal regions which contain the 7-dehydrocholesterol[55]. Since 7-dehydrocholesterol in organic solvents undergoes photoisomerization to produce pre-vitamin D_3 which later thermoequilibrates to form vitamin D_3, it seems likely that this is the mechanism of formation of the antirachitic substance in skin induced by ultraviolet light. Experiments have been carried out which show that ultraviolet irradiation of skin will produce antirachitic material. Recently vitamin D_3 has been isolated from rachitic rat skin irradiated with ultraviolet light and positively identified by mass spectrometry[56,57]. Others have suggested that pre-vitamin D_3 is the first product of the irradiation of skin[58,59]. To what extent the skin can produce vitamin D is not entirely settled either. Bekemeier[60] has reported production of vitamin D in the skin of pigs. Recently in the author's laboratory, 12.8 IU/g has been demonstrated in rats upon 15 min irradiation with a high intensity ultraviolet lamp. This production rate of 51.2 IU h^{-1} g^{-1} seems possible on a limited exposure. Certainly sunlight can significantly increase the circulating levels of 25-OH-D_3 [44,61].

It might be mentioned parenthetically that fish accumulate large amounts of vitamin D in their livers[13]. This is also found in some sharks, which do not possess significant amounts of calcified skeleton. The question of what the vitamin D is doing there and how it originates remains open. Attempts to demonstrate that fish possess a non-photochemical method of producing vitamin D_3 have not yet been successful[62]. Although results by Bills suggest that there must be non-photochemical vitamin D production in marine life[63], those results are also not conclusive. This also remains an interesting and potentially important biological problem to pursue.

Metabolism of vitamin D (Figure 5)

Following its absorption or synthesis in the skin as much as 60–80% of the vitamin D is taken up by the liver[29,30,45,64]. In the liver, the vitamin undergoes hydroxylation[65,66] on carbon 25 to yield 25-OH-D_3. This reaction takes place in the endoplasmic reticulum and requires NADPH, Mg^{2+}, molecular oxygen and a cytoplasmic factor[67]. The enzyme concerned is a mixed-function mono-oxygenase dependent on cytochrome P-450[68,69]. This system has recently been solubilized and reconstituted, showing it to be a two component system[70] (Figure 6). In addition to the microsomal system, a mitochondrial 25-hydroxylase has been described[71]. This system is a three component mixed-function mono-oxygenase that has been solubilized and reconstituted[72]. It is not specific for vitamin D since it hydroxylates cholesterol. Furthermore, it has a K_m of 10^{-6} M for vitamin D, whereas the microsomal system has a K_m of 10^{-8} M. It is likely that the microsomal system operates at physiological concentrations of vitamin D, whereas the mitochondrial system operates at pharmacological doses.

It seems certain that the major if not sole 25-hydroxylation takes place in the liver under physiologic conditions. Although 25-hydroxylation does take place in intestinal homogenates of chicks[73–75], little extrahepatic 25-hydroxylation appears to take place in mammals[64].

The 25-OH-D_3 appears in the blood from the liver and is the major circulating metabolite of vitamin D in plasma, rivalling vitamin D itself[76,77]. The normal levels in blood of this metabolite are 15–35 ng/ml[78–80].

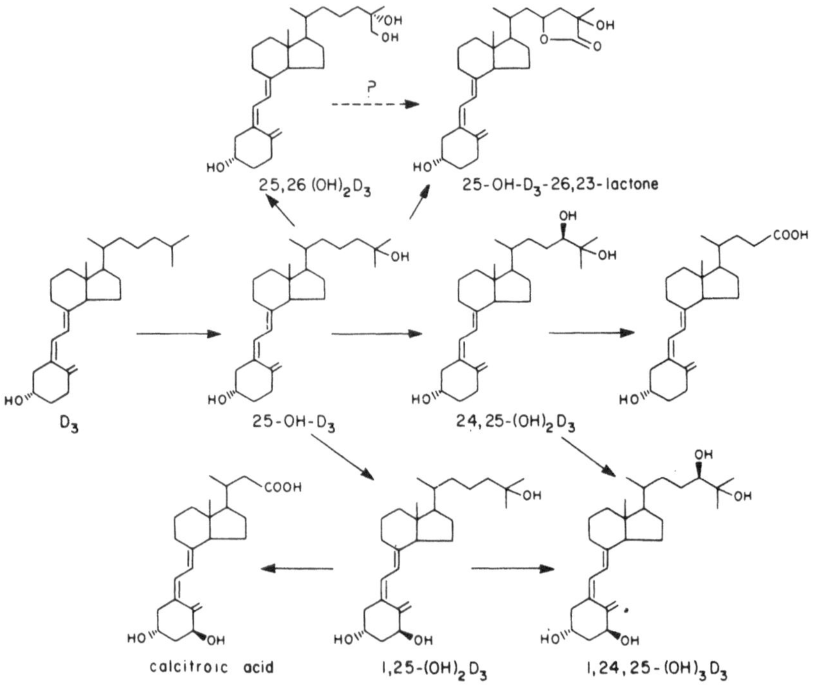

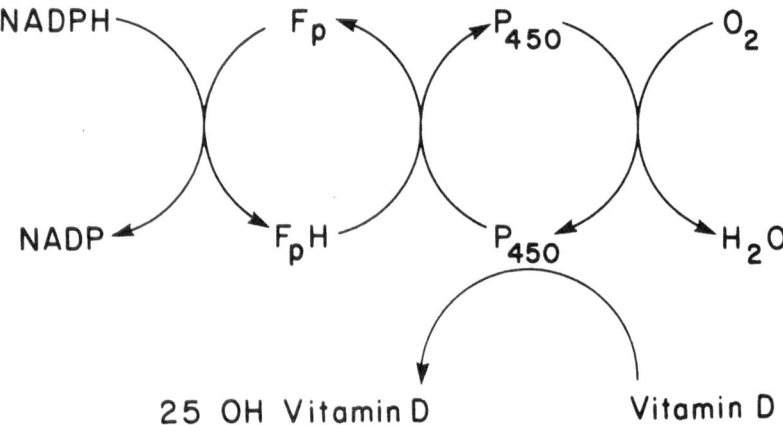

Figure 5 Pathway of vitamin D metabolism as is currently understood. The major pathway of activation is vitamin $D_3 \rightarrow$ 25-OH-$D_3 \rightarrow$ 1,25-(OH)$_2$D$_3$. The other known metabolic conversions are of unknown physiological significance

Figure 6 Mechanism of the liver microsomal catalysed 25-hydroxylation of vitamin D·

The 25-OH-D$_3$ is transported on the specific α-globulin to the kidney, where it undergoes further hydroxylation on either carbon 1, carbon 24 or carbon 26. To produce its known biological effects on intestine and bone, it must be hydroxylated on carbon 1 to yield 1,25-dihydroxyvitamin D$_3$ (1,25-(OH)$_2$D$_3$)[81–83]. The C-1 hydroxylation takes place exclusively in kidney tissue and more specifically in mitochondria[84,85,86]. This reaction has been conclusively shown to be a three component mixed function mono-oxygenase using a specific cytochrome P-450 to catalyse the hydroxylation[87–89]. The three components have been solubilized and reconstituted into an active 1-hydroxylase. The components are a flavoprotein called renal ferredoxin reductase, an iron sulphur protein, renal ferredoxin and a cytochrome P-450. In intact tissue, Krebs cycle substrate oxidation catalyses the energy-dependent transhydrogenation of internal NADP with NADH, which provides the reducing equivalents for the hydroxylation through the mechanism[90] shown in Figure 7.

Clear evidence has been provided that 1,25-(OH)$_2$D$_3$ is a metabolically active form of vitamin D in intestinal calcium transport[82], bone calcium mobilization[83] and phosphate transport of intestine[91]. The possible necessity for its further metabolism, before it can act on intestinal calcium transport, has also been shown to be remote[92–94]. However, it has recently been demonstrated that 1,25-(OH)$_2$D$_3$ undergoes side chain oxidation very rapidly after its administration to yield calcitroic acid[51,95,96] (Figure 6). Calcitroic acid constitutes 40–60% of the intestinal ^{3}H derived from 1,25-(OH)$_2$D$_3$ at the time it responds. However calcitroic acid has minimal biological activity *in vivo*[97] suggesting it to be on the pathway of degradation.

As will be shown in a later section, the need for calcium or for phosphorus

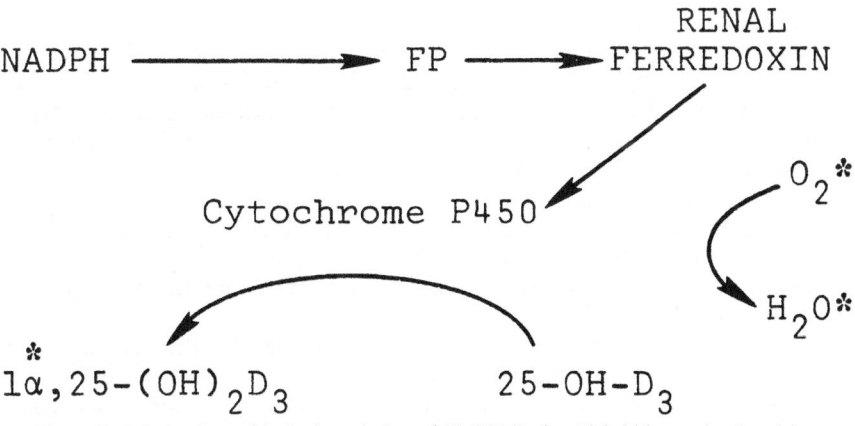

Figure 7 Mechanism of 1α-hydroxylation of 25-OH-D$_3$ in chick kidney mitochondria

stimulates the synthesis of $1,25\text{-}(OH)_2D_3$ in the kidney. However, if serum calcium and phosphorus levels are normal, the synthesis of $1,25\text{-}(OH)_2D_3$ diminishes in animals given vitamin D, and instead the kidney mitochondria hydroxylate the 25-OH-D_3 on carbon 24 to produce 24,25-dihydroxyvitamin D_3 $(24,25\text{-}(OH)_2D_3)$[98]. The 24-hydroxylase has many properties similar to those of 1-hydroxylase[99]. It is a mixed function mono-oxygenase[100] and recent work suggests it also is a cytochrome P-450 system (Ghazarian, personal communication). The 24-hydroxylase is obviously more widely distributed than the 1-hydroxylase since nephrectomy does not eliminate 24-hydroxylation[101,102] and in fact, it can be found in intestine[103] and cartilage[104]. The exact function of the $24,25\text{-}(OH)_2D_3$ is not as yet known, but it is a major dihydroxyvitamin D metabolite found in man[105] and rats[106]; it is biologically active in rats[107,108]. To stimulate the intestine and bone, it must first be hydroxylated to 1,24,25-trihydroxyvitamin D_3 $(1,24,25\text{-}(OH)_3D_3)$[109]. This metabolite has only 60% of the intestinal calcium transport activity of $1,25\text{-}(OH)_2D_3$[110]. In cultures it is about one-tenth as active as $1,25\text{-}(OH)_2D_3$ in bone resorption[111]. Unfortunately, its significance is not yet known, although it has been detected as a normal metabolite in rats[102]. It has been suggested that $24R,25\text{-}(OH)_3D_3$ has special activity in mineralization of bone[112,114], in suppression of parathyroid gland size[115] and in embryonic development in chicks[116]. However, these are suggestions and work with 24,24-difluoro-25-hydroxyvitamin D_3 does not support these suggestions[113], at least with respect to bone and intestine.

$24,25\text{-}(OH)_2D_3$ is rapidly converted to a water-soluble metabolite 25,26,27-trisnor-vitamin D_3 carboxylic acid[117]. Currently this author favours the concept that 24-hydroxylation is a mechanism for inactivation of the vitamin D molecule. In support of this it has been shown in the chick that $24R,25\text{-}(OH)_2D_3$ is relatively inactive and is rapidly degraded and excreted[118].

Another metabolite of vitamin D_3 has been isolated in pure form and identified as 25,26-dihydroxyvitamin D_3 $(25,26\text{-}(OH)_2D_3)$[119], the significance of this metabolite is unknown. It has some calcium transport activity in intestine but has little effect on bone[120]. Because nephrectomy prevents its activity on intestine, most likely it must be hydroxylated on C-1 to act. Its site of production is the kidney but not exclusively so[121].

A new metabolite of vitamin D_3 has recently been isolated and identified as 25-hydroxyvitamin D_3-26,23-lactone (25-OH-D_3-26,23-lactone)[122]. Its activity is unknown but it is synthesized in large amounts under circumstances of increased vitamin D administration[122,123], its function, if any, is unknown. Its appearance in the blood of patients with kidney stones suggests it to be of considerable importance.

$25,26\text{-}(OH)_2D_3$ and the 26,23-lactone are converted to $1,25,26\text{-}(OH)_2D_3$ and $1\alpha,25$-dihydroxy-26,23-lactone respectively in small amounts in vivo[124]. These metabolites are much less active than $1,25\text{-}(OH)_2D_3$ on the known systems responsive to vitamin D_3.

Other metabolites of vitamin D_3 have been discovered, but they have not been identified[125]. Although much has been learned about vitamin D metabolism, much still remains to be learned and this area will remain active for some years to come.

Vitamin D$_2$

Vitamin D$_2$ is also metabolized to 25-hydroxyvitamin D$_2$ (25-OH-D$_2$)[126] and subsequently to 1,25-dihydroxyvitamin D$_2$ (1,25-(OH)$_2$D$_2$) or 24,25-dihydroxyvitamin D$_2$ (24,25-(OH)$_2$D$_2$) in a scheme completely analogous to the vitamin D$_3$ sequence[127,128]. Of some interest is that chicks respond poorly to vitamin D$_2$ because they rapidly metabolize it to products which are excreted[129]. In support of this, isolated target tissues from chicks do not discriminate against 1,25-(OH)$_2$D$_2$[130]. The discrimination appears to result from the rapid conversion of 25-hydroxylated vitamin D$_2$ compounds to the corresponding 25-glucuronide followed by biliary elimination[49].

REGULATION OF VITAMIN D METABOLISM

Role of vitamin D and its metabolites

From the previous section it is indeed obvious that the active forms of vitamin D are synthesized exclusively in the kidney and have their function in intestine and bone. One might, therefore, surmise that the active form of vitamin D can be considered a hormone. As a hormone, it follows that its biosynthesis or secretion must be regulated in a feed-back fashion by the substances it seeks to affect. This section will demonstrate that the production of the active forms of vitamin D is in fact regulated by serum calcium, serum phosphorus, the parathyroid hormone, the sex hormones and growth hormone and by vitamin D itself.

The first demonstration that the formation of 1,25-(OH)$_2$D$_3$ is regulated took place immediately after the isolation and identification of this important metabolite. In that initial study, Boyle et al.[106] demonstrated that vitamin D-deficient rats produce large amounts of 1,25-(OH)$_2$D$_3$ regardless of their dietary calcium and phosphate intake. On the other hand, animals primed with vitamin D showed a depressed production of 1,25-(OH)$_2$D$_3$ with increasing dietary calcium and enhanced production of 24,25-(OH)$_2$D$_3$. This finding in the rat was reaffirmed in the chick by studies of Omdahl et al.[131] In every case, vitamin D-deficient animals apparently lacked the ability to make 24,25-(OH)$_2$D$_3$. Thus among other factors vitamin D apparently induces or makes possible the synthesis of the 24,25-(OH)$_2$D$_3$. More recently it has been shown that 1,25-(OH)$_2$D$_3$ itself is the active form in stimulating 24-hydroxylation[132]. Evidence has been presented that the 1,25-(OH)$_2$D$_3$ probably induces the appearance of the 24-hydroxylase[133], and as its activity is stimulated, the activity of the 25-OH-D$_3$-1-hydroxylase is diminished. Whether 1,25-(OH)$_2$D$_3$ itself has any other role besides induction of the 24-hydroxylase in the regulation of vitamin D metabolism remains unknown, although previous work had shown that the 1,25-(OH)$_2$D$_3$ is a product inhibitor of the 1α-hydroxylase enzyme of the kidney[86]. The regulation of the hydroxylases by 1,25-(OH)$_2$D$_3$ involves processes mediated by the cell nucleus[134]. 1,25-(OH)$_2$D$_3$ suppresses 25-OH-D$_3$ 1α-hydroxylase and stimulates the 24R-hydroxylase when added to cultures of chick or monkey kidney cells[135-137]. The mechanism however remains unknown.

Regulation of vitamin D metabolism by calcium

Dietary calcium suppresses the synthesis of $1,25\text{-}(OH)_2D_3$ while stimulating the synthesis of the $24,25\text{-}(OH)_2D_3$[106]. Thus as the diet is made low in calcium, the synthesis and secretion of a calcium mobilizing hormone, $1,25\text{-}(OH)_2D_3$, increases. This important observation led to the disclosure[138] that the $1,25\text{-}(OH)_2D_3$ might in part represent Nicolaysen's endogenous factor, a hormone that was postulated to be secreted by the skeleton and that would direct the intestine to absorb calcium[139]. Thus the well known ability of animals and man to adapt to dietary calcium could well be accounted for on the basis of regulation of $1,25\text{-}(OH)_2D_3$ synthesis. To establish this idea both rats and chicks have been shown to lose their ability to adapt to dietary calcium when given a constant exogenous supply of $1,25\text{-}(OH)_2D_3$, whereas their ability to adapt to dietary calcium is clearly evident in animals given an exogenous source of the immediate precursor, $25\text{-}OH\text{-}D_3$[15, 16]. Thus it seems likely that $1,25\text{-}(OH)_2D_3$ represents at least in large measure the endogenous factor which Nicolaysen was seeking years ago.

It is, however, difficult to imagine how the kidney enzyme system might sense the dietary calcium levels. A study was carried out to test the ability of animals *in vivo* to synthesize $1,25\text{-}(OH)_2D_3$, relative to their serum calcium concentration, which is $9.5\,\text{mg}/100\,\text{ml}$ in the author's exoperimental animals, that there is a very close relationship between the synthesis of the vitamin D metabolites and the serum calcium concentration. At normal serum calcium concentration, which is $9.5\,\text{mg}/100\,\text{ml}$ in the auhor's experimental animals, both $1,25\text{-}(OH)_2D_3$ and $24,25\text{-}(OH)_2D_3$ are made in approximately equal amounts. However, even a slight hypocalcaemia stimulates $1,25\text{-}(OH)_2D_3$ synthesis. As the animals become normal to hypercalcaemic, the synthesis of

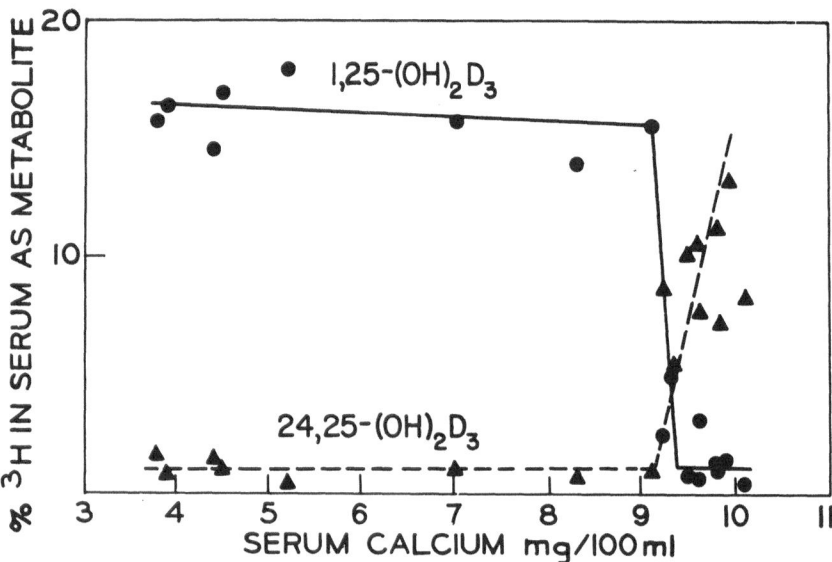

Figure 8 The relationship of serum calcium concentration to the accumulation of either $1,25\text{-}(OH)_2D_3$ or $24,25\text{-}(OH)_2D_3$ from $25\text{-}OH\text{-}D_3$ in the plasma of rats

this hormonal substance is shut down. Under these circumstances 24,25-$(OH)_2D_3$ is made. Thus the need for calcium is translated through hypocalcaemia, which is in turn involved in the stimulation of 1,25-$(OH)_2D_3$ synthesis. This relationship has been confirmed in other laboratories[140, 141], and has led to the suggestion that calcium ions themselves might be the regulatory agent. However, if calcium itself is involved at the molecular level in the regulation, it must function in a manner more complex than as an inhibitor of the 1-hydroxylase. With cultures of kidney cells a stimulation of 24-hydroxylase by increased ambient calcium concentration has been observed[135]. In addition, the 1-hydroxylase is suppressed[136, 137].

Regulation by parathyroid hormone

Because the serum calcium level can be shown to be closely involved in the negative regulation of synthesis of 1,25-$(OH)_2D_3$, it was reasonable to suspect that the parathyroid gland and the parathyroid hormone might be involved in the calcaemic regulation. It is already known that the parathyroid glands monitor serum calcium concentration and secrete parathyroid hormone in response to hypocalcaemia[142]. Therefore, the parathyroid hormone might be the actual agent which stimulates synthesis of 1,25-$(OH)_2D_3$. This concept was clearly demonstrated[143], confirmed[144, 145], and reconfirmed[141]. It seems almost certain that the hypocalcaemic control of 1,25-$(OH)_2D_3$ synthesis is via the parathyroid glands, and that in this instance it is the parathyroid hormone which in some unknown way stimulates synthesis of 1,25-$(OH)_2D_3$ and shuts down the synthesis of the 24,25-$(OH)_2D_3$. This mechanism appears to involve an adenyl cyclase mechanism[146] and can be demonstrated in cultures[136, 137].

Regulation of vitamin D metabolism by phosphate

It is well known that severe hypophosphataemia brings about a marked stimulation of intestinal calcium absorption[147, 148]. At least a large segment of this stimulation results from the stimulation of 1,25-$(OH)_2D_3$ synthesis[148]. Hypophosphataemia in the absence of thyroparathyroid glands will stimulate 1,25-$(OH)_2D_3$ accumulation[149]. In fact a relationship can be shown between serum inorganic phosphate concentration and 1,25-$(OH)_2D_3$ accumulation provided that the thyroparathyroid complex is removed (Figure 9). Serum inorganic phosphate under these circumstances can be regulated by dietary deprivation and by means of glucose loading of the animals. These animals, after they have adapted to such treatment for a period of at least 1 week, show a clear relationship between serum inorganic phosphate concentration and 1,25-$(OH)_2D_3$ accumulation[148] (Figure 9). Normal serum phosphorus in experimental rats is about 9–10 mg/100 ml. At this level without the parathyroid glands, the animals make entirely 24,25-$(OH)_2D_3$. On the other hand, as serum inorganic phosphate is lowered to levels below 8 mg/100 ml, the animals accumulate 1,25-$(OH)_2D_3$. Although the stimulation of 25-OH-D_3-1-hydroxylase has been questioned by Henry et al.[141], accumulation of 1,25-$(OH)_2D_3$ in blood of phosphate deprived animals has been shown[150].

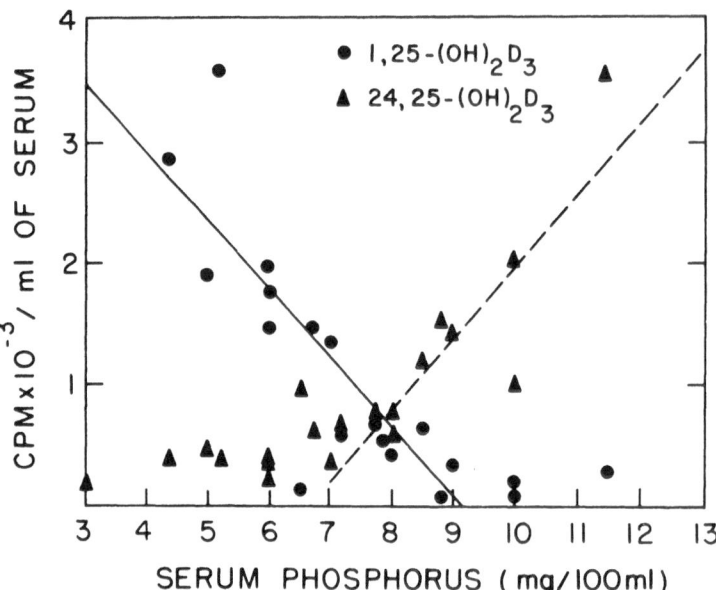

Figure 9 The relationship of serum inorganic phosphorus concentration to the accumulation of 1,25-$(OH)_2D_3$ or 24,25-$(OH)_2D_3$ from 25-OH-D_3 in thyroparathyroidectomized rats. Rats were fed a variety of diets and their serum inorganic phosphorus concentration was adjusted by means of dietary restriction of phosphorus or by means of glucose loading. All rats were thyroparathyroidectomized prior to the carrying out of the experiment

Further a stimulation of 1-hydroxylase by phosphate deprivation has also been shown, although it is much less dramatic than calcium deprivation[151]. Thus hypophosphataemia or the need for phosphate causes accumulation of 1,25-$(OH)_2D_3$. As will be shown in a later section the 1,25-$(OH)_2D_3$ not only has its functions in calcium metabolism, but it also plays a direct role in the metabolism of phosphate. Thus it seems reasonable to assume that serum phosphate should in some way control 1,25-$(OH)_2D_3$ synthesis. There is evidence, however, that phosphate depletion itself stimulates calcium absorption even in the presence of excess 1,25-$(OH)_2D_3$[16].

Molecular mechanism of regulation of the renal hydroxylases of 25-OH-D_3

Regulation of vitamin D metabolism in response to parathyroid hormone or phosphate depletion does not occur rapidly but requires several hours, if not days, to be accomplished[143,149]. This is not consistent with an ionic inhibition or activation of existing hydroxylases, as has been suggested by several groups on the basis of reported inhibition of 1α-hydroxylase of mitochondria by addition of calcium or phosphate to the incubation medium. Calcium inhibition *in vitro* of the 1α-hydroxylase is known to occur provided the required reducing equivalents are from oxidation of Krebs cycle substrates[152,153]. However, similar *in vitro* inhibition by calcium can also be obtained for the 24-hydroxylase despite the fact that high calcium *in vivo* stimulates 24,25-$(OH_2)D_3$ production. Furthermore, if one supplies an external source of NADPH then even up to 10 mM calcium will not inhibit the reaction of either the 1-hydroxylase or the 24-hydroxylase[90]. It seems likely that *in vitro* calcium inhibition of the incubated intact mitochondria with Krebs cycle substrates results from an interference of oxidative phosphory-lation. The resultant lack of high energy intermediates would retard the energy dependent transhydrogenation and the generation of reducing equivalents for the hydroxylases. Other similar arguments can be made for the direct effects of inorganic phosphate.

The halflife of the 1α-hydroxylase is of the order of 2–4 h[154]. A possible regulatory mechanism might, therefore, involve the synthesis and degradation of the hydroxylases. Thus it is possible that intracellular calcium and or phosphorus might well regulate the synthesis of the hydroxylases, or the degradation. So far this mechanism has not been adequately examined, and thus the molecular mechanism which underlies the regulation phenomenon described has not been settled and must remain a very active field of investigation.

THE INTERACTION BETWEEN VITAMIN D AND THE PARATHYROID HORMONE

From the work of Harrison *et al.*[155] and later Rasmussen *et al.*[156] it has become evident that a vitamin D-deficient animal is resistant to even large amounts of exogenous parathyroid hormone. Thus the hypercalcaemic activity of the parathyroid hormone is absent in the vitamin D-deficient animal. However, there is some controversy as to whether the parathyroid hormone induced phosphate diuresis is vitamin D-dependent or not[157]. Certainly it is less dependent upon vitamin D than the calcium mobilizing activity of the parathyroid hormone[158]. More recently, Forte *et al.*[159] have shown this system to be independent of vitamin D in normocalcaemic animals. In addition, there has been a controversy as to whether parathyroid hormone plays a direct role in stimulating intestinal calcium transport. Evidence for and against this has been put forth by a variety of investigators, suggesting that a small difference in experimental protocol gave substantially different results.

With the understanding that the parathyroid hormone plays an important role in the regulation of synthesis of 1,25-$(OH)_2D_3$ it seemed possible to clarify the interrelationship between these two important calcium homeostatic agents. It has been possible to demonstrate that the 1,25-$(OH)_2D_3$ induced bone calcium mobilization requires the presence of the parathyroid hormone[160]. It had been previously shown that the parathyroid hormone induced bone calcium mobilization requires the presence of vitamin D[156]. On the other hand, 1,25-$(OH)_2D_3$ stimulates intestinal calcium transport equally well whether the parathyroid hormone is present or not, and in fact the parathyroid hormone does not in any way directly enhance intestinal calcium transport[160]. These results are supported by the findings that radioactive parathyroid hormone does not bind to intestine, whereas it does bind to kidney, bone and liver *in vivo*[161].

As a result of these findings, the calcium homeostatic mechanism must be revised (Figure 10). It seems likely that the hypocalcaemic stimulus induces the secretion of parathyroid hormone. The parathyroid hormone causes a phosphate diuresis in the kidney and stimulates synthesis of $1,25\text{-}(OH)_2D_3$. The parathyroid hormone and the $1,25\text{-}(OH)_2D_3$ act at the bone site co-operatively to stimulate mobilization of calcium from bone. In kidney, both $1,25\text{-}(OH)_2D_3$ and parathyroid hormone increase renal reabsorption of calcium[162–164]. On the other hand, $1,25\text{-}(OH)_2D_3$ acts directly on intestine to stimulate intestinal calcium absorption. These mechanisms restore serum calcium to normal values, shutting off parathyroid hormone secretion[165].

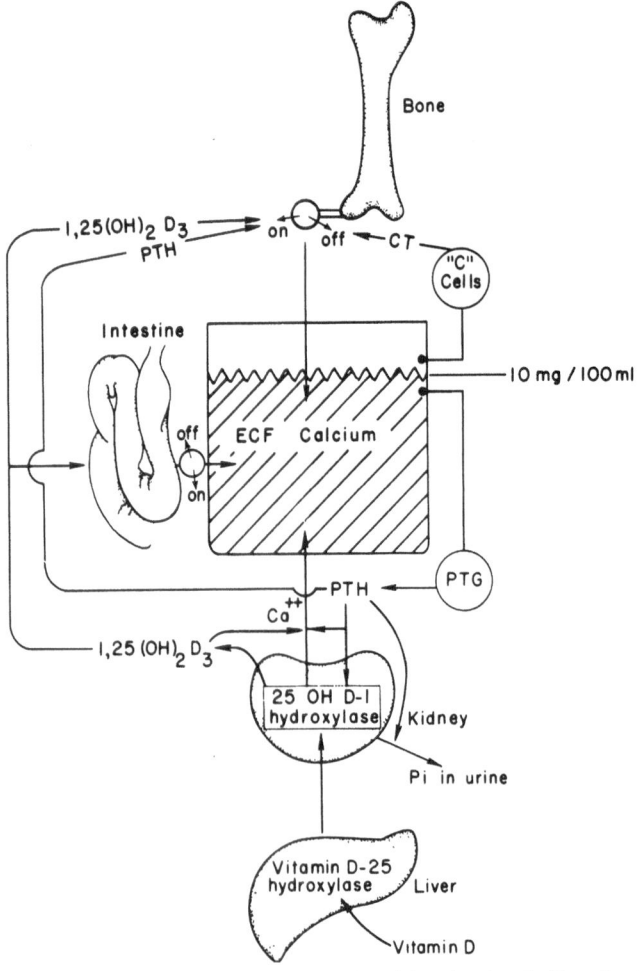

Figure 10 The calcium homeostatic mechanism involving the vitamin D endocrine system

It is disturbing that the synthesis and secretion of 1,25-$(OH)_2D_3$ can be stimulated by hypocalcaemic stimulus on one hand and hypophosphataemic stimulus on the other. This is further compounded by the fact that the 1,25-$(OH)_2D_3$ not only stimulates intestinal calcium transport, but stimulates intestinal phosphate transport as well[91,166]. It seems as though a single hormone with dual functions and dual stimuli for secretion could not specifically correct the original stimulus. However, the specificity of function at the physiologic level can easily be shown if the sequence of events following each stimulus is considered. Figure 11 demonstrates that the hypocalcaemic stimulus results in parathyroid hormone secretion which turns on the synthesis of 1,25-$(OH)_2D_3$. Due to the presence of the parathyroid hormone, bone calcium can be mobilized by 1,25-$(OH)_2D_3$ and calcium reabsorption is increased in the kidney. However, phosphate absorption and mobilization is also increased by 1,25-$(OH)_2D_3$. Parathyroid hormone, however, causes a large phosphate diuresis which negates the phosphataemic effect of the 1,25-$(OH)_2D_3$, resulting in a net increase in serum calcium and no change in serum inorganic phosphate[165].

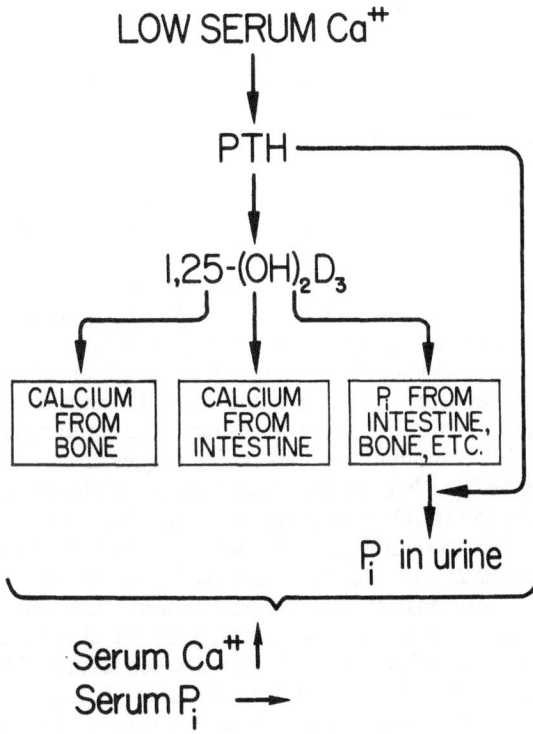

Figure 11 Sequence of events following low calcium stimulation of 1,25-$(OH)_2D_3$ production

The hypophosphataemic stimulus shown in Figure 12 demonstrates that in this case $1,25\text{-}(OH)_2D_3$ synthesis is stimulated in the absence of parathyroid hormone secretion, and in fact under hypophosphataemic conditions, parathyroid hormone secretion is likely to be suppressed. Without parathyroid hormone, $1,25\text{-}(OH)_2D_3$ does not mobilize calcium from bone. It can stimulate intestinal calcium transport, but the absence of the parathyroid hormone allows for calcium excretion in the urine. The $1,25\text{-}(OH)_2D_3$ in addition stimulates phosphate mobilization and because parathyroid hormone is absent, the phosphate mobilized is not excreted into the urine. The net effect under these circumstances is a rise in serum phosphate and little or no change in serum calcium. Thus $1,25\text{-}(OH)_2D_3$ can serve both as a calcium mobilizing hormone and as a phosphate mobilizing hormone, with a marked degree of physiologic specificity by its physiologic interaction with the parathyroid hormone system.

REGULATION OF THE RENAL VITAMIN D HYDROXYLASES BY THE SEX HORMONES

One of the most demanding of calcium sysytems is that which is found in egg-laying birds who protect their eggs by laying down a shell of calcium carbonate. It is known that prior to the egg-laying process, calcium is assimilated and deposited in the bone in the form of a histologically discernible form called medullary bone[167]. This deposition occurs at the time that the oviduct develops and other factors necessary for egg production are stimulated by the sex hormones. At the time the egg is produced calcium must be mobilized from medullary bone for deposit with the egg, and later for deposit of calcium carbonate as egg shell. It can be clearly demonstrated that at the time egg production is occurring, the 25-OH-D_3-1-hydroxylase is very high as measured directly on homogenates of chicken or quail kidneys[168,169]. Male birds of the same age and on the same diet, on the other hand, produce primarily $24,25\text{-}(OH)_2D_3$. If oestradiol is injected into the mature male, within 6 h the 24-hydroxylase is suppressed and the 25-OH-D_3-1-hydroxylase is stimulated. This stimulation is very specific for oestrogen and requires the presence of testosterone or progesterone or both. Thus immature males or immature females will not respond to a single injection of oestradiol, but will respond if they are treated at the same time with testosterone or progesterone or both. Castrate male birds will also respond to a combination of testosterone and oestradiol. A combination of oestradiol, progesterone and testosterone will produce 25-OH-D_3-1-hydroxylase at extremely high levels. The time course of response of the 25-OH-D_3-1-hydroxylase to an injection of oestradiol in mature Japanese quail is shown in Figure 13. The elevation of serum calcium follows the stimulation of the 25-OH-D_3-1-hydroxylase. In continuing investigations it has been possible to demonstrate that, preceding the mobilization of medullary bone for egg formation, there is a stimulation of the 25-OH-D_3-1-hydroxylase presumably by the sex hormones[170]. The elevated serum $1,25\text{-}(OH)_2D_3$ brings about the mobilization of calcium from medullary bone, which is then used to deposit with egg yolk on one hand and used to form egg shells on the other. Once the egg has been laid, the bird again reforms medullary bone in preparation for the

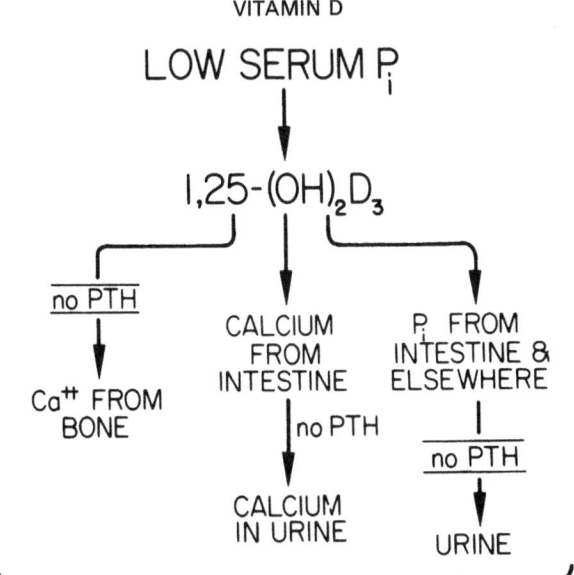

Figure 12 Sequence of events following low serum phosphorus stimulation of 1,25-(OH)₂D₃ production. Note in this case that 1,25-(OH)₂D₃ results in a rise in serum phosphorus with little change in serum calcium

next cycle whereby an egg is produced. It now appears that the 25-OH-D₃-1-hydroxylase is modulated in preparation for the calcium needs in egg-shell formation. Thus when medullary bone formation is progressing the 25-OH-D₃-1-hydroxylase is low, but when medullary bone is being mobilized for egg production the 25-OH-D₃-1-hydroxylase is high. The intricate detail and nature of how the 25-OH-D₃-1-hydroxylase is stimulated or suppressed during the egg laying cycle is not fully understood, although it is clear that the sex hormones play a major role in this regulation.

Because of the role of the sex hormones in regulating 25-OH-D₃-1-hydroxylase in laying birds, it is of obvious interest to investigate whether the sex hormones can regulate production of 1,25-(OH)₂D₃ in mammals. Such work might shed light on the bone disease osteoporosis which afflicts postmenopausal women. Unfortunately we do not know at this stage whether the 25-OH-D₃-1-hydroxylase in mammals is regulated by the sex hormones,

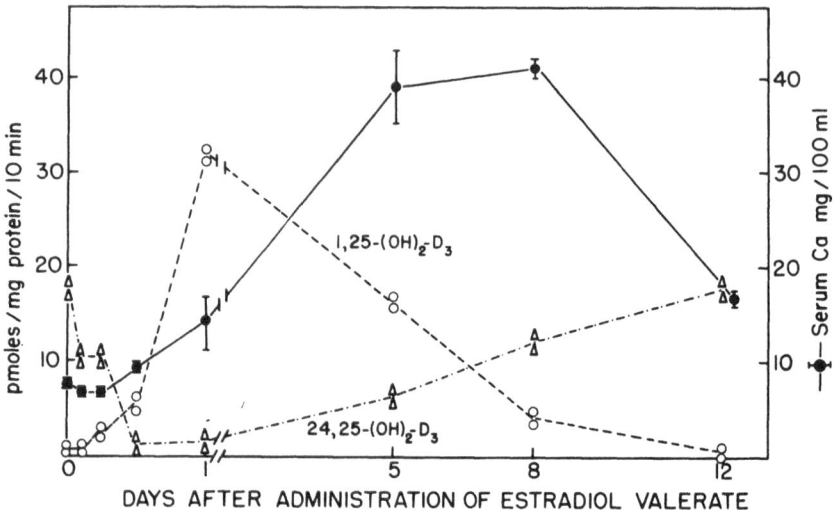

Figure 13 Time course of response of the 25-OH-D$_3$-1-hydroxylase, the 25-OH-D$_3$-24-hydroxylase and serum calcium concentration to an injection of oestradiol valerate to mature male Japanese quail. Note that the rise in the hydroxylase activity precedes the rise in serum calcium concentration

although increased serum levels of 1,25-(OH)$_2$D$_3$ in postmenopausal women given oestrogen has been demonstrated[171]. One can expect additional work in this area during the next few years which may help to clarify this important area.

MECHANISM OF VITAMIN D ACTION

Overall physiological function of vitamin D

The mineralization of bone can be regarded as the final end-effect of the mechanism of action of vitamin D. Although this final end-effect has been the stimulus for much work in the area of mineralization process, so far there is no clear evidence which would directly involve a function of vitamin D on the mineralization process[15]. In fact, it appears that the major action of vitamin D is to elevate plasma calcium and phosphate levels to supersaturation, which in turn is necessary for the normal mineralization of bone. In the absence of vitamin D the plasma is regarded as undersaturated, which accounts in large measure for the lack of mineralization. The question whether vitamin D may function at the mineralization site, however, must remain open inasmuch as at the present time it cannot be excluded.

Vitamin D brings about the elevation of plasma calcium and phosphate to supersaturation by two well known mechanisms, and two others which are perhaps less well known. The best known mechanism is that vitamin D is essential for normal absorption of calcium[15]. It has been believed that phosphate is the ion which accompanies calcium in this process, but in addition it has recently been shown that vitamin D activates a phosphate transport reaction of the intestine which is independent of calcium transport[91,172,173]. These two mechanisms then pump calcium and phosphate from the intestinal lumen to the extracellular fluid compartment. Another well established mechanism is the mobilization of calcium and hence phosphate from previously formed bone. This mechanism was originally discovered by Carlsson[174] and has been confirmed many times by several investigators. This mechanism would appear to decalcify bone rather than to calcify it; however, it must be regarded as another mechanism whereby calcium and phosphate can be contributed to the extracellular fluid pool, which in turn is necessary for the mineralization of newly forming bone.

Finally, vitamin D is believed to increase renal reabsorption of calcium[163,175]. However, whether vitamin D actually plays a direct role in renal reabsorption of phosphate has not been entirely settled, although recent evidence suggests that vitamin D does not improve renal reabsorption of phosphate[162,176].

Intestinal calcium transport

The vitamin D stimulated intestinal calcium absorption is an active process in which metabolic energy is used to support the transfer of calcium from lumen of intestine to the serosal fluid against an electro-chemical potential gradient[177,178]. The exact mechanism whereby this transfer takes place remains largely unknown. Schachter and his colleagues have put forth the idea that vitamin D stimulates both the entry of calcium into the intestinal cells across the brush border and also the exit of calcium across the basal-lateral membrane[179]. Wasserman and Kallfelz[180] have provided evidence that vitamin D increases the flux of calcium from lumen to blood and blood to lumen. Martin and DeLuca[181] have shown that the primary site of vitamin D action is in the brush border surface, and that vitamin D does not influence the ratios of calcium flux from lumen to plasma and plasma to lumen, in agreement with the studies of Wasserman. Adams *et al.*[182] demonstrated that if the intestinal brush border membrane is rendered permeable to calcium with the antibiotic filipin, then the vitamin D-deficient intestine can transport calcium in a manner similar to the intestines from animals given vitamin D. Thus it seems clear that a major site of action of vitamin D is at the brush border surface. The nature of the change remains unsettled.

Taylor and Wasserman[183] first described a specific calcium binding protein which appears in the intestine of chicks following vitamin D administration. There has been much work on the calcium binding protein which in the case of the chick binds 4 moles of calcium per mole of protein[184]. The protein has a molecular weight of somewhere in the neighbourhood of 28 000 in the case of chick, and around 8–12 000 in the case of mammalian species[185,186]. There is a rough correlation between the appearance of the calcium binding protein and the ability to transport calcium across intestine[187]; however, the actual participation of this protein in the calcium transport process has not been established. Harmeyer and DeLuca[188] demonstrated that the appearance of the calcium binding protein in the intestine does not correlate well with calcium transport. More recently Spencer et al.[189] have come to the same conclusion in studies with 1,25-$(OH)_2D_3$. Thus it is unlikely that the calcium binding protein is the calcium transport carrier induced by vitamin D.

In embryonic organ cultures of intestine, 1,25-$(OH)_2D_3$, 25-OH-D_3, 1α-hydroxyvitamin D_3 (1α-OH-D_3) and vitamin D itself all induce the formation of the calcium binding protein[190]. However, the concentration of 1,25-$(OH)_2D_3$ required is much less than that of vitamin D. It would appear from the results of Corradino[190], therefore, that the 1,25-$(OH)_2D_3$ functions at least in part by inducing the formation of the calcium binding protein. However, in the young growing animal it is not entirely clear whether the transport response to 1,25-$(OH)_2D_3$ involves induction and new protein synthesis. In the case of the rat, predosing with actinomycin D does not prevent the intestinal calcium transport response to 1,25-$(OH)_2D_3$, while at the same concentration and in the same animals the 1,25-$(OH)_2D_3$ induced bone calcium mobilization is blocked[191,192]. On the other hand, Norman and his colleagues have reported that dosing every 2 h with actinomycin D can prevent the 1,25-$(OH)_2D_3$ induced increase in intestinal calcium transport in the chick[193]. In the author's laboratory, the results with chick have been equivocal and in circumstances where the chick survives actinomycin treatment, 1,25-$(OH)_2D_3$ does induce intestinal calcium absorption. Recent work by Morrissey et al.[194] and Bickle et al.[195] support the work of Tanaka et al. Whether new protein synthesis is required for 1,25-$(OH)_2D_3$ induced intestinal calcium transport in growing animals has not, therefore, been entirely settled.

Mention should be made of the calcium dependent adenosine triphosphatase of the brush border. Because of the necessity of metabolic energy for intestinal calcium transport, and because the brush border is the site of vitamin D function, a vitamin D dependent calcium adenosine triphosphatase activity was looked for. This activity could be demonstrated easily both in the chick and the rat and has since been studied extensively[196,197]. There is some evidence that the calcium dependent ATPase is identical with intestinal alkaline phosphatase, but this has not, as yet, been proved[198]. It is uncertain whether this complex plays a role in intestinal calcium absorption. Its time course of appearance does not correlate well with the elevation of intestinal calcium transport. However, the same can be said for the calcium binding protein of Wasserman and Taylor. In short, very little can yet be concluded as to what is the molecular mechanism of calcium transport across intestinal membrane.

Because 1,25-$(OH)_2D_3$ is similar to a steroid hormone chemically and biologically, it is expected that 1,25-$(OH)_2D_3$ works in the intestine and bone by a mechanism similar to that which has been suggested for oestrogen and other steroid hormones[199]. Namely that the 1,25-$(OH)_2D_3$ binds to a cytoplasmic receptor protein which is then transferred into the nucleus, where it undergoes a molecular weight change, and where it somehow induces the transcription of messenger RNA of a specific gene(s), which in turn codes for proteins responsible for intestinal calcium transport[200-203] (Figure 14). In agreement with such an hypothesis, the existence of a 3.7S receptor protein in the intestine of chicks has been demonstrated[201,204]. Furthermore, a 3.2S

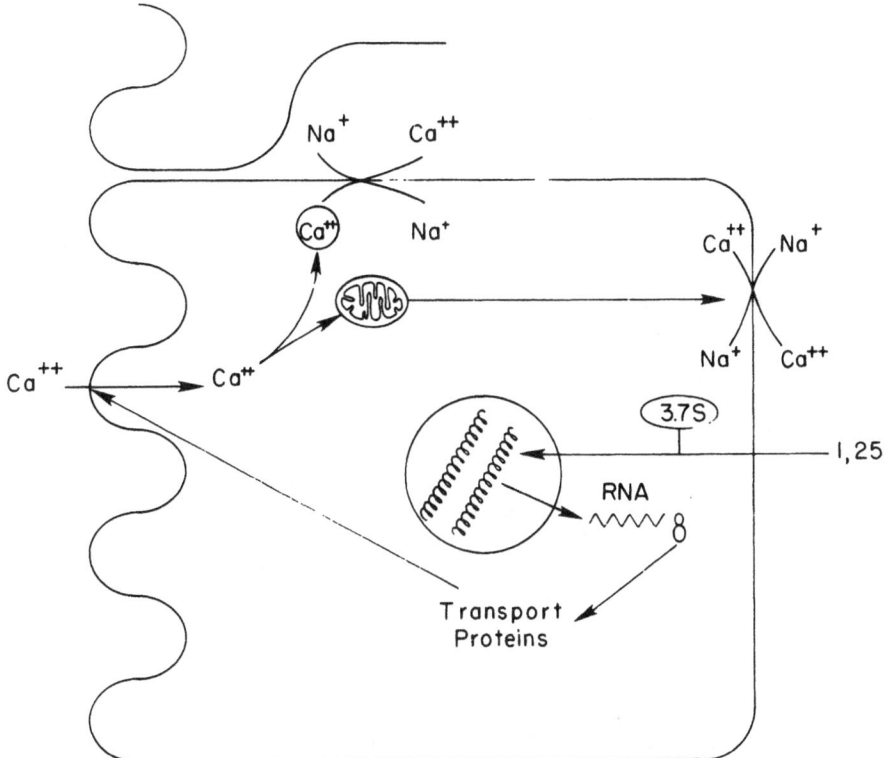

Figure 14 Postulated mechanisms whereby 1,25-(OH)$_2$D$_3$ initiates intestinal calcium transport. 1,25-(OH)$_2$D$_3$ interacts with a 3.7S receptor which stimulates production of messenger RNA coding for calcium transport proteins. These proteins which are unknown at the present time stimulate the passage of calcium across the microvillus brush border where it then accumulates either in mitochondria or in vessicles immediately under the terminal web. These then release their calcium at the basal-lateral membrane by means of a sodium dependent calcium extrusion process

receptor for 1,25-(OH)$_2$D$_3$ has been found in bone and rat intestine[130,205,206]. The transfer of the receptor 1,25-(OH)$_2$D$_3$ complex to intestinal nuclear chromatin has been suggested[199,207]. Nuclear location of ^{3}H-1,25-(OH)$_2$D$_3$ in intestine has recently been demonstrated[208,209] by autoradiography and using high specific activity 1,25-(OH)$_2$-[26,27-^{3}H]D$_3$. Thus a nuclear function of 1,25-(OH)$_2$D$_3$ in intestine and bone is likely, but its exact nature is unknown.

Intestinal phosphate transport

Harrison and Harrison[210] attempted to show that vitamin D plays an important role in phosphate metabolism by suggesting that it is involved in the renal tubular reabsorption of phosphate. They recognized at the time that this phenomenon might be secondary to changes in parathyroid hormone secretion. Although this has proved to be the case, the idea that vitamin D functions in phosphate metabolism must be regarded as an important one. It is known that an important component of the reversal of rachitic and osteomalacic lesions is the elevation of serum inorganic phosphate[211,212]. Although this had been thought to be secondary to the intestinal calcium transport mechanism, more recent work has shown it to be quite independent. Harrison and Harrison first studied intestinal phosphate transport in the distal small intestine[172]. They could show that vitamin D increased this transport and that the system appeared to be different from the intestinal calcium transport mechanism. However, they were unable to demonstrate that the process could take place in the absence of calcium. More recent work from Kowarski and Schachter[213] and from Wasserman and Taylor[173] has shown that there is a calcium independent phosphate transport mechanism which is responsive to vitamin D. The uptake of phosphate is sodium dependent, whereas intestinal calcium uptake is sodium independent[214]. The system requires glucose and is stimulated by $1,25\text{-}(OH)_2D_3$ as well as $25\text{-}OH\text{-}D_3$, but not $24,25\text{-}(OH)_2D_3$ [91,166]. Nephrectomy prevents the response to physiologic amounts of $25\text{-}OH\text{-}D_3$ but does not prevent the response to the $1,25\text{-}(OH)_2D_3$ compound, suggesting that $1,25\text{-}(OH)_2D_3$ is the active form in that system as well. The phosphate transport reaction is an active process and has been carefully studied[166]. Little else is known about the phosphate transport reaction and much work remains to be done to understand this system.

Bone calcium mobilization system

Vitamin D-deficient animals placed on a low calcium diet develop a severe hypocalcaemia. The administration of vitamin D_3 to these animals results in an elevation of serum calcium concentration to normal. Since the diet is essentially devoid of calcium, the rise in serum calcium must come from some other source. The only source large enough to sustain such an elevation is the skeleton, and hence this represents a measure of the vitamin D induced bone calcium mobilization. This conclusion has been verified by means of ^{45}Ca-labelled bone mineral[174] and by tissue culture experiments[215]. In the latter system the $1,25\text{-}(OH)_2D_3$ is about 1000–5000 times more effective[216–218] than the $25\text{-}OH\text{-}D_3$. Vitamin D_3 itself has little or no activity in inducing bone calcium mobilization. In *in vivo* experiments it can be shown that the $1,25\text{-}(OH)_2D_3$ is about 10 times more effective than vitamin D_3 and about twice as effective as $25\text{-}OH\text{-}D_3$ in this system[219]. However, of great significance is the fact that nephrectomy, which prevents 1-hydroxylation of $25\text{-}OH\text{-}D_3$, prevents bone calcium mobilization response to $25\text{-}OH\text{-}D_3$ and vitamin D_3, whereas it does not prevent the bone mineral mobilization response to the $1,25\text{-}(OH)_2D_3$ compound, providing strong evidence that $1,25\text{-}(OH)_2D_3$ is the metabolically active form in this system as well as in the intestine[83]. Radioactive $1,25\text{-}(OH)_2D_3$ has been used to demonstrate that it is not further metabolized before it causes calcium mobilization from bone[92,93].

The mechanism whereby $1,25\text{-}(OH)_2D_3$ brings about mobilization of calcium from bone is not known. It is not at all clear whether this involves osteoclastic resorption, osteocytic osteolysis or osteoblastic mediated transfer of calcium from bone fluid to extracellular fluid. It is likely that $1,25\text{-}(OH)_2D_3$

does increase osteoclastic bone resorption but the remainder of the sequence is still unknown. It is certain, however, that actinomycin D given prior to 1,25-$(OH)_2D_3$ will block mobilization of calcium from bone, whereas when it is given after 1,25-$(OH)_2D_3$ it can no longer block that system, suggesting that transcription of DNA is involved in this response[192]. A 3.7S receptor for 1,25-$(OH)_2D_3$ has been demonstrated in bone of chicks and a 3.2S receptor in the bone of rats[220, 221].

Of some interest is that parathyroid hormone and 1,25-$(OH)_2D_3$ independently stimulate resorption of bone in culture[216]. This is in contrast to the situation *in vivo*, in which both are required for the mobilization of calcium from bone. There have been many attempts at explaining the disparity of the results, but so far this has remained unanswered. The idea that the cultures retain residual parathyroid hormone and 1,25-$(OH)_2D_3$ cannot be excluded. However, a more likely explanation is that the culture system does not measure the action of 1,25-$(OH)_2D_3$ in calcium homeostasis but rather the initial event in bone remodelling[222], while the *in vivo* experiments measure the calcium homeostatic machinery involving the osteoblastic membrane barrier.

DISEASES OF BONE AS A CONSEQUENCE OF DEFECTS IN VITAMIN D METABOLISM
Renal osteodystrophy

Perhaps the greatest number of patients who show a clear defect in vitamin D metabolism are those suffering from chronic renal failure. Certainly in late stages of chronic renal failure there is an absence of 1,25-$(OH)_2D_3$ and other 1-hydroxylated forms of vitamin D[84,223,224]. It is well known that patients suffering from chronic renal failure develop severe bone disease which has at least three components; one is osteomalacia, another is osteitis fibrosa due to secondary hyperparathyroidism, and a third is osteosclerosis. The osteomalacia is likely to result from a defective supply of the active form of vitamin D, which results in the failure of mineral mobilization and deposition in bone. The development of secondary hyperparathyroidism, however, is much more complex. Bricker *et al.*[225] have suggested that the secondary hyperparathyroidism results from nephron destruction causing a small but real rise in serum inorganic phosphate. This rise in serum inorganic phosphate suppresses ionized calcium causing hypersecretion of parathyroid hormone. The increased parathyroid hormone causes the remaining nephrons to reabsorb less phosphate. This cycle persists, resulting in massive secondary hyperparathyroidism. However, Tanaka and DeLuca have shown that not only serum inorganic phosphate plays a role in synthesis of 1,25-$(OH)_2D_3$, but that the renal cortical levels of inorganic phosphate may be the actual regulator of the 1,25-$(OH)_2D_3$ synthesis[149]. Thus it seems possible that as nephrons are destroyed the increased reabsorption of phosphate which occurs in the remaining nephrons may cause a high renal cortical level of inorganic phosphate which would repress 1,25-$(OH)_2D_3$ synthesis. Thus very early in the development of the disease a rise in inorganic phosphate may shut off synthesis of this hormone, resulting in defective utilization of calcium and hence secondary hyperparathyroidism. In any case, there is no doubt that a major component of the bone disease associated with chronic renal failure is a defective synthesis of $1,25\text{-}(OH)_2D_3$, and therefore, it is reasonable that results are now rapidly accumulating to show that $1,25\text{-}(OH)_2D_3$ and its synthetic analogue, $1\alpha\text{-}OH\text{-}D_3$, are effective in the treatment of 90 % of the cases of bone disease associated with the disturbance[226-232].

Hypoparathyroidism and pseudohypoparathyroidism

The discussion on regulation of vitamin D metabolism has illustrated the importance of the parathyroid hormone in the synthesis of $1,25\text{-}(OH)_2D_3$ in response to a hypocalcaemic stimulus. Clearly hypoparathyroid patients should lack the ability to make $1,25\text{-}(OH)_2D_3$ in response to hypocalcaemia. Although this has not yet been proved, it is well known that small physiologic doses of $1,25\text{-}(OH)_2D_3$ and low doses of $1\alpha\text{-}OH\text{-}D_3$ plus dietary calcium produce a marked response in serum calcium concentration[233,234]. These patients are managed quite well with such small doses as 1 μg of $1,25\text{-}(OH)_2D_3$ per day and 2–4 μg of $1\alpha\text{-}OH\text{-}D_3$ per day.

Pseudohypoparathyroid patients are a complex group, in which there is failure of end-organ responsiveness to parathyroid hormone. It is likely that these patients cannot make $1,25\text{-}(OH)_2D_3$ in response to a hypocalcaemic stimulus, in spite of the fact that they secrete parathyroid hormone. These patients[234] also respond to low doses of $1\alpha\text{-}OH\text{-}D_3$ and $1,25\text{-}(OH)_2D_3$.

Vitamin D dependency autosomal recessive resistant rickets type I

This disease is one in which children who carry the genetic defect develop severe rickets in the face of normal intakes of vitamin D. Their disease can be prevented or completely cured by the administration of 50 000–100 000 units of vitamin D_3 daily. This disease now appears to be a metabolic defect in the 1α-hydroxylase of $25\text{-}OH\text{-}D_3$. It seems likely that this enzyme is defective, having perhaps a high Michaelis constant for the substrate $25\text{-}OH\text{-}D_3$. Children suffering from this disease can be cured with physiologic doses of $1,25\text{-}(OH)_2D_3$ of 1 μg/day[235]. Somewhat higher levels of $1\alpha\text{-}OH\text{-}D_3$ are required[236,237]. However, there are cases which show some degree of resistance, which means that there may be more to the disease than a simple defect in the 1α-hydroxylase system. Recently low plasma levels of $1,25\text{-}(OH)_2D_3$ in children with the disease have been shown, supporting the conclusion of a genetic block in the 1-hydroxylase system[238].

Hypophosphataemic vitamin D resistant rickets

This is an X-linked dominant disease in which severe rickets develops together with a severe hypophosphataemia. Treatments of these rachitic children have varied from introduction of large amounts of phosphate to the introduction of large amounts of vitamin D. In all cases, treatments have been only partially successful. With the development of our understanding of vitamin D metabolism it was naturally conceived that this disease may represent a defect in vitamin D metabolism. Although this may still be the case, it is clear that no metabolites of vitamin D have yet proved successful in the treatment of the disease state. The best current idea concerning its aetiology is that the genetic disease results in a phosphate leak in a variety of organs, the most important being the kidney, but which may be obvious in the intestine and the salivary gland[239,240]. Besides a renal loss of phosphate, these patients have a reduced calcium absorption[241] and low levels of $1,25\text{-}(OH)_2D_3$ in their blood[238,242]. Treatment is best accomplished with frequent doses of oral phosphate (1.5 g/day given in five or more doses) and $1,25\text{-}(OH)_2D_3$ to improve calcium absorption and perhaps bone mineralization[243,244].

Vitamin D dependency rickets type II

There have been three independent observations of an autosomal recessive disease in which affected siblings exhibit alopecia, rickets and high levels of plasma $1,25\text{-}(OH)_2D_3$ [245-247] suggesting an end-organ defect in the vitamin D system. It is likely but not proved that these patients have target organ resistance to $1,25\text{-}(OH)_2D_3$.

Dilantin and phenobarbital induced bone disease

In some surveys as many as 30% of patients on long term dilantin and phenobarbital treatment for epilepsy develop bone disease as measured by a decrease in bone density and other parameters[248]. Although there has been disagreement from some groups concerning the incidence of disease among such patients, it seems clear that there is at least a fraction of this population which is at risk. Work by Stamp et al.[249] and by MacLaren and Lifshitz[250] has shown that this disease is accompanied by low circulating levels of $25\text{-}OH\text{-}D_3$. Hahn and collaborators have suggested that phenobarbital and dilantin might induce the destruction of vitamin D and its metabolites in the liver[251]. On the other hand, the suggestion has been made that the phenobarbital and dilantin interfere with the 25-hydroxylation of vitamin D_3. Both are consistent with available information and it is clear that physiologic amounts of $25\text{-}OH\text{-}D_3$ will correct the bone lesions. However, it is of some interest that larger doses of vitamin D_3 will also correct the defect.

Osteoporosis: steroid induced and postmenopausal

Patients treated with large amounts of glucocorticoids often develop severe osteoporosis. This may in part result from a block in the intestinal absorption of calcium or a defect in vitamin D metabolism[252-254]. Nevertheless, treatment of these patients with $25\text{-}OH\text{-}D_3$ or $1,25\text{-}(OH)_2D_3$ reverses their bone lesions (T. J. Hahn and R. Chesney, personal communication).

Postmenopausal women with osteoporosis have low rates of intestinal calcium absorption which cannot be stimulated by ordinary vitamin D given at low doses. However, $1,25\text{-}(OH)_2D_3$ will increase intestinal calcium absorption[171]. They also have reduced levels of $1,25\text{-}(OH)_2D_3$ in their plasma[255]. It is possible that inappropriate amounts of $1,25\text{-}(OH)_2D_3$ are made to meet the calcium needs of postmenopausal patients. Treatment with $1,25\text{-}(OH)_2D_3$ may be useful in correcting at least some of the defects seen in this disease. Certainly a failure to absorb appropriate amounts of calcium results in loss from the skeleton, in an attempt to prevent hypocalcaemia. Over a 30-year period, this could substantially contribute to the development of osteoporosis.

Summary of clinical uses of vitamin D metabolites

There are many disease states which bear consideration in terms of vitamin D metabolite therapy, and the role of possible defects in vitamin D metabolism in their aetiology. It is clear that much new information will be forthcoming in this important new and developing area of the therapeutics of bone disease. This will be enhanced by the synthesis of vitamin D analogues which will have presumably specific biological properties.

VITAMIN D TOXICITY

Vitamin D is known to be toxic in large amounts. Exactly what level of vitamin D is toxic in human beings is a matter of debate. As little as 2000 units has been suggested[19], but it is likely that this dose would be toxic only in the case of individuals who are unusually sensitive to vitamin D. It seems likely that vitamin D toxicity will be experienced at dosages above 5000 units per day. The recommended daily intake of vitamin D is 200 units per day[19]. Thus the safety factor is quite large, and individuals with normal dietary levels of vitamin D need not worry about toxicity. However, for people who take large amounts of vitamins there is a great concern that toxic levels can be achieved. It is this author's view that intakes of vitamin D above 400 units per day should be avoided unless specifically prescribed by a physician treating a pathological state. Even when such treatment is being used, it is important that periodically these patients should have serum calcium and phosphorus and urinary calcium measurements taken, to be sure that vitamin D toxicity is not being attained. As long as serum calcium levels remain within the normal range, vitamin D toxicity will not be observed.

Vitamin D toxicity symptoms include nausea, lack of appetite, polyuria, itchiness of skin (pruritus), renal failure, cardiovascular involvement and ultimately, death. Death is usually the result of nephrocalcinosis, heart and aortic calcification along with subcutaneous deposits of calcium and phosphorus. Although vitamin D toxicity is not common, it is an unnecessary condition which can be avoided by merely being aware of the potential toxicity.

If toxicity due to vitamin D is observed, as shown by the above symptoms, and by chemical evidence of hypercalcaemia and hypercalciuria, treatment should be sought to immediately correct the hypercalcaemia. This can be brought about by the administration of a low calcium diet and the administration of a furosemide diuretic which should help to bring calcium to within the normal range. If the hypercalcaemia returns upon withdrawal of the furosemide, it may be necessary to treat the patient with a glucocorticoid, such as prednisone, to keep the serum calcium concentration in the normal range for a matter of 2–3 months, whereupon prednisone therapy can be carefully terminated with close control of serum calcium concentration.

It is indeed surprising, with the elaborate controls on the functional metabolism of vitamin D, that vitamin D toxicity can even occur. However, as pointed out in a previous section, it is clear that the receptor proteins and thus the targets of intestine and bone will respond to *large* amounts of 25-OH-D_3. Inasmuch as the 25-hydroxylase feedback regulation can be overcome with *large* amounts of vitamin D, and *large* amounts of 25-OH-D_3 have indeed been noted in animals receiving large amounts of vitamin D[123], it seems likely that 25-OH-D_3 is the agent which brings about vitamin D toxicity. It seems likely that under conditions of hypervitaminosis D the large amounts of circulating 25-OH-D_3 will interact with the $1,25\text{-(OH)}_2\text{D}_3$ receptors of intestine and bone and initiate intestinal calcium absorption, bone calcium mobilization and probably intestinal phosphate absorption, giving rise to hypercalcaemia and unwanted calcification of kidney, heart, aorta and other sites.

CONCLUSION

It is now clear that vitamin D, in a manner analogous to cholesterol, serves as a building block for at least one and possibly more hormones which play important physiologic roles in the regulation of divalent cation and inorganic phosphate metabolism. Other possible functions of vitamin D may be uncovered as the requirements for the calcium and phosphate metabolism role are met.

Vitamin D, which is generated either in the skin or which is taken in the diet, is converted primarily in the liver to the 25-hydroxy derivative. The 25-OH-D_3 proceeds via a specific transport protein to the kidney, where it undergoes either 1-hydroxylation or 24-hydroxylation depending upon the physiologic state of the organism. When the subject requires calcium, as translated by hypocalcaemia, the parathyroid glands secrete parathyroid hormone which among its other physiologic functions stimulates synthesis of $1,25\text{-(OH)}_2\text{D}_3$. The $1,25\text{-(OH)}_2\text{D}_3$ then proceeds to the active sites where it mobilizes calcium from intestine and bone. Under conditions of hypophosphataemia, $1,25\text{-(OH)}_2\text{D}_3$ is also made, which in turn mobilizes phosphate from intestine and elsewhere. When serum calcium and phosphate are normal, little or no $1,25\text{-(OH)}_2\text{D}_3$ is made. Instead, 24-hydroxylation of 25-OH-D_3 takes place. The exact role of 24-hydroxylation remains unknown. The complex vitamin D endocrine system which exists in the kidney plays a central role in calcium homeostasis and phosphate metabolism. Clear defects in the system result in a variety of bone diseases which can be corrected by the administration of the missing form of vitamin D. Exactly how the active forms of vitamin D function at the target tissues remains unknown and is a current area of intensive investigation.

ACKNOWLEDGEMENTS

Some of the original investigations reported in this chapter are supported by a program–project grant no. AM-14881 from the National Institutes of Health, and by the Harry Steenbock Research Fund of the Wisconsin Alumni Research Foundation.

References

1. Smerdon, G. T. (1950). *Daniel Whistler and the English disease.* A translation and biographical note. *J. Hist. Med.,* **5,** 397
2. Mellanby, E. (1919). An experimental investigation on rickets. *Lancet,* **1,** 407
3. Mellanby, E. (1919). A further determination of the part played by accessory food factors in the aetiology of rickets. *J. Physiol.,* **52,** liii
4. McCollum, E. V., Simmonds, N. and Pitz, W. (1916). The relation of the unidentified dietary factors, the fat-soluble A, and water-soluble B, of the diet to the growth-promoting properties of milk. *J. Biol. Chem.,* **27,** 33
5. McCollum, E. V., Simmonds, N., Becker, J. E. and Shipley, P. G. (1922). Studies on experimental rickets. XXI. An experimental demonstration of the existence of a vitamin which promotes calcium deposition. *J. Biol. Chem.,* **53,** 293
6. Huldshinsky, K. (1919). Heilun von Rachitis durch Künstliche Höhensonne. *Dtsch Med. Wochenschr.,* **45,** 712
7. Steenbock, H. and Black, A. (1924). Fat-soluble vitamins. XVII. The induction of growth-promoting and calcifying properties in a ration by exposure to ultraviolet light. *J. Biol. Chem.,* **61,** 405
8. Hess, A. F., Weinstock, M. and Helman, F. D. (1925). The antirachitic value of irradiated phytosterol and cholesterol. *J. Biol. Chem.,* **63,** 305
9. Askew, F. A., Bourdillon, R. B., Bruce, H. M., Jenkins, R. G. C. and Webster, T. A. (1931). The distillation of vitamin D. *Proc. R. Soc.,* **B107,** 76
10. Windaus, A., Linsert, O. and Lüttringhaus, A. (1932). Crystalline-vitamin D_2. *Ann.,* **492,** 226
11. Windaus, A., Schenck, F. and von Werder, F. (1936). Über des antirachitisch wirksame Bestrahlungs-produkt aus 7-dehydro-Cholesterin. *Hoppe-Seylers Z. Physiol. Chem.,* **241,** 100
12. Lun, J. and DeLuca, H. F. (1966). Biologically active metabolite of vitamin D_3 from bone, liver and blood serum. *J. Lipid Res.,* **7,** 739
13. Sebrell, W. H., Jr. and Harris, R. S. (1954). Vitamin D group. In Sebrell, W. H., Jr. and Harris, R. S. (eds.) *The Vitamins.* Vol. II, pp. 131–266. (New York: Academic Press)
14. Frost, H. M. (1966). Bone Dynamics in Osteoporosis and Osteomalacia. *Henry Ford Hospital Surgical Monograph Series,* (Springfield: C. A. Thomas)
15. Omdahl, J. L. and DeLuca, H. F. (1973). Regulation of vitamin D metabolism and function. *Physiol. Rev.,* **53,** 327
16. Ribovich, M. L. and DeLuca, H. F. (1975). The influence of dietary calcium and phosphorus on intestinal calcium transport in rats given vitamin D metabolites. *Arch. Biochem. Biophys.,* **170,** 529
17. Dent, C. E. and Smith, R. (1969). Nutritional osteomalacia. *Q. J. Med.,* **38,** 195
18. Holmes, A. M., Enoch, B. A., Taylor, J. L. and Jones, M. E. (1973). Occult rickets and osteomalacia amongst the Asian immigrant population. *Q. J. Med.,* **42,** 125
19. *Recommended Dietary Allowances.* (1974). 8th Edn. (Washington, DC: National Academy of Sciences)
20. Crowfoot, D. and Dunitz, J. D. (1948). Structure of calciferol. *Nature (London),* **162,** 608
21. Trinh-Toan, DeLuca, H. F. and Dahl, L. F. (1976). Solid-state conformations of vitamin D_3. *J. Org. Chem.,* **41,** 3477
22. DeLuca, H. F. and Schnoes, H. K. (1976). Metabolism and mechanism of action of vitamin D. *Ann. Rev. Biochem.,* **45,** 631
23. DeLuca, H. F., Paaren, H. E. and Schnoes, H. K. (1979). Vitamin D and calcium metabolism. In Dewar, M. J. S., Hafner, K., Heilbronner, E., Ito, S., Lehn, J.-M., Niedenzu,

K., Rees, C. W., Shäfer, K., Wittig, G. and Boschke, F. L. (eds.) *Topics in Current Chemistry.* pp. 1–65. (Berlin: Springer-Verlag)

24. Fieser, L. F. and Fieser, M. (1959). Vitamin D. In Fieser, L. F. and Fieser, M. (eds.) *Steroids.* pp. 90–168. (New York: Reinhold Publishing Corp.)

25. Shoppee, C. W. (1964). *Chemistry of the Steroids.* 2nd ed., pp. 63–75. (London: Butterworths)

26. Windaus, A. and Trautman, G. (1937). Crystalline vitamin D_4. *Hoppe-Seylers Z. Physiol. Chem.,* **247,** 185

27. DeLuca, H. F., Weller, M., Blunt, J. W. and Neville, P. F. (1968). Synthesis, biological activity. and metabolism of 22,23-^{3}H-vitamin D_4. *Arch. Biochem. Biophys.,* **124,** 122

28. Schachter, D., Finkelstein, J. D. and Kowarski, S. (1964). Metabolism of vitamin D. I. Preparation of radioactive vitamin D and its intestinal absorption in the rat. *J. Clin. Invest.,* **43,** 787

29. Norman, A. W. and DeLuca, H. F. (1963). The preparation of H^3-vitamins D_2 and D_3 and their localization in the rat. *Biochemistry,* **2,** 1160

30. Kodicek, E. (1956). Metabolic studies on vitamin D. In Wolstenholme, G. W. E. and O'Connor, C. M. (eds.). *Ciba Foundation Symposium on Bone Structure and Metabolism.* pp. 161–174. (Boston: Little, Brown and Co.)

31. Greaves, J. D. and Schmidt, C. L. A. (1933). The role played by bile in the absorption of vitamin D in the rat. *J. Biol. Chem.,* **102,** 101

32. Avioli, L. V., Lee, S. W., McDonald, J. E., Lund, J. and DeLuca, H. F. (1967). Metabolism of vitamin D_3-^{3}H in human subjects: Distribution in blood, bile feces, and urine. *J. Clin. Invest.,* **46,** 983

33. Rikkers, H. and DeLuca, H. F. (1967). An *in vivo* study of the carrier proteins of ^{3}H-vitamins D_3 and D_4 in rat serum. *Am. J. Physiol.,* **213,** 380

34. Rikkers, H., Kletzien, R. and DeLuca, H. F. (1969). Vitamin D binding globulin in the rat: Specificity for the vitamin D. *Proc. Soc. Exp. Biol. Med.,* **130,** 1321

35. DeCrousaz, P., Blanc, B. and Antener, I. (1965). Vitamin D activity in normal human serum and serum proteins. *Helv. Odontol. Acta,* **9,** 151

36. Haddad, J. G. and Walgate, J. (1976). 25-Hydroxyvitamin D transport in human plasma. *J. Biol. Chem.,* **251,** 4803

37. Imawari, M., Kida, K. and Goodman, D. S. (1976). The transport of vitamin D and its 25-hydroxy metabolite in human plasma. *J. Clin. Invest.,* **58,** 514

38. Bouillon, R., Van Baelen, H., Rombauts, W. and DeMoor, P. (1976). The purification and characterisation of the human-serum binding protein for the 25-hydroxycholecalciferol (transcalciferin). Identity with group-specific component. *Eur. J. Biochem.,* **66,** 285

39. Botham, K. M., Ghazarian, J. G., Kream, B. E. and DeLuca, H. F. (1976). Isolation of a potent inhibitor of 25-hydroxyvitamin D_3-1-hydroxylase from rat serum. *Biochemistry,* **15,** 2130

40. Daiger, S. P., Schanfield, M. S. and Cavalli-Sforza, L. L. (1975). Group-specific component (Gc) proteins bind vitamin D and 25-hydroxyvitamin D. *Proc. Natl. Acad. Sci. USA,* **72,** 2076

41. Belsey, R., DeLuca, H. F. and Potts, J. R., Jr. (1971). Competitive binding assay for vitamin D and 25-OH vitamin D. *J. Clin. Endocrinol. Metab.,* **33,** 554

42. Haddad, J. G., Jr., Min, C., Mendelsohn, M., Slatopolsky, E. and Hahn, T. J. (1977). Competitive protein-binding radioassay of 24,25-dihydroxyvitamin D in sera from normal and anephric subjects. *Arch. Biochem. Biophys.,* **182,** 390

43. Taylor, C. M., DeSilva, P. and Hughes, S. E. (1977). Competitive protein-binding assay for 24,25-dihydroxycholecalciferol. *Calc. Tissue Res.,* **22,** 40

44. Shepard, R. M., Horst, R. L., Hamstra, A. J. and DeLuca, H. F. (1979). Determination of vitamin D and its metabolites in plasma from normal and anephric man. *Biochem. J.,* **182,** 55

45. Neville, P. F. and DeLuca, H. F. (1966). The synthesis of [1,2-^{3}H] vitamin D_3 and the tissue localization of a 0.25 μg (10 IU) dose per rat. *Biochemistry,* **5,** 2201

46. Gray, R. W., Weber, H. P., Dominguez, J. H. and Lemann, J., Jr. (1974). The metabolism of vitamin D_3 and 25-hydroxyvitamin D_3 in normal and anephric humans. *J. Clin. Endocrinol. Metab.,* **39,** 1045

47. Bell, P. A. and Kodicek, E. (1969). Investigations on metabolites of vitamin D in rat bile. Separation and partial identification of a major metabolite. *Biochem. J.,* **115,** 663

48. Higaki, M., Takahashi, M., Suzuki, T. and Sahashi, Y. (1965). Metabolic activities of vitamin D in animals. IV. Distribution of vitamin D sulfokinase in animal tissues and its isolation. *J. Vitaminol.*, **11**, 266
49. LeVan, L. W., Schnoes, H. K. and DeLuca, H. F. (1980). Isolation and identification of 25-hydroxyvitamin D_2 25-glucuronide: A biliary metabolite of vitamin D_2 in the chick. *Biochemistry*, **20**, 222
50. Onisko, B. L., Esvelt, R. P., Schnoes, H. K. and DeLuca, H. F. (1980). Metabolites of $1\alpha,25$-dihydroxyvitamin D_3 in rat bile. *Biochemistry*, **19**, 4124
51. Esvelt, R. P., Schnoes, H. K. and DeLuca, H. F. (1979). Isolation and characterization of 1α-hydroxy-tetranor-vitamin D-23-carboxylic acid: A major metabolite of 1,25-dihydroxyvitamin D_3. *Biochemistry*, **18**, 3977
52. Windaus, A. and Bock, F. (1937). Über das Provitamin aus dem Sterin der Schweineschwarte. *Z. Physiol. Chem.*, **245**, 168
53. Idler, D. R. and Baumann, C. A. (1952). Skin sterols. II. Isolation of $\Delta7$-cholesterol. *J. Biol. Chem.*, **195**, 623
54. Windaus, A., Lettre, H. and Schenck, F. (1935). 7-Dehydrocholesterol. *Ann.*, **520**, 98
55. Daniels, F., Jr. (1964). In Field, J. (ed.). *Handbook of Physiological Adaptation to Environment.* p. 969 (Baltimore: Williams and Wilkins)
56. Esvelt, R. P., Schnoes, H. K. and DeLuca, H. F. (1978). Vitamin D_3 from rat skins irradiated *in vitro* with ultraviolet light. *Arch. Biochem. Biophys.*, **188**, 282
57. Holick, M. F., Richtand, N. M., McNeill, S. C., Holick, S. A., Frommer, J. E., Henley, J. W. and Potts, J. T., Jr. (1979). Isolation and identification of previtamin D_3 from the skin of rats exposed to ultraviolet irradiation. *Biochemistry*, **18**, 1003
58. Petrova, E. A., Nikulicheva, S. I. and Lazareva, N. P. (1976). Formation of precholecalciferol *in vivo. Vopr. Pitaniya*, **5**, 50
59. Holick, M. F. and Clark, M. B. (1978). The photobiogenesis and metabolism of vitamin D. *Fed. Proc.*, **37**, 2567
60. Bekemeier, H. (1958). Versuche zur maximalen antirachitischen UV-Aktivierung isolierter menschlicher Haut. *Acta Biol. Med. Ger.*, **1**, 756
61. Haddad, J. G. and Stamp, T. C. B. (1974). Circulating 25-hydroxyvitamin D in man. *Am. J. Med.*, **57**, 57
62. Blondin, G. A., Kulkarni, B. D. and Nes, W. R. (1967). A study of the origin of vitamin D from 7-dehydrocholesterol in fish. *Comp. Biochem. Physiol.*, **20**, 379
63. Bills, C. E. (1954). Vitamin D group. In Sebrell, W. H., Jr. and Harris, R. S. (eds.). *The Vitamins.* Vol. II, Chapter 6, pp. 132–223. (New York: Academic Press)
64. Olson, E. B., Jr., Knutson, J. C., Bhattacharyya, M. H. and DeLuca, H. F. (1976). The effect of hepatectomy on the synthesis of 25-hydroxyvitamin D_3. *J. Clin. Invest.*, **57**, 1213
65. Ponchon, G., Kennan, A. L. and DeLuca, H. F. (1969). "Activation" of vitamin D by the liver. *J. Clin. Invest.*, **48**, 2032
66. Horsting, M. and DeLuca, H. F. (1969). *In vitro* production of 25-hydroxycholecalciferol. *Biochem. Biophys. Res. Commun.*, **36**, 251
67. Bhattacharyya, M. H. and DeLuca, H. F. (1974). Subcellular location of rat liver calciferol-25-hydroxylase. *Arch. Biochem. Biophys.*, **160**, 58
68. Madhok, T. C., Schnoes, H. K. and DeLuca, H. F. (1978). Incorporation of oxygen-18 into the 25-position of cholecalciferol by hepatic cholecalciferol 25-hydroxylase. *Biochem. J.*, **175**, 479
69. Madhok, T. C. and DeLuca, H. F. (1979). Characteristics of the rat liver microsomal enzyme system converting cholecalciferol into 25-hydroxycholecalciferol. Evidence for the participation of cytochrome P-450. *Biochem. J.*, **184**, 491
70. Yoon, P. S. and DeLuca, H. F. (1980). Resolution and reconstitution of soluble components of rat liver microsomal vitamin D_3 25-hydroxylase. *Arch. Biochem. Biophys.*, **203**, 529
71. Björkhem, I. and Holmberg, I. (1978). Assay and properties of a mitochondrial 25-hydroxylase active on vitamin D_3. *J. Biol. Chem.*, **253**, 842
72. Pedersen, J. I., Holmberg, I. and Björkhem, I. (1979). Reconstitution of vitamin D_3 25-hydroxylase activity with a cytochrome P-450 preparation from rat liver mitochondria. *FEBS Lett.*, **98**, 394
73. Tucker, G., III, Gagnon, R. E. and Haussler, M. R. (1973). Vitamin D_3-25-hydroxylase: Tissue occurrence and apparent lack of regulation. *Arch. Biochem. Biophys.*, **155**, 47

74. Bhattacharyya, M. H. and DeLuca, H. F. (1974). The regulation of calciferol-25-hydroxylase in the chick. *Biochem. Biophys. Res. Commun.*, **59**, 734

75. Holick, S. A., Holick, M. F., Tavela, T. E., Schnoes, H. K. and DeLuca, H. F. (1976). Metabolism of 1α-hydroxyvitamin D_3 in the chick. *J. Biol. Chem.*, **251**, 1025

76. Ponchon, G. and DeLuca, H. F. (1969). Metabolites of vitamin D_3 and their biologic activity. *J. Nutr.*, **99**, 157

77. Stanbury, S. W., Mawer, E. B., Lumb, G. A., Hill, L. F., Holman, C. A., Jones, M. and Van Den Berg, C. J. (1972). Some aspects of vitamin D metabolism in man. In Taylor, S. (ed.). *Endocrinology 1971*. pp. 487–499. (London: Heinemann Medical)

78. Belsey, R., Clark, M. B., Bernat, M., Glowacki, J., Holick, M. F., DeLuca, H. F. and Potts, J. T., Jr. (1974). The physiologic significance of plasma transport of vitamin D and metabolites. *Am. J. Med.*, **57**, 50

79. Haddad, J. G. and Hahn, T. J. (1973). Natural and synthetic sources of circulating 25-hydroxyvitamin D in man. *Nature (London)*, **244**, 515

80. Eisman, J. A., Shepard, R. M. and DeLuca, H. F. (1977). Determination of 25-hydroxyvitamin D_2 and 25-hydroxyvitamin D_3 in human plasma using high-pressure liquid chromatography. *Anal. Biochem.*, **80**, 298

81. Holick, M. F., Schnoes, H. K., DeLuca, H. F., Suda, T. and Cousins, R. J. (1971). Isolation and identification of 1,25-dihydroxycholecalciferol. A metabolite of vitamin D active in intestine. *Biochemistry*, **10**, 2799

82. Boyle, I. T., Miravet, L., Gray, R. W., Holick, M. F. and DeLuca, H. F. (1972). The response of intestinal calcium transport to 25-hydroxy and 1,25-dihydroxy vitamin D in nephrectomized rats. *Endocrinology*, **90**, 605

83. Holick, M. F., Garabedian, M. and DeLuca, H. F. (1972). 1,25-Dihydroxycholecalciferol: Metabolite of vitamin D_3 active on bone in anephric rats. *Science*, **176**, 1146

84. Fraser, D. R. and Kodicek, E. (1970). Unique biosynthesis by kidney of a biologically active vitamin D metabolite. *Nature (London)*, **228**, 764

85. Gray, R., Boyle, I. and DeLuca, H. F. (1971). Vitamin D metabolism: The role of kidney tissue. *Science*, **172**, 1232

86. Gray, R. W., Omdahl, J. L., Ghazarian, J. G. and DeLuca, H. F. (1972). 25-Hydroxycholecalciferol-1-hydroxylase: Subcellular location and properties. *J. Biol. Chem.*, **247**, 7528

87. Ghazarian, J. G., Schnoes, H. K. and DeLuca, H. F. (1973). Mechanism of 25-hydroxycholecalciferol-1α-hydroxylation. Incorporation of oxygen-18 into the 1α position of 25-hydroxycholecalciferol. *Biochemistry*, **12**, 2555

88. Ghazarian, J. G., Jefcoate, C. R., Knutson, J. C., Orme-Johnson, W. H. and DeLuca, H. F. (1974). Mitochondrial cytochrome P_{450}: A component of chick kidney 25-hydroxy-cholecalciferol-1α-hydroxylase. *J. Biol. Chem.*, **249**, 3026

89. Pedersen, J. I., Ghazarian, J. G., Orme-Johnson, N. R. and DeLuca, H. F. (1976). Isolation of chick renal mitochondrial ferredoxin active in the 25-hydroxyvitamin D_3-1α-hydroxylase system. *J. Biol. Chem.*, **251**, 3933

90. Ghazarian, J. G. and DeLuca, H. F. (1974). 25-Hydroxycholecalciferol-1-hydroxylase: A specific requirement for NADPH and a hemoprotein component in chick kidney mitochondria. *Arch. Biochem. Biophys.*, **160**, 63

91. Chen, T. C., Castillo, L., Korycka-Dahl, M. and DeLuca, H. F. (1974). Role of vitamin D metabolites in phosphate transport of rat intestine. *J. Nutr.*, **104**, 1056

92. Frolik, C. A. and DeLuca, H. F. (1971). 1,25-Dihydroxycholecalciferol: the metabolite of vitamin D responsible for increased intestinal calcium transport. *Arch. Biochem. Biophys.*, **147**, 143

93. Frolik, C. A. and DeLuca, H. F. (1972). Metabolism of 1,25-dihydroxycholecalciferol in the rat. *J. Clin. Invest.*, **51**, 2900

94. Wong, R. G., Myrtle, J. F., Tsai, H. C. and Norman, A. W. (1972). Studies on calciferol metabolism. V. The occurrence and biological activity of 1,25-dihydroxy-vitamin D_3 in bone. *J. Biol. Chem.*, **247**, 5728

95. Kumar, R., Harnden, D. and DeLuca, H. F. (1976). Metabolism of 1,25-dihydroxyvitamin D_3: Evidence for side-chain oxidation. *Biochemistry*, **15**, 2420

96. Harnden, D., Kumar, R., Holick, M. F. and DeLuca, H. F. (1976). Side chain metabolism of 25-hydroxy-[26,27-^{14}C]vitamin D_3 and 1,25-dihydroxy-[26,27-^{14}C] vitamin D_3 *in vivo*. *Science*, **193**, 493

97. Esvelt, R. P. and DeLuca, H. F. (1980). Calcitroic acid: Biological activity and tissue distribution studies. *Arch. Biochem. Biophys.*, **206**, 403

98. Holick, M. F., Schnoes, H. K., DeLuca, H. F., Gray, R. W., Boyle, I. T. and Suda, T. (1972). Isolation and identification of 24,25-dihydroxycholecalciferol: A metabolite of vitamin D_3 made in the kidney. *Biochemistry*, **11**, 4251

99. Knutson, J. C. and DeLuca, H. F. (1974). 25-Hydroxyvitamin D_3-24-hydroxylase: Subcellular location and properties. *Biochemistry*, **13**, 1543

100. Madhok, T. C., Schnoes, H. K. and DeLuca, H. F. (1977). Mechanism of 25-hydroxyvitamin D_3-24-hydroxylation: Incorporation of oxygen-18 into the 24 position of 25-hydroxyvitamin D_3. *Biochemistry*, **16**, 2142

101. Garabedian, M., Pavlovitch, H., Fellot, C. and Balsan, S. (1974). Metabolism of 25-hydroxyvitamin D_3 in anephric rats: A new active metabolite. *Proc. Natl. Acad. Sci. USA*, **71**, 554

102. Tanaka, Y., Castillo, L., DeLuca, H. F. and Ikekawa, N. (1977). The 24-hydroxylation of 1,25-dihydroxyvitamin D_3. *J. Biol. Chem.*, **252**, 1421

103. Kumar, R., Schnoes, H. K. and DeLuca, H. F. (1978). Rat intestinal 25-hydroxyvitamin D_3- and $1\alpha,25$,dihydroxyvitamin D_3-24-hydroxylase. *J. Biol. Chem.*, **253**, 3804

104. Garabedian, M., DuBois, M. B., Corvol, M. T., Pezant, E. and Balsan, S. (1978). Vitamin D and cartilage. I. *In vitro* metabolism of 25-hydroxycholecalciferol by cartilage. *Endocrinology*, **102**, 1262

105. Horst, R. L., Shepard, R. M., Jorgensen, N. A. and DeLuca, H. F. (1979). The determination of 24,25-dihydroxyvitamin D and 25,26-dihydroxyvitamin D in plasma from normal and nephrectomized man. *J. Lab. Clin. Med.*, **93**, 277

106. Boyle, I. T., Gray, R. W. and DeLuca, H. F. (1971). Regulation by calcium of *in vivo* synthesis of 1,25-dihydroxycholecalciferol and 21,25-dihydroxycholecalciferol. *Proc. Natl. Acad. Sci. USA*, **68**, 2131

107. Boyle, I. T., Omdahl, J. L., Gray, R. W. and DeLuca, H. F. (1973). The biological activity and metabolism of 24,25-dihydroxyvitamin D_3. *J. Biol. Chem.*, **248**, 4174

108. Tanaka, Y., DeLuca, H. F., Ikekawa, N., Morisaki, M. and Koizumi, N. (1975). Determination of stereochemical configuration of the 24-hydroxyl group of 24,25-dihydroxyvitamin D_3 and its biological importance. *Arch. Biochem. Biophys.*, **170**, 620

109. Holick, M. F., Kleiner-Bossaller, A., Schnoes, H. K., Kasten, P. M., Boyle, I. T. and DeLuca, H. F. (1973). 1,24,25-Trihydroxyvitamin D_3: A metabolite of vitamin D_3 effective on intestine. *J. Biol. Chem.*, **248**, 6691

110. Castillo, L., Tanaka, Y., DeLuca, H. F. and Ikekawa, N. (1978). On the physiological role of 1,24,25-trihydroxyvitamin D_3. *Min. Electrol. Metab.*, **1**, 198

111. Stern, P. H., DeLuca, H. F. and Ikekawa, N. (1975). Bone resorbing activities of 24-hydroxy stereoisomers of 24-hydroxyvitamin D_3 and 24,25-dihydroxyvitamin D_3. *Biochem. Biophys. Res. Commun.*, **67**, 965

112. Rasmussen, H. and Bordier, P. (1978). Vitamin D and bone. *Metabol. Bone Dis. Rel. Res.*, **1**, 7

113. Tanaka, Y., DeLuca, H. F., Kobayashi, Y., Taguchi, T., Ikekawa, N. and Morisaki, M. (1979). Biological activity of 24,24-difluoro-25-hydroxyvitamin D_3. Effect of blocking of 24-hydroxylation on the functions of vitamin D. *J. Biol. Chem.*, **254**, 7163

114. Goodwin, D., Noff, D. and Edelstein, S. (1978). 24,25-Dihydroxyvitamin D is a metabolite of vitamin D essential for bone formation. *Nature (London)*, **276**, 517

115. Henry, H. L., Taylor, A. N. and Norman, A. W. (1977). Response of chick parathyroid glands to the vitamin D metabolites 1,25-dihydroxyvitamin D_3 and 24,25-dihydroxyvitamin D_3. *J. Nutr.*, **107**, 1918

116. Henry, H. L. and Norman, A. W. (1978). Vitamin D: Two dihydroxylated metabolites are required for normal chicken egg hatchability. *Science*, **201**, 835

117. DeLuca, H. F. and Schnoes, H. K. (1979) Recent developments in the metabolism of vitamin D. In Norman, A. W., Schaefer, K., Herrath, D. V., Grigoleit, H. G., Coburn, J. W., DeLuca, H. F., Mawer, E. B. and Suda, T. (eds.) *Vitamin D: Basic Research and Its Clinical Application*. pp. 445–458. (Berlin: Walter de Gruyter Co.)

118. Holick, M. F., Baxter, L. A., Schraufrogel, P. K., Tavela, T. E. and DeLuca, H. F. (1976). Metabolism and biological activity of 24,25-dihydroxyvitamin D_3 in the chick. *J. Biol. Chem.*, **251**, 397

119. Suda, T., DeLuca, H. F., Schnoes, H. K., Tanaka, Y. and Holick, M. F. (1970). 25,26-Dihydroxycholecalciferol, a metabolite of vitamin D_3 with intestinal calcium transport activity. *Biochemistry*, **9**, 4776

120. Lam, H. Y., Schnoes, H. K. and DeLuca, H. F. (1975). Synthesis and biological activity of 25,26-dihydroxycholcalciferol. *Steroids*, **25**, 247

121. Tanaka, Y., Shepard, R. M., DeLuca, H. F. and Schnoes, H. K. (1978). The 26-hydroxylation of 25-hydroxyvitamin D_3 *in vitro* by chick renal homogenates. *Biochem. Biophys. Res. Commun.*, **83**, 7

122. Wichmann, J. K., DeLuca, H. F., Schnoes, H. K., Horst, R. L., Shepard, R. M. and Jorgensen, N. A. (1979). 25-Hydroxyvitamin D_3 26,23-lactone: A new *in vivo* metabolite of vitamin D. *Biochemistry*, **18**, 4775

123. Shepard, R. M. and DeLuca, H. F. (1980). Plasma concentrations of vitamin D and its metabolites in the rat as influenced by vitamin D_3 or 25-hydroxyvitamin D_3 intakes. *Arch. Biochem. Biophys.*, **202**, 43

124. Tanaka, Y., Wichmann, J. K., Paaren, H. E., Schnoes, H. K. and DeLuca, H. F. (1980). The role of kidney tissue in the production of 25-hydroxyvitamin D_3-26,23-lactone and $1\alpha,25$-dihydroxyvitamin D_3-26,23-lactone. *Proc. Natl. Acad. Sci. USA*, **77**, 6411

125. Ribovich, M. L. and DeLuca, H. F. (1977). Effect of dietary calcium and phosphorus on vitamin D_3 metabolism. *Arch. Biochem. Biophys.*, **188**, 145

126. Suda, T., DeLuca, H. F., Schnoes, H. K. and Blunt, J. W. (1969). The isolation and identification of 25-hydroxyergocalciferol. *Biochemistry*, **8**, 3515

127. Jones, G. and DeLuca, H. F. (1974). Isolation and identification of 1,25-dihydroxyvitamin D_2. *Biochemistry*, **14**, 1250

128. Jones, G., Schnoes, H. K., LeVan, L. and DeLuca, H. F. (1980). Isolation and identification of 24-hydroxyvitamin D_2 and 24,25-dihydroxyvitamin D_2. *Arch. Biochem. Biophys.*, **202**, 450

129. Imrie, M. H., Neville, P. F., Snellgrove, A. W. and DeLuca, H. F. (1967). Metabolism of vitamin D_2 and vitamin D_3 in the rachitic chick. *Arch. Biochem. Biophys.*, **120**, 525

130. Parkes, C. O. and DeLuca, H. F. (1979). The influence of substitution at C_{24} on the calcium-binding protein-stimulating activity of vitamin D metabolites in chick embryonic duodenum. *Arch. Biochem. Biophys.*, **194**, 271

131. Omdahl, J. L., Gray, R. W., Boyle, I. T., Knutson, J. and DeLuca, H. F. (1972). Regulation of metabolism of 25-hydroxycholecalciferol by kidney tissue *in vitro* by dietary calcium. *Nature New Biol.*, **237**, 63

132. Tanaka, Y. and DeLuca, H. F. (1974). Stimulation of 24,25-dihydroxyvitamin D_3 production by 1,25-dihydroxyvitamin D_3. *Science*, **183**, 1198

133. Tanaka, Y., Lorenc, R. S. and DeLuca, H. F. (1975). The role of 1,25-dihydroxyvitamin D_3 and parathyroid hormone in the regulation of chick renal 25-hydroxyvitamin D_3-24-hydroxylase. *Arch. Biochem. Biophys.*, **171**, 521

134. Larkins, R. G., MacAuley, S. J. and MacIntyre, I. (1974). Feedback control of vitamin D metabolites by nuclear action of 1,25-dihydroxyvitamin D_3 on the kidney. *Nature (London)*, **252**, 412

135. Juan, D. and DeLuca, H. F. (1977). The regulation of 24,25-dihydroxyvitamin D_3 production in cultures of monkey kidney cells. *Endocrinology*, **101**, 1184

136. Henry, H. L. (1979). Response of chick kidney cell cultures to 1,25-dihydroxyvitamin D_3. In Norman, A. W., Schaefer, K., Herrath, D. v., Grigoleit, H. G., Coburn, J. W., DeLuca, H. F., Mawer, E. B. and Suda, T. (eds.). *Vitamin D: Basic Research and Its Clinical Application*. pp. 467–474. (Berlin: Walter de Gruyter)

137. Trechsel, U., Bonjour, J.-P. and Fleisch, H. (1979). Regulation of the metabolism of 25-hydroxyvitamin D_3 in primary cultures of chick kidney cells. *J. Clin. Invest.*, **64**, 206

138. Boyle, I. T., Gray, R. W., Omdahl, J. L. and DeLuca, H. F. (1972). Calcium control of the *in vivo* biosynthesis of 1,25-dihydroxyvitamin D_3: Nicolaysen's endogenous factor. In Taylor, S. (ed.). *Endocrinology 1971*. pp. 468–476. (London: Heinemann Medical)

139. Nicolaysen, R., Eeg-Larsen, N. and Malm, O. J. (1953). Physiology of calcium metabolism. *Physiol. Rev.*, **33**, 424

140. Galante, L., MacAuley, S. J., Colston, K. W. and MacIntyre, I. (1972). Effect of parathyroid extract on vitamin D metabolism. *Lancet*, **1**, 985

141. Henry, H. L., Midgett, R. J. and Norman, A. W. (1974). Regulation of 25-hydroxyvitamin D_3-1-hydroxylase *in vivo*. *J. Biol. Chem.*, **249**, 7584
142. Rasmussen, H. (1974). Parathyroid hormone, calcitonin, and the calciferols. In Williams, R. H. (ed.). *Textbook of Endocrinology*. 5th edn., pp. 660–773. (Philadelphia: W. B. Saunders)
143. Garabedian, M., Holick, M. F., DeLuca, H. F. and Boyle, I. T. (1972). Control of 25-hydroxycholecalciferol metabolism by the parathyroid glands. *Proc. Natl. Acad. Sci. USA*, **69**, 1673
144. Fraser, D. R. and Kodicek, E. (1973). Regulation of 25-hydroxycholecalciferol-1-hydroxylase activity in kidney by parathyroid hormone. *Nature New Biol.*, **241**, 163
145. Hill, L. F. and Mawer, E. B. (1972). The interrelationships between vitamin D, parathyroid hormone and calcitonin. Abstract presented at the *Annual General Meeting of the Medical Research Society*, December, 1972
146. Suda, T., Horiuchi, N., Fukushima, M., Nishii, Y. and Ogata, E. (1977). Regulation of the metabolism of vitamin D_3 and 25-hydroxyvitamin D_3. In Norman, A. W., Schaefer, K., Coburn, J. W., DeLuca, H. F., Fraser, D., Grigoleit, H. G. and Herrath, D. v. (eds.). *Vitamin D: Biochemical, Chemical and Clinical Aspects Related to Calcium Metabolism*. pp. 201–210. (Berlin: Walter de Gruyter)
147. Morrisey, R. L. and Wasserman, R. H. (1971). Calcium absorption and calcium-binding protein in chicks on differing calcium and phosphorus intakes. *Am. J. Physiol.*, **220**, 1509
148. Tanaka, Y., Frank, H. and DeLuca, H. F. (1973). Intestinal calcium transport: Stimulation by low phosphorus diets. *Science*, **181**, 564
149. Tanaka, Y. and DeLuca, H. F. (1973). The control of 25-hydroxyvitamin D metabolism by inorganic phosphorus. *Arch. Biochem. Biophys.*, **154**, 566
150. Hughes, M. R., Brumbaugh, P. F., Haussler, M. R., Wergedal, J. E. and Baylink, D. J. (1975). Regulation of serum $1\alpha,25$-dihydroxyvitamin D_3 by calcium and phosphate in the rat. *Science*, **190**, 578
151. Baxter, L. A. and DeLuca, H. F. (1976). Stimulation of 25-hydroxyvitamin D_3-1α-hydroxylase by phosphate depletion. *J. Biol. Chem.*, **251**, 3158
152. Ghazarian, J. G., Tanaka, Y. and DeLuca, H. F. (1975). The biochemistry of the chick kidney mitochondrial 25-hydroxyvitamin D_3-1α-hydroxylase and its regulation. In Talmage, R. V., Owen, M. and Parsons, J. A. (eds.) *Calcium Regulating Hormones*. pp. 381–390. (Amsterdam: Excerpta Medica)
153. DeLuca, H. F. (1975). Minireview: Regulation of vitamin D metabolism. *Life Sci.*, **17**, 1351
154. Tanaka, Y., Chen, T. C. and DeLuca, H. F. (1972). Dependence of 25-hydroxy-cholecalciferol-1-hydroxylase regulation on RNA and protein synthesis. *Arch. Biochem. Biophys.*, **152**, 291
155. Harrison, H. C., Harrison, H. E. and Park, E. A. (1958). Vitamin D and citrate metabolism. Effect of vitamin D in rats fed diets adequate in both calcium and phosphorus. *Am. J. Physiol.*, **192**, 432
156. Rasmussen, H., DeLuca, H., Arnaud, C., Hawker, C. and von Stedingk, M. (1963). The relationship between vitamin D and parathyroid hormone. *J. Clin. Invest.*, **42**, 1940
157. Harrison, H. E. and Harrison, H. C. (1964). The interaction of vitamin D and parathyroid hormone on calcium phosphorus and magnesium homeostasis in the rat. *Metabolism*, **13**, 952
158. Arnaud, C., Rasmussen, H. and Anast, C. (1966). Further studies on the interrelationship between parathyroid hormone and vitamin D. *J. Clin. Invest.*, **45**, 1955
159. Forte, L. R., Nickols, G. A. and Anast, C. S. (1976). Renal adenylate cyclase and the interrelationship between parathyroid hormone and vitamin D in the regulation of urinary phosphate and adenosine cyclic 3′,5′-monophosphate excretion. *J. Clin. Invest.*, **57**, 559
160. Garabedian, M., Tanaka, Y., Holick, M. F. and DeLuca, H. F. (1974). Response of intestinal calcium transport and bone calcium mobilization to 1,25-dihydroxyvitamin D_3 in thyroparathyroidectomized rats. *Endocrinology*, **94**, 1022
161. Zull, J. E. and Repke, D. W. (1972). The tissue localization of tritiated parathyroid hormone in thyroparathyroidectomized rats. *J. Biol. Chem.*, **247**, 2195
162. Steele, T. H., Engle, J. E., Tanaka, Y., Lorenc, R. S., Dudgeon, K. L. and DeLuca, H. F. (1975). Phosphatemic action of 1,25-dihydroxyvitamin D_3. *Am. J. Physiol.*, **229**, 489
163. Sutton, R. A. L. and Dirks, J. H. (1978). Renal handling of calcium. *Fed. Proc.*, **37**, 2112
164. Kleeman, C. R., Bernstein, D., Rockney, R., Dowling, J. T. and Maxwell, M. H. (1961).

Studies on the renal clearance of diffusible calcium and the role of the parathyroid glands in its regulation. In Green, R. O. and Talmage, R. V. (eds.) *The Parathyroids*. pp. 353–387. (Springfield: C. C. Thomas)

165. DeLuca, H. F. (1974). Vitamin D: The vitamin and the hormone. *Fed. Proc.*, **33**, 2211

166. Walling, M. W. (1977). Effects of 1α,25-dihydroxyvitamin D_3 on active intestinal inorganic phosphate absorption. In Norman, A. W., Schaefer, K., Coburn, J. W., DeLuca, H. F., Fraser, D., Grigoleit, H. G. and Herrath, D. v. (eds.). *Vitamin D: Biochemical, Chemical and Clinical Aspects Related to Calcium Metabolism*. pp. 321–330. (Berlin: Walter de Gruyter)

167. Bell, D. J. and Freeman, B. M. (1971). *Physiology and Biochemistry of the Domestic Fowl.* In Bell, D. J. and Freeman, B. M. (eds.). Vol. 3. (London: Academic Press)

168. Tanaka, Y., Castillo, L. and DeLuca, H. F. (1976). Control of the renal vitamin D hydroxylases in birds by the sex hormones. *Proc. Natl. Acad. Sci. USA*, **73**, 2701

169. Castillo, L., Tanaka, Y., DeLuca, H. F. and Sunde, M. L. (1977). The stimulation of 25-hydroxyvitamin D_3-1α-hydroxylase by estrogen. *Arch. Biochem. Biophys.*, **179**, 211

170. Castillo, L., Tanaka, Y., Wineland, M. J., Jowsey, J. O. and DeLuca, H. F. (1979). Production of 1,25-dihydroxyvitamin D_3 and formation of medullary bone in the egg-laying hen. *Endocrinology*, **104**, 1598

171. Gallagher, J. C., Riggs, B. L., Eisman, J., Hamstra, A., Arnaud, S. B. and DeLuca, H. F. (1979). Intestinal calcium absorption and serum vitamin D metabolites in normal subjects and osteoporotic patients. Effect of age and dietary calcium. *J. Clin. Invest.*, **64**, 729

172. Harrison, H. E. and Harrison, H. C. (1961). Intestinal transport of phosphate: Action of vitamin D, calcium, and potassium. *Am. J. Physiol.*, **201**, 1007

173. Wasserman, R. H. and Taylor, A. N. (1973). Intestinal absorption of phosphate in the chick: Effect of vitamin D_3 and other parameters. *J. Nutr.*, **103**, 586

174. Carlsson, A. (1952). Tracer experiments on the effect of vitamin D on the skeletal metabolism of calcium and phosphorus. *Acta Physiol. Scand.*, **26**, 212

175. Gran, F. C. (1960). The retention of parenterally injected calcium in rachitic dogs. *Acta Physiol. Scand.*, **50**, 132

176. Bonjour, J.-P., Preston, C. and Fleisch, H. (1977). Effect of 1,25-dihydroxyvitamin D_3 on renal handling of P_i in thyroparathyroidectomized rats. *J. Clin. Invest.*, **60**, 1419

177. Wasserman, R. H., Kallfelz, F. A. and Comar, C. L. (1961). Active transport of calcium by rat duodenum *in vivo. Science*, **133**, 883

178. Schachter, D. (1963). Vitamin D and the active transport of calcium by the small intestine. In Wasserman, R. H. (ed.). *The Transfer of Calcium and Strontium Across Biological Membranes*. pp. 197–210. (New York: Academic Press)

179. Schachter, D., Kowarski, S., Finkelstein, J. D. and Wang Ma, R. (1966). Tissue concentration differences during active transport of calcium by intestine. *Am. J. Physiol.*, **211**, 1131

180. Wasserman, R. H. and Kallfelz, F. A. (1962). Vitamin D_3 and unidirectional fluxes across rachitic chick duodenum. *Am. J. Physiol.*, **203**, 221

181. Martin, D. L. and DeLuca, H. F. (1969). Influence of sodium on calcium transport by the rat small intestine. *Am. J. Physiol.*, **216**, 1351

182. Adams, T. H., Wong, R. G. and Norman, A. W. (1970). Studies on the mechanism of action of calciferol. II. Effects of the polyene antibiotic, filipin, on vitamin D-mediated calcium transport. *J. Biol. Chem.*, **245**, 4432

183. Taylor, A. N. and Wasserman, R. H. (1967). Vitamin D_3-induced calcium-binding protein: Partial purification, electrophoretic visualization, and tissue distribution. *Arch. Biochem. Biophys.*, **119**, 536

184. Wasserman, R. H., Bar, A., Corradino, R. A., Taylor, A. N. and Peterlik, M. (1975). Calcium absorption and calcium binding protein synthesis in the chick: Evidence for a 1,25-dihydroxycholecalciferol-like factor in *Solanum malacoxylon*. In Talmage, R. V., Owen, M. and Parsons, J. A. (eds.). *Calcium Regulating Hormones*. pp. 318–329. (Amsterdam: Excerpta Medica)

185. Drescher, D. and DeLuca, H. F. (1971). Vitamin D stimulated calcium binding protein from rat intestinal mucosa. Purification and some properties. *Biochemistry*, **10**, 2302

186. Bruns, E. H. and Avioli, L. V. (1975). The activity and the synthesis of CaBP during vitamin D replacement in the rachitic rat. In Talmage, R. V., Owen, M. and Parsons, J. A. (eds.). *Calcium Regulating Hormones*. pp. 336–345. (Amsterdam: Excerpta Medica)

187. Ebel, J. G., Taylor, A. N. and Wasserman, R. H. (1969). Vitamin D induced calcium binding protein of intestinal mucosa in relation to vitamin D dose level and lag period. *Am. J. Clin. Nutr.*, **22**, 431

188. Harmeyer, J. and DeLuca, H. F. (1969). Calcium-binding protein and calcium absorption after vitamin D administration. *Arch. Biochem. Biophys.*, **133**, 247

189. Spencer, R., Charman, M., Wilson, P. W. and Lawson, D. E. M. (1978). The relationship between vitamin D-stimulated calcium transport and intestinal calcium-binding protein in the chicken. *Biochem. J.*, **170**, 93

190. Corradino, R. A. (1973). Embryonic chick intestine in organ culture: Response to vitamin D₃ and its metabolites. *Science*, **179**, 402

191. Tanaka, Y., DeLuca, H. F., Omdahl, J. and Holick, M. F. (1971). Mechanism of action of 1,25-dihydroxycholecalciferol on intestinal calcium transport. *Proc. Natl. Acad. Sci. USA*, **68**, 1286

192. Tanaka, Y. and DeLuca, H. F. (1971). Bone mineral mobilization activity of 1,25-dihydroxycholecalciferol, a metabolite of vitamin D. *Arch. Biochem. Biophys.*, **146**, 574

193. Tsai, H. C., Midgett, R. J. and Norman, A. W. (1973). Studies on calciferol metabolism. VII. The effects of actinomycin D and cycloheximide on the metabolism, tissue and subcellular localization and action of vitamin D₃. *Arch. Biochem. Biophys.*, **157**, 339

194. Morrissey, R. L., Zolock, D. T., Bikle, D. D., Empson, R. N., Jr. and Bucci, T. J. (1978). Intestinal response to 1α,25-dihydroxycholecalciferol. I. RNA polymerase, alkaline phosphatase, calcium and phosphorus uptake *in vitro*, and *in vivo* calcium transport and accumulation. *Biochim. Biophys. Acta*, **538**, 23

195. Bikle, D. D., Zolock, D. T., Morrissey, R. L. and Herman, R. H. (1978). Independence of 1,25-dihydroxyvitamin D₃-mediated calcium transport from *de novo* RNA and protein synthesis. *J. Biol. Chem.*, **253**, 484

196. Martin, D. L., Melancon, M. J., Jr. and DeLuca, H. F. (1969). Vitamin D stimulated, calcium-dependent adenosine triphosphatase from brush borders of rat small intestine. *Biochem. Biophys. Res. Commun.* **35**, 819

197. Melancon, M. J., Jr. and DeLuca, H. F. (1970). Vitamin D stimulation of calcium-dependent adenosine triphosphatase in chick intestinal brush borders. *Biochemistry*, **9**, 1658

198. Haussler, M. R., Nagode, L. A. and Rasmussen, H. (1970). Induction of intestinal brush border alkaline phosphatase by vitamin D and identity with Ca-ATPase. *Nature (London)*, **228**, 1199

199. O'Malley, B. W. and Means, A. R. (1974). Female steroid hormones and target cell nuclei. *Science*, **183**, 610

200. Brumbaugh, P. F. and Haussler, M. R. (1973). 1α,25-Dihydroxyvitamin D₃ receptor: Competitive binding of vitamin D analogs. *Life Sciences*, **13**, 1737

201. Brumbaugh, P. F. and Haussler, M. R. (1974). 1α,25-Dihydroxycholecalciferol receptors in intestine. II. Temperature-dependent transfer of the hormone to chromatin via a specific cytosol receptor. *J. Biol. Chem.*, **249**, 1258

202. Brumbaugh, P. F. and Haussler, M. R. (1974). 1α,25-Dihydroxycholecalciferol receptors in intestine. I. Association of 1α,25-dihydroxycholecalciferol with intestinal mucosa chromatin. *J. Biol. Chem.*, **249**, 1251

203. Brumbaugh, P. F. and Haussler, M. R. (1975). Nuclear and cytoplasmic binding components for vitamin D metabolites. *Life Sciences*, **16**, 353

204. Kream, B. E., Reynolds, R. D., Knutson, J. C., Eisman, J. A. and DeLuca, H. F. (1976). Intestinal cytosol binders of 1,25-dihydroxyvitamin D₃ and 25-hydroxyvitamin D₃. *Arch. Biochem. Biophys.*, **176**, 779

205. Kream, B. E., Eisman, J. A. and DeLuca, H. F. (1977). Intestinal cytosol binders for 1,25-dihydroxyvitamin D₃: Use in a competitive binding protein assay. In Norman, A. W., Schaefer, K., Coburn, J. W., DeLuca, H. F., Fraser, D., Grigoleit, H. G. and Herrath, D. v. (eds.) *Vitamin D: Biochemical, Chemical and Clinical Aspects Related to Calcium Metabolism*, pp. 501–510. (Berlin: Walter de Gruyter, Inc.)

206. Kream, B. E., Yamada, S., Schnoes, H. K. and DeLuca, H. F. (1977). A specific cytosol binding protein for 1,25-dihydroxyvitamin D₃ in rat intestine. *J. Biol. Chem.*, **252**, 4501

207. Procsal, D. A., Okamura, W. H. and Norman, A. W. (1975). Structural requirements for the interaction of 1α,25-(OH)₂-vitamin D₃ with its chick intestinal receptor system. *J. Biol. Chem.*, **250**, 8382

208. Zile, M., Bunge, E. C., Barsness, L., Yamada, S., Schnoes, H. K. and DeLuca, H. F. (1978). Localization of 1,25-dihydroxyvitamin D_3 in intestinal nuclei *in vivo*. *Arch. Biochem. Biophys.*, **186**, 15

209. Stumpf, W. E., Sar, M., Reid, F. A., Tanaka, Y. and DeLuca, H. F. (1979). Target cells for 1,25-dihydroxyvitamin D_3 in intestinal tract, stomach, kidney, skin, pituitary and parathyroid. *Science*, **206**, 1188

210. Harrison, H. E. and Harrison, H. C. (1941). The renal excretion of inorganic phosphate in relation to the action of vitamin D and parathyroid hormone. *J. Clin. Invest.*, **20**, 47

211. Fraser, D., Kooh, S. W. and Scriver, C. R. (1967). Hyperparathyroidism as the cause of hyperaminoaciduria and phosphaturia in human vitamin D deficiency. *Pediatr. Res.*, **1**, 425

212. Tanaka, Y. and DeLuca, H. F. (1974). Role of 1,25-dihydroxyvitamin D_3 in mainaining serum phosphorus and curing rickets. *Proc. Natl. Acad. Sci. USA*, **71**, 1040

213. Kowarski, S. and Schachter, D. (1969). Effects of vitamin D on phosphate transport and incorporation into mucosal constituents of rat intestinal mucosa. *J. Biol. Chem.*, **244**, 211

214. Taylor, A. N. (1974). *In vitro* phosphate transport in chick ileum: Effect of cholecalciferol, calcium, sodium, and metabolic inhibitors. *J. Nutr.*, **104**, 489

215. Trummel, C. L., Raisz, L. G., Blunt, J. W. and DeLuca, H. F. (1969). 25-Hydroxycholecalciferol: Stimulation of bone resorption in tissue culture. *Science*, **163**, 1450

216. Raisz, L. G., Trummel, C. L., Holick, M. F. and DeLuca, H. F. (1972). 1,25-Dihydroxycholecalciferol: A potent stimulator of bone resorption in tissue culture. *Science*, **175**, 768

217. Reynolds, J. J., Holick, M. F. and DeLuca, H. F. (1973). The role of vitamin D metabolites in bone resorption. *Calc. Tiss. Res.*, **12**, 295

218. Stern, P. H., Trummel, C. L., Schnoes, H. K. and DeLuca, H. F. (1975). Bone resorbing activity of vitamin D metabolites and congeners *in vitro*: Influence of hydroxyl substituents in the A ring. *Endocrinology*, **97**, 1552

219. Tanaka, Y., Frank, H. and DeLuca, H. F. (1973). Biological activity of 1,25-dihydroxyvitamin D_3 in the rat. *Endocrinology*, **92**, 417

220. Kream, B. E., Jose, M., Yamada, S. and DeLuca, H. F. (1977). A specific high-affinity binding macromolecule for 1,25-dihydroxyvitamin D_3 in fetal bone. *Science*, **197**, 1086

221. Mellon, W. S. and DeLuca, H. F. (1980). A specific 1,25-dihydroxyvitamin D_3 binding macromolecule in chicken bone. *J. Biol. Chem.*, **255**, 4081

222. Rasmussen, H. and Bordier, P. (1974). *Physiological and Cellular Basis of Metabolic Bone Disease*. (Baltimore: Williams & Wilkins)

223. Haussler, M. R., Baylink, D. J., Hughes, M. R., Brumbaugh, P. F., Wergedal, J. E., Shen, F. H., Nielsen, R. L., Counts, S. J., Bursac, K. M. and McCain, T. (1976). The assay of $1\alpha,25$-dihydroxyvitamin D_3: Physiologic and pathologic modulation of circulating hormone levels. *Clin. Endocrinol.*, **5**, 151s

224. Eisman, J. A., Hamstra, A. J., Kream, B. E. and DeLuca, H. F. (1976). A sensitive, precise and convenient method for determination of 1,25-dihydroxyvitamin D in human plasma. *Arch. Biochem. Biophys.*, **176**, 235

225. Bricker, N. S., Slatopolsky, E., Reiss, E. and Avioli, L. V. (1969). Calcium, phosphorus and bone in renal disease and transplantation. *Arch. Intern. Med.*, **123**, 543

226. Brickman, A. S., Coburn, J. W., Massry, S. G. and Norman, A. W. (1974). 1,25-Dihydroxyvitamin D_3 in normal man and patients with renal failure. *Ann. Intern. Med.*, **80**, 161

227. Brickman, A. S., Sherrard, D. J., Jowsey, J., Singer, F. R., Baylink, D. J., Maloney, N., Massry, S. G., Norman, A. W. and Coburn, J. W. (1974). 1,25-Dihydroxycholecalciferol. Effect on skeletal lesions and plasma parathyroid hormone levels in uremic osteodystrophy. *Arch. Intern. Med.*, **134**, 883

228. Silverberg, D. S., Bettcher, K. B., Dossetor, J. B., Holick, M. F., Overton, T. R. and DeLuca, H. F. (1975). Effect of 1,25-dihydroxycholecalciferol in renal osteodystrophy. *Can. Med. Assoc. J.*, **112**, 190

229. Chesney, R. W., Moorthy, A. V., Eisman, J. E., Jax, D. K., Mazess, R. B. and DeLuca, H. F. (1978). Increased growth after long-term oral $1\alpha,25$-vitamin D_3 in childhood renal osteodystrophy. *N. Engl. Med. J.*, **298**, 238

230. Chan, J. C. M. and DeLuca, H. F. (1977). Growth velocity in a child on prolonged hemodialysis. Beneficial effect of 1α-hydroxyvitamin D_3. *J. Am. Med. Assoc.*, **238**, 2053

231. Chan, J. C. M., Oldham, S. B. and DeLuca, H. F. (1977). Effectiveness of 1α-hydroxyvitamin D in children with renal osteodystrophy associated with hemodialysis. *J. Pediatr.*, **90**, 820

232. Chan, J. C. M. and DeLuca, H. F. (1979). Calcium and parathyroid disorders in children. Chronic renal failure and treatment with calcitriol. *J. Am. Med. Assoc.*, **241**, 1242

233. Kooh, S. W., Fraser, D., DeLuca, H. F., Holick, M. F., Belsey, R. E., Clark, M. B. and Murray, T. M. (1975). Treatment of hypoparathyroidism and pseudohypoparathyroidism with metabolites of vitamin D: Evidence for impaired conversion of 25-hydroxyvitamin D to 1α,25-dihydroxyvitamin D. *N. Engl. J. Med.*, **293**, 840

234. Neer, R. M., Holick, M. F., DeLuca, H. F. and Potts, J. T., Jr. (1975). Effects of 1α-hydroxyvitamin D_3 and 1,25-dihydroxyvitamin D_3 on calcium and phosphorus metabolism in hypoparathyroidism. *Metabolism*, **24**, 1403

235. Fraser D., Kooh, S. W., Kind, H. P., Holick, M. F., Tanaka, Y. and DeLuca, H. F. (1973). Pathogenesis of hereditary vitamin D dependent rickets: An inborn error of vitamin D metabolism involving defective conversion of 25-hydroxy-vitamin D to 1α,25-dihydroxyvitamin D. *N. Engl. J. Med.*, **289**, 817

236. Balsan, S., Garabedian, M., Sorgniard, R., Dommergues, J. P., Courtecuisse, V., Holick, M. F. and DeLuca, H. F. (1975). Metabolites and analogs of vitamin D: Therapeutic effects in D-deficiency and "pseudo-deficiency" rickets. In Norman, A. W., Schaefer, K., Grigoleit, H. G., Herrath, D. v. and Ritz, E. (eds.). *Vitamin D and Problems Related to Uremic Bone Disease.* pp. 247–258. (Berlin, New York: Walter de Gruyter)

237. Reade, T. M., Scriver, C. R., Glorieux, F. H., Nogrady, B., Delvin, E., Poirier, R., Holick, M. F. and DeLuca, H. F. (1975). Response to crystalline 1α-hydroxyvitamin D_3 in vitamin D dependency. *Pediatr. Res.*, **9**, 593

238. Scriver, C. R., Reade, T. M., DeLuca, H. F. and Hamstra, A. J. (1978). Serum 1,25-$(OH)_2D$ levels in normal subjects and in patients with hereditary rickets or bone disease. *N. Engl. J. Med.*, **299**, 976

239. Scriver, C. R. (1974). Rickets and the pathogenesis of impaired tubular transport of phosphate and other solutes. *Am. J. Med.*, **57**, 43

240. O'Doherty, P. J. A., DeLuca, H. F. and Eicher, E. M. (1977). Lack of effect of vitamin D and its metabolites on intestinal phosphate transport in familial hypophosphatemia of mice. *Endocrinology*, **101**, 1325

241. Williams, T. F., Winter, R. W. and Burnett, C. H. (1966). Familial (hereditary) vitamin D-resistant rickets with hypophosphatemia. In Stanbury, J. B., Wyngaarden, J. B. and Fredrickson, D. S. (eds.). *The Metabolic Basis of Inherited Disease.* pp. 1179–1204. (New York: McGraw-Hill)

242. Chesney, R. W., Mazess, R. B., Rose, P., Hamstra, A. J. and DeLuca, H. F. (1980). Supranormal 25-hydroxyvitamin D and subnormal 1,25-dihydroxyvitamin D. Their role in X-linked hypophosphatemic rickets. *Am. J. Dis. Child.*, **134**, 140

243. Glorieux, F. H., Scriver, C. R., Reade, T. M., Goldman, H. and Roseborough, A. (1972). Use of phosphate and vitamin D to prevent dwarfism and rickets in X-linked hypophosphatemia. *N. Engl. J. Med.*, **287**, 481

244. Glorieux, F. H., Bordier, J. P., Marie, P., Travers, R., Delvin, E. E. and Pettifor, J. M. (1979). The response of bone to oral phosphate salts (Pi), ergocalciferol (D_2) and/or 1α,25-dihydroxycholecalciferol (1,25-DHCC) in familial hypophosphatemia (FH). In Norman, A. W., Schaefer, K., Herrath, D. v., Grigoleit, H.-G., Coburn, J. W., DeLuca, H. F., Mawer, E. B. and Suda, T. (eds.) *Vitamin D: Basic Research and Its Clinical Application*, pp. 1163–1165. (Berlin: Walter de Gruyter)

245. Bell, N. H., Hamstra, A. J. and DeLuca, H. F. (1978). Vitamin D-dependent rickets Type II: Resistance of target organs to 1,25-dihydroxyvitamin D. *N. Engl. J. Med.*, **298**, 996

246. Rosen, J. F., Fleischman, A. R., Finberg, L. and DeLuca, H. F. (1978). A new type of rickets: Unresponsiveness of bone and intestine to high levels of endogenously synthesized 1,25-dihydroxyvitamin D_3. *Am. Pediatr. Soc.*, abstract

247. Marx, S. J., Speigel, A. M., Brown, E. M., Gardner, D. G., Downs, R. W., Jr., Attie, M., Hamstra, A. J. and DeLuca, H. F. (1978). A familial syndrome of decrease in sensitivity to 1,25-dihydroxyvitamin D. *J. Clin. Endocrinol.*, **47**, 1303

248. Kruse, R. (1968). Osteopathien bei antiepileptischer Langzeittherapie. *Monatsschr. Kinderheilkd.*, **116**, 378

249. Stamp, T. C. B., Round, J. M., Rowe, J. F. and Haddad, J. G. (1972). Plasma levels and

therapeutic effect of 25-hydroxycholecalciferol in epileptic patients taking anticonvulsant drugs. *Br. Med. J.*, **4**, 9

250. MacLaren, N. and Lifshitz, F. (1973). Vitamin D-dependency rickets in institutionalized, mentally retarded children on long term anticonvulsant therapy. II. The response to 25-hydroxycholecalciferol and to vitamin D_3. *Pediatr. Res.*, **7**, 914

251. Hahn, J. J., Brige, S. J., Scharp, C. R. and Avioli, L. V. (1972). Phenobarbital-induced alterations in vitamin D metabolism. *J. Clin. Invest.*, **51**, 741

252. Favus, M. J., Kimberg, D. V., Millar, G. N. and Gershon, E. (1973). Effects of cortisone administration on the metabolism and localization of 25-hydroxycholecalciferol in the rat. *J. Clin. Invest.*, **52**, 1328

253. Chesney, R. W., Mazess, R. B., Hamstra, A. J. and DeLuca, H. F. (1978). Reduction of serum-1,25-dihydroxyvitamin D_3 in children receiving glucocorticoids. *Lancet*, **2**, 1123

254. Carre, M., Ayigbede, O., Miravet, L. and Rasmussen, H. (1974). The effect of prednisolone upon the metabolism and action of 25-hydroxy and 1,25-dihydroxyvitamin D_3. *Proc. Natl. Acad. Sci. USA*, **71**, 2996

255. Gallagher, J. C., Riggs, B. L. and DeLuca, H. F. (1980). Effect of estrogen on calcium absorption and serum vitamin D metabolites in postmenopausal osteoporosis. *J. Clin. Endocrinol. Metab.*, **51**, 1359

6
Vitamin A deficiency and blindness in children

S. G. SRIKANTIA

INTRODUCTION

Human vitamin A deficiency has a global distribution, and is a major public health problem in several developing countries. Its importance lies in the fact that severe forms of the deficiency contribute to an unknown but large extent to irreversible blindness in young children, although it has been roughly estimated that about 100 000 serious cases are seen every year throughout the world[1,2]. The disease has been extensively investigated and the aetiological factors that are responsible for the widespread prevalence are well understood. It is unfortunate that in spite of this, hypovitaminosis A has not received the attention which it should from the public health point of view.

EPIDEMIOLOGY
Global incidence

Vitamin A deficiency, like protein energy malnutrition (PEM), is usually a manifestation of a poor socioeconomic environment. Also, it is a public health problem only in those areas of the world where β-carotene (provitamin A) is the source of dietary vitamin A. It is rarely seen in communities when diets provide more than 50% of the vitamin as preformed vitamin A, which is present only in foods of animal origin.

It is an important cause of preventable blindness in many Asian countries such as Bangla Desh, Burma, Sri Lanka, Pakistan, India, The Philippines, Vietnam, Korea and Thailand. It is frequently seen in several countries in the Middle East and Africa – Iran, Iraq, Jordan, The Lebanon, Libya, Sudan, Tanganiyaka and UAR. Brazil, El Salvador, Guatemala, Mexico and Haiti are other countries from which cases of keratomalacia have been reported.

Age and sex incidence

Age plays an important role not only in the prevalence of vitamin A deficiency, but also in the nature and severity of ocular lesions which are the only clinical manifestations. The reasons for this are, as yet, not known. Although vitamin A deficiency can occur at any age, it is seen most frequently in children of preschool and school age. The incidence of mild forms progressively increases with increasing age, it thus being higher in school children than in pre-school children. However, the great majority of severe forms which affect vision are seen in the age groups 1 and 3 years – an observation of considerable public health importance. During the first year of life, severe forms are rare because of breast feeding, and the few cases that are seen are among infants who are bottle-fed and are marasmic. The reason for the serious corneal manifestation which leads to blindness being confined to the younger child has not, as yet, been satisfactorily explained. It cannot be explained either by differences in the dietary intake or on the basis of superadded infection. It has, however, a marked association with the severe forms of protein malnutrition such as kwashiorkor and marasmus.

The incidence of mild and moderate vitamin A deficiency signs shows a clear cut sex difference, it being higher in boys than in girls. Below 5 years of age, the proportion is 60:40, which rises to 85:15 at 10 years of age. Such a sex difference is not seen in the incidence of the severe forms – keratomalacia[3]. Serum levels of vitamin A tend to be higher in young girls than in boys, although adult men have higher levels than do adult women. The simultaneous administration of oestradiol and testosterone to immature pullets has been found to substantially increase vitamin A levels in plasma, suggesting that sex hormones can influence vitamin A metabolism[4]. Further studies are obviously needed to elucidate the mechanism involved.

AETIOLOGY OF VITAMIN A DEFICIENCY
Dietary intake

Not all children whose dietary intakes are low show signs of deficiency, although children who do have signs invariably have low intakes. Therefore, it is clear that factors other than the immediate intake of the vitamin have a significant role. The vitamin A nutritional status of the mother during pregnancy and lactation, delayed introduction of supplementary foods during infancy and frequent attacks of infections are among such factors. Dietary intake of vitamin A by pregnant women in poor communities is low and circulating levels of the vitamin progressively fall during pregnancy[5,6]. Levels of serum vitamin A in infants born to such mothers[5] are usually below 15 μg/dl, and the liver stores[7] below 10 μg/dl of plasma[8] and 35 μg/g in the liver of their well nourished counterparts[9,10]. Infants born to mothers whose vitamin A nutritional status is unsatisfactory, thus start life with a handicap of inadequate vitamin A stores.

Vitamin A in breast milk

During early infancy, vitamin A needs are met exclusively from breast milk.

The concentration of vitamin A in milk of mothers whose dietary intakes of the vitamin are satisfactory[11], is over 50 μg/dl as against a value of 25 μg/dl or less in the milk of mothers whose vitamin A intakes are low[12, 13]. The growth and nutritional status of breast-fed infants is satisfactory during the first 4–6 months of life, and no signs of vitamin A deficiency have ever been recorded in such infants even from communities where vitamin A deficiency is widespread. Even when breast feeding is prolonged and the introduction of food supplements is delayed, signs of deficiency are rare as long as the child gets some breast milk, indicating that the small amounts of the vitamin which milk provides are enough to prevent clinical manifestations.

Supplementary foods and diets which older infants and young children receive in poor communities are invariably vegetable based and contain β-carotene and not preformed vitamin A. The intake of vitamin A on such diets has been found to be around 50 % or less of the recommended allowances[14, 15]. The low fat content of these diets may have an aetiological role, since it is recognised that among factors known to influence absorption of β-carotene, fat is an important one.

Role of infections and parasitic infestations

Keratomalacia is often precipitated by an infective episode, such as measles, chicken pox, bronchopneumonia and a bout of dysentery or diarrhoea. Infections can play a role in the development of vitamin A deficiency in a number of ways. An acute infective episode not only leads to a marked reduction in food intake but also leads to several metabolic alterations. Circulating levels of vitamin A fall during infection, which, however, return to pre-infection levels without dietary supplements of vitamin A[16–18]. The extent of the fall is influenced by the degree of pyrexia and age of the subject. The mechanism of this fall is not known, but obviously is not secondary to a reduction in liver stores. It is most likely to be mediated through alterations in the transport of the vitamin from liver to serum. This possibility is supported by the finding that the concentration of retinol binding protein (RBP), which is the specific carrier protein, is lowered in subjects with infective hepatitis[19].

Absorption of vitamin A is considerably impaired during infections, irrespective of the nature of the infection. Absorption of a physiological dose of tritiated retinyl acetate ranged from 30–70 % in children with respiratory tract infections and diarrhoea, as against over 95 % in normal children, and returned to normal values once the infection was controlled[20]. In communities where vitamin A deficiency is widespread, chronic recurrent infections are the rule, and in situations where the diet contains low amounts of the vitamin, in the form of β-carotene, these infective episodes can seriously aggravate vitamin A deficiency. Hepatic stores of vitamin A in subjects dying of chronic infections have been reported to be as low as 6–24 μg/g, in contrast to over 45 μg/g in subjects who died from accidents[16,18]. Similar observations have been made in infants.

There are also reports which show that parasitic infestations, particularly with ascariasis and giardiasis, interfere with vitamin A absorption[21, 23].

ROLE OF PROTEIN ENERGY MALNUTRITION (PEM) IN VITAMIN A DEFICIENCY

PEM and vitamin A deficiency are the two most commonly seen deficiency diseases in young children in several parts of the developing world. The prevalence of ocular signs of vitamin deficiency is often several fold higher in children with severe PEM than in the community, and the severe forms are almost always seen in children with kwashiorkor and marasmus. Levels of serum vitamin A in severe PEM are lower than in apparently normal children. On the basis of these observations, it has been stated that there is a very close inter-relationship between vitamin A and some other nutrients.

Data obtained from studies on experimental animals have suggested that PEM may interfere with the intestinal absorption of preformed vitamin A, conversion of β-carotene to vitamin A, hepatic storage and transport of the vitamin and also utilization at the tissue level. Studies carried out in the human, however, have not always confirmed these observations. Absorption of very large doses of vitamin A in children with kwashiorkor have been reported to be both impaired[24] and normal[25], when assessed by the extent of increase in serum vitamin A levels following the vitamin A load. However, using labelled vitamin A, the absorption of physiological amounts of the vitamin has been found to be unimpaired in children with severe PEM[20]. The protein nutritional status does not appear to be critical in the metabolism of β-carotene. In parts of West Africa, red palm oil, which is a rich source of β-carotene, is included in habitual diets. In such populations, although PEM is widespread, ocular signs of vitamin A deficiency are extremely rare[26]. A similar observation has been reported among Javanese children, who ate cassava but had good amounts of β-carotene in their diets[27]. These findings show that even in severe PEM, the conversion of β-carotene to vitamin A is adequate, and that the vitamin A so formed is absorbed and utilized. In children suffering from mild–moderate PEM, among whom ocular signs of deficiency are present, absorption and utilization of β-carotene has been found to be satisfactory, as assessed by serum vitamin A levels and disappearance of clinical signs[28].

During the post-absorptive state, vitamin A circulates in plasma attached to a specific carrier protein – retinol binding protein (RBP). The concentration of this protein has been reported to be low both in children suffering from PEM and from vitamin A deficiency[29–31]. Low levels of serum vitamin A in severe PEM has been attributed to an impaired synthesis of RBP in the liver. Children with kwashiorkor treated with adequate protein and calorie diets, which do not contain vitamin A, have been found to show elevated levels of vitamin A and RBP in circulation. On the basis of these findings, it has been suggested that low levels of vitamin A in PEM may reflect a defective hepatic synthesis of RBP rather than a deficiency of vitamin A *per se*. Recent studies have, however, shown that even in severely malnourished children with corneal lesions, although serum vitamin A levels were very low, the concentration of RBP did not fall to the same extent. Moreover, following the administration of vitamin A, there was a significant and rapid increase of both vitamin A and RBP levels within 4 hours before any change in protein nutrition could occur[31]. These findings are similar to those made in vitamin A deficient children. Vitamin A deficiency *per se* has been found to interfere with the release of RBP from the liver, even when that organ has adequate amounts of the carrier protein[32].

Although it has been claimed that signs of vitamin A deficiency respond better when vitamin A and protein are given together, it has been the general experience that even the severe forms of vitamin A deficiency can be reversed rapidly and completely by the administration of vitamin A alone without the administration of any other nutrient including protein. This suggests that utilization of the vitamin is satisfactory even in severe PEM – an observation in line with the finding that if diets contain enough vitamin A, children with kwashiorkor do not develop ocular signs.

Thus, dietary inadequacy of vitamin A seems to play an overriding role in the development of vitamin A deficiency signs. Although there is evidence for the metabolic inter-relationship between protein and vitamin A, the balance of evidence does not suggest a critical role for protein in the widespread prevalence of vitamin A deficiency. Diets of children who suffer from PEM are inadequate with respect to a number of nutrients including vitamin A, and this alone is sufficient to explain the high incidence, without having to invoke a role for protein. This, however, does not mean that improvement of protein status will have no effect on vitamin A status. In the prevention and control of vitamin A deficiency in a malnourished population, appreciation of this fact is important.

CLINICAL MANIFESTATIONS

In man, clinical manifestations of vitamin A deficiency are exclusively ocular. The term xerophthalmia is used to indicate collectively, all eye lesions due to vitamin A deficiency. It includes night blindness, conjunctival xerosis, Bitot spots, corneal xerosis and keratomalacia. There are excellent descriptions of these manifestations elsewhere[33]. A brief account of the salient features is given below.

Night blindness

Night blindness is the first functional evidence due to rod dysfunction. Its presence in young children is difficult to establish since it is subjective. It is important to recognize that night blindness can also arise from severe anaemia as well as ascorbic acid and niacin deficiencies, although they are rare.

Conjunctival lesions

Dryness, wrinkling, thickening, unwettability and loss of transparency of the bulbar conjunctiva, particularly against the palpebral feature, are characteristic of conjunctival xerosis. Pigmentation often accompanies these changes. Early stages are hard to identify, although it has now been suggested that they can be easily identified by a simple dye technique. The reliability of this method, however, is the subject of some controversy.

The Bitot spot is more easily recognized. When typical, it is a triangular, raised, silver-grey, foamy plaque, raised above the conjunctival surface, most often seen on the temporal side. There are many variants of this typical lesion.

Conjunctival lesions do not interfere with vision and have been considered as manifestations of mild and moderate vitamin A deficiency of a chronic nature.

Corneal lesions

The blinding effects of vitamin A deficiency are due to corneal damage. Conjunctival lesions are almost always present by the time the cornea is involved. The cornea shows dryness, loses its shiny, transparent nature and becomes hazy. This stage of corneal xerosis is completely reversible with appropriate treatment; but if neglected, corneal xerosis rapidly leads to softening, ulceration and colliquative necrosis with destruction of the anterior part of the eye ball. This is irreversible. Loss of vision depends upon the degree and site of corneal involvement.

BIOCHEMICAL ASPECTS OF VITAMIN A DEFICIENCY

Serum levels of vitamin A have been widely used for purposes of assessing vitamin A nutritional status. Levels below 10 μg/dl have been considered as indicating deficiency, levels between 10 and 19 μg/dl as low, between 20 and 29 μg/dl as acceptable and levels above 50 μg/dl as high[34]. While this may be acceptable for population groups, its use in individual cases must be made with caution, since the degree of correlation between serum vitamin A levels and the presence or absence of ocular signs is very low. The validity of using serum vitamin A levels as a reliable biochemical index of vitamin A status has been extensively reviewed[35].

The precise role of vitamin A in vision is well understood as a result of the pioneering work of Wald and Morton, but very little is known regarding its role in non-visual metabolic processes, several of which have been reported to be altered in experimentally induced vitamin A deficiency in animals. Several of these biochemical systems have been examined to determine whether vitamin A acts as a coenzyme. No evidence for such a role has been found[36]. That vitamin A may act as a membrane active compound regulating transfer of metabolites across membranes, and by influencing membrane stability, has been long suggested. This has been reviewed by Roels et al.[37] The most important and specific effect of vitamin A appears to be concerned with the synthesis of glycoproteins. Its role in glycosyl transfer reactions has also been recently reviewed[38, 39].

The excretion of two lysozomal enzymes – aryl sulphatase and acid phosphate – in urine of children with ocular signs of vitamin A deficiency, was found to show considerable reduction following the administration of a daily dose of 10 000 IU of vitamin A for 1–2 weeks[40]. Similarly, in children with kwashiorkor who usually have signs of vitamin A deficiency, a loading dose of vitamin A brought about a marked reduction in urinary excretion of aryl sulphatase[41], suggesting that vitamin A deficiency is associated with altered lysozomal stability.

The role of vitamin A in sulphate metabolism has been extensively studied in experimental animals with conflicting reports. However, in man there is evidence that vitamin A deficiency may modify sulphate metabolism. Vitamin A deficient children excrete low amounts of total and sulphated mucopolysaccharides, which are restored to normal with specific vitamin A therapy[42]. Homogenates of colonic mucosa of vitamin A deficient children have been found to incorporate ^{35}S less effectively into mucopolysaccharides than do extracts from normal children, and treatment with vitamin A corrected this abnormality[43]. More recently, it has been demonstrated that in both vitamin A deficient children and vitamin A deficient rats, plasma somatomedin activity as measured by sulphate uptake by rat cartilage is significantly lowered, and returned to normal after the administration of vitamin A[44]. Sulphate uptake by vitamin A deficient rat cartilage was low even in the presence of normal somatomedin activity in the incubation medium[44]. Further studies are obviously needed to elucidate the mechanisms involved.

In experimentally induced vitamin A deficiency both in man and in animals, anaemia and hypoferraemia have been observed[45]. Xerophthalmia and anaemia co-exist in children of poor communities, and in a recent study carried out to investigate the possible interrelationship between the two diseases, it was observed that the mean haemoglobin level in children who had serum vitamin A levels below 20 μg/dl, was slightly but significantly lower than in those with vitamin A levels above 20 μg/dl[46]. Absorption of iron in vitamin A deficient children was found not to be impaired[47], suggesting that either the mobilization of iron from the stores or utilization of iron is impaired. The former possibility is supported by results of animal studies, which have shown that vitamin A deficiency is associated with increased amounts of iron in the liver[48]. The extent to which vitamin A deficiency has a role in the widespread prevalence of iron deficiency anaemia is, however, not clear.

The interrelationship between vitamin A and vitamin E has long been shown in animals. There is little information whether this is also valid for man. In a recent study, no correlation was found between circulating levels of vitamin A and vitamin E in children; daily supplements of 100 mg of vitamin E for 2 weeks resulted in a clear cut rise in serum vitamin A levels both in normal and vitamin A deficient children[49]. The amount of vitamin E used was large, and whether at physiological levels of intake there is any relationship between the two vitamins is not known.

Among factors reported to modify RBP synthesis and, therefore, vitamin A levels, is zinc. Supplements of zinc given to undernourished children who have vitamin A deficiency signs were not associated with any change either in RBP or vitamin A levels, although they had low levels of zinc[50]. It is possible that the children studied did not have a zinc deficiency of a severity which affected RBP metabolism.

TREATMENT OF VITAMIN A DEFICIENCY

Night blindness and conjunctival manifestations respond satisfactorily to daily oral doses of 1000 μg of vitamin A. In a small proportion of older children and in adults Bitot spots persist, in spite of large doses of vitamin A.

Corneal xerosis can progress to keratomalacia within hours with loss of vision and must, therefore, be regarded as a medical emergency. It is generally believed that the intramuscular administration of vitamin A is more effective than the oral route in such cases. This is not entirely true, since the response depends upon the type of vitamin A preparation used. Intramuscular administration of even large amounts of vitamin A in an oil base, fail to increase serum vitamin A levels[25, 51–53]. Although corneal manifestations do improve in many children in spite of this, in some, eye signs have been found to deteriorate. In contrast, the intramuscular administration of a water miscible preparation was invariably associated with elevated serum vitamin A levels within hours, and the clinical response was uniformly good[25, 51–54]. Since it is of paramount importance to rapidly raise serum vitamin A levels so that enough vitamin reaches the cornea, the intramuscular administration of an oily preparation is clearly unsuitable, and only a water miscible preparation should be used. Oral administration of either oily or water miscible vitamin A preparations have been found to be effective, but the parenteral use of the water miscible preparation is the method of choice, since associated gastroenteritis may interfere with intestinal absorption.

PREVENTION AND CONTROL

Dietary inadequacy of vitamin A is the single most important aetiological factor in the development of xerophthalmia. The most rational approach for its control and prevention is, therefore, to ensure that diets contain enough vitamin A.

Foods of animal origin containing vitamin A are expensive and, therefore, beyond the reach of those among whom vitamin A deficiency is a problem. Alternate less expensive sources of β-carotene are available. Green leafy vegetables such as amaranth and spinach contain enough β-carotene, to raise levels of serum vitamin A significantly when as little as 25–30 g are consumed daily[55]. Encouraging the consumption of green leafy vegetables, without introducing any other change in the diets can, therefore, make an impact on the extent of the problem. The inclusion of small amounts of edible fats will further improve the situation. The latter may, however, not be a practicable recommendation, since in countries where edible oils and fats are in short supply, this food item is one of the most expensive. In many communities, green leafy vegetables are often not included in the diets of young children, for reasons other than availability, and an intensive programme of nutrition education would be necessary to bring about the necessary change in the attitude towards green leafy vegetables. Additional interim methods are, therefore, needed to reduce vitamin A morbidity.

Massive dose approach

Vitamin A can be stored in the liver and released when the need arises. One of the ways of ensuring that vitamin A deficiency does not develop, is to build up hepatic stores of the vitamin by periodic administration of the vitamin. This has been attempted in the past through the distribution of vitamin A capsules at frequent intervals to segments of the population at high risk, but this has had very limited impact because of many practical limitations, such as coverage and regularity of intake. The use of a massive dose of vitamin A given preferably once a year has been suggested as a public health measure for the control of blindness due to vitamin A deficiency in children. Practical aspects which need to be examined in this context are (1) the size of the dose, (2) the type of preparation to be used, (3) the route of administration and (4) the frequency with which it has to be administered. The dose must be large enough to be useful and yet not too large to lead to acute vitamin A toxicity. The type of preparation and the route of administration should permit as large a hepatic storage as possible. The frequency must be kept to a minimum.

In a series of studies carried out in India, the administration of a single large dose of 200 000 IU of an oily preparation of vitamin A was found to result in the retention of 50 % of this amount[20]. Satisfactory levels of vitamin A in blood were maintained for periods up to 6 months[56] although in another study it was found that elevated levels were maintained for only shorter periods[54]. In the latter situation, pre-school children had been maintained on a special diet which provided only 30 μg of vitamin A daily – a level much lower than that present in the habitual diet. Results of community studies in rural areas using an annual single massive oral dose showed that the incidence of signs of acute toxicity was not of a magnitude to pose any problems[57]. Following the administration of the massive dose, the urinary excretion of two lysozomal enzymes – aryl sulphatase and acid phosphate – showed only a transient increase in 50 % of the children studied[38], indicating that there was no significant lysozomal instability, which is known to occur in acute hypervitaminosis A. Based on these findings, a vitamin A prophylaxis programme at the national level has been implemented in India, wherein children between the ages of 1 and 4 years, who are at risk, receive orally, 200 000 IU of an oily preparation of vitamin A once every 6 months. This is implemented with the existing health infrastructure (the primary health centre), and an evaluation of this programme has shown that it has brought down the incidence of xerophthalmia by about 70 % as found in an earlier pilot study[56]. Two other Asian countries, Bangla Desh[58] and Indonesia[59], have also implemented a similar vitamin A prophylaxis programme on a large scale, with essentially similar results.

Fortification of foods

Fortification of suitable foods with vitamin A is another approach, which has been attempted. In Guatemala, vitamin A has been added to refined sugar, which is used almost universally[60]. It has been shown in both experimental animal and human studies that the use of this fortified sugar is associated with elevated levels of vitamin A in serum[61,62]. Attempts to use common salt as a vehicle for vitamin A in India have not been promising. With the type of crude salt used and the way it is stored in Indian rural homes, more than 80 % of the added vitamin A has been found to be lost within 3–4 weeks after its addition. Also, the cost factor is an important consideration. The cost in Guatemala was 7 cents (US) per year per inhabitant.

The extent of reduction in the prevalence of ocular signs of vitamin A deficiency, particularly Bitot spots, after the implementation of the programme has been used to evaluate its effectiveness. It is not always easy to obtain satisfactory baseline data on the prevalence of deficiency signs particularly in large scale operations, and this has often posed problems for evaluation. A simple and reliable method is now available by which the effectiveness can be measured, even in the absence of baseline data[64]. This method makes use of the well documented relationship between age on the one hand and the incidence of ocular signs on the other.

Vitamin A deficiency continues to be a major public health problem in spite of the extensive information there is available about the disease. Although the methods of prophylaxis described here do make an impact, they must perhaps be considered as short term measures to minimize morbidity until such time that the problem can be solved by raising the socioeconomic levels of the population and by improving the dietary intake of the vitamin.

Addition of retinyl palmitate to sugar administered to Guatemalan children resulted after one or two years in a highly significant rise in serum vitamin A values in 76 % of the subjects[63].

References

1. Oomen, H. A. P. C., McLaren, D. S. and Escapini, H. (1964). Epidemiology and public health aspects of hypovitaminosis A – A global survey on xerophthalmia. *Trop. Geogr. Med.*, **16**, 271
2. McLaren, D. S. (1966), Present knowledge of the role of vitamin A in health and disease. *Trans. R. Soc. Trop. Med. Hyg.*, **60**, 436
3. Srikantia, S. G. (1975). Human vitamin A deficiency. In Bourne, G. H. (ed.). *World Review of Nutrition and Dietetics.* pp. 181–231 (Basel: S. Karger)
4. Chapman, D. G., Gluck, M., Common, R. H. and Maw, W. A. (1949). The influence of gonadal hormones on the serum vitamin A of the immature pullet. *Can. J. Res.*, **27**, 37
5. Venkatachalam, P. S., Bhavani, B. and Gopalan, C. (1962). Studies on vitamin A nutritional status of mothers and infants in poor communities in India. *J. Pediatr.*, **61**, 262
6. Badr El Din, M. K. and Hammad, S. (1966). Serum vitamin A in infancy and childhood in the malnourished. *J. Trop. Pediatr.*, **12**, 63
7. Leela, I. and Apte, S. V. (1972). Nutrient stores in human fetal livers. *Br. J. Nutr.*, **27**, 313
8. Lewis, J. M., Bodansky, O., Lithenfield, M. C. C. and Schneider, H. (1947). Supplements of vitamin A and carotene during pregnancy: Their effects on the levels of serum vitamin A in the blood of mothers and new born. *Am. J. Dis. Child.*, **73**, 142
9. Smith, B. M. and Malthus, E. M. (1962). Vitamin A content of human liver from autopsies in New Zealand. *Br. J. Nutr.*, **16**, 213
10. Tisher, K. D., Carr, C. J., Huff, J. E. and Hubner, T. E. (1970). Dark adaptation and night vision. *Fed. Proc.*, **29**, 1605
11. Kon, S. K. and Mawson, E. H. (1950). Human milk. *Med. Res. Councl. Spl. Rep. Ser.* **269**, (London: HMSO)
12. Belavady, B. and Gopalan, C. (1959). Chemical composition of human milk in poor Indian women. *Ind. J. Med. Res.*, **47**, 234

13. Patwardhan, V. N. (1969). Hypovitaminosis A and epidemiology of xerophthalmia. *Am. J. Clin. Nutr.*, **22**, 1106
14. Report of a Technical Group Meeting (1970). *Hypovitaminosis A in the Americas* (Washington: Pan American Health Organization)
15. Studies on pre-school children (1974). *Ind. Counc. Med. Res. Tech. Rep. Ser.*, **26**, 17 (New Delhi: ICMR)
16. Moore, T. (1937). Vitamin A and carotene: The vitamin A reserve of the adult human being in health and disease. *Biochem. J.*, **31**, 155
17. Popper, H. and Steigmann, F. (1943). The clinical significance of plasma vitamin A level. *J. Am. Med. Assoc.*, **123**, 1108
18. Jacobs, A. L., Leifner, Z. A., Moore, T. and Sharman, I. M. (1954). Vitamin A in rheumatic fever. *Am. J. Clin. Nutr.*, **2**, 155
19. Smith, F. R., Raz, A. and Goodman, D. S. (1970). Radioimmunoassay of human plasma retinol binding protein. *J. Clin. Invest.*, **49**, 1754
20. Sivakumar, B. and Reddy, V. (1975). Absorption of labelled vitamin A in children during infection. *Br. J. Nutr.*, **27**, 299
21. Ketsampes, C. P., McCoord, A. B. and Philips, W. A. (1944). Vitamin A absorption in ten cases of giardiasis. *Am. J. Dis. Child.*, **67**, 189
22. Mgasena, S. (1969). A study of serum vitamin A levels in patients suffering from parasitic disease in Thailand. *Proc. First. South East Asian Seminar on Nutrition*, Djakarta.
23. Sivakumar, B. and Reddy, V. (1975). Absorption of vitamin A with ascariasis. *J. Trop. Med. Hyg.*, **78**, 114
24. Arroyave, G., Viteri, F., Behar, M. and Scrimshaw, N. S. (1959). Impairment of intestinal absorption of vitamin A palmitate in severe protein calorie malnutrition. *Am. J. Clin. Nutr.*, **7**, 185
25. Vinodini Reddy and Srikantia, S. G. (1966). Serum vitamin A in kwashiorkor. *Am. J. Clin. Nutr.*, **18**, 105
26. Scragg, J. and Rubidge, C. (1960). Kwashiorkor in African children in Durban. *Br. Med. J.*, **2**, 1979
27. Oomen, H. A. P. C. (1969). Clinical epidemiology of xerophthalmia in man. *Am. J. Clin. Nutr.*, **22**, 1098
28. Pereira, S. M. and Begum, A. (1968). Studies on the prevention of vitamin A deficiency. *Ind. J. Med. Res.*, **56**, 362
29. Smith, F. R., Goodman, D. S., Arroyave, G. and Viteri, F. (1973). Serum vitamin A, retinol binding protein and prealbumin concentrations in protein calorie malnutrition. *Am. J. Clin. Nutr.*, **26**, 982
30. Venkataswamy, G., Glover, J., Cobby, M. and Pirie, A. (1977). Retinol binding protein in serum of xerophthalmic malnourished children before and after treatment at a nutrition centre.
31. Vinodini Reddy, Mohan Ram, M. and Raghuramulu, N. (1979). Retinol binding protein and vitamin A levels in malnourished children. *Acta Ped. Scand.* (In press)
32. Muto, Y., Smith, J. E., Milch, P. O. and Goodman, D. S. (1972). Regulation of retinol binding protein metabolism by vitamin A status in the rat. *J. Biol. Chem.*, **247**, 2542
33. McLaren, D. S., Oomen, H. A. P. C. and Escapini, H. (1966). Ocular manifestations of vitamin A deficiency in man. *Bull. WHO*, **34**, 357
34. Interdepartmental Committee on Nutrition for National Defence (1963). *Manual for Nutrition Surveys*, 2nd Edn., p. 235 (Bethesda: NIH)
35. Pearson, W. N. (1967). Blood and urinary vitamin levels as potential indices of body stores. *Am. J. Clin. Nutr.*, **20**, 514
36. Rogers, W. E. (1969). Re-examination of coenzyme activities thought to show evidence of a coenzyme role for vitamin A. *Am. J. Clin. Nutr.*, **22**, 1003
37. Roels, O. A., Anderson, O. R., Lui, N. S. T., Shah, D. O. and Tront, M. E. (1969). Vitamin A and membranes. *Am. J. Clin. Nutr.*, **22**, 1020
38. DeLuca, L. M. (1977). The direct involvement of vitamin A in glycosyl transfer reactions of mammalian membranes. In Marson, P. L., Diczfalusy, Glover, J. and Olson, R. E. (eds.). *Vit. Horm.*, **35**, 1
39. Wolf, G. (1977). Retinol linked sugars in glycoprotein synthesis. *Nutr. Rev.*, **35**, 97
40. Vinodini Reddy and Mohan Ram, M. (1971). Urinary excretion of lysozomal enzymes in hypovitaminosis and hypervitaminosis in children. *Ind. J. Vit. Nutr. Res.*, **41**, 321

41. Ittyrah, T. R., Dumm, M. E. and Bachhawat, B. K. (1967). Urinary excretion of lysozymal arylsulphatases in kwashiorkor. *Clin. Chim. Acta*, **17**, 405

42. Mohanram, M. and Reddy, V. (1971). Urinary excretion of acid mucopolysaccharides in kwashiorkor and vitamin A deficient children. *Clin. Chim. Acta*, **34**, 93

43. Mohanram, M. and Reddy, V. (1973). Incorporation of ^{35}S sulphate into mucopolysaccharides of colon in vitamin A deficient children. *Int. J. Vit. Nutr. Res.*, **43**, 56

44. Mohan, P. S. and Kamala Jaya Rao (1979). Personal communication.

45. Hodges, R. E., Sauberlich, H. E., Canham, J. E., Wallace, D. L., Rucker, R. B., Mejia, L. A. and Mohanram, M. (1978). Hematopoietic studies in vitamin A deficiency. *Am. J. Clin. Nutr.*, **31**, 876

46. Mohanram, M., Kulkarni, K. A. and Reddy, V. (1977). Haematological studies in vitamin A deficient children. *Int. J. Vit. Nutr. Res.*, **47**, 389

47. Mohanram, M. and Reddy, V. (1977). Iron absorption in vitamin A deficient children. *Ann. Rep. Natl. Inst. Nut.*, **60**

48. Mejia, L. A., Hodges, R. E., Mohanram, M., Rucker, R. B., Arroyave, G. and Viteri, F. (1976). Anaemia in vitamin A deficiency. *Clin. Res.*, **24**, 315

49. Jagadeesan, V. and Reddy, V. (1979). Interrelationship between vitamins E and A: A clinical study. *Clin. Chim. Acta* (In press)

50. Shingwekar, Mohanram, M. and Reddy, V. (1979). Effect of zinc supplementation on plasma levels of vitamin A and retinol binding protein in malnourished children. *Clin. Chim. Acta* (In press)

51. Kramer, B., Sobel, A. E. and Gottifried, S. P. (1947). Serum vitamin A levels in children: A comparison following the oral and intramuscular administration of vitamin A in oily and aqueous mediums. *Am. J. Dis. Child.*, **73**, 543

52. McLaren, D. S., Shirajian, E., Tehalian, M. and Khoury, G. (1965). Xerophthalmia in Jordan. *Am. J. Clin. Nutr.*, **17**, 117

53. Pereira, S. M., Begum, A., Issac, T. and Dumm, M. E. (1967). Vitamin A theory in children with kwashiorkor. *Am. J. Clin. Nutr.*, **20**, 297

54. McLaren, D. S. (1967). Vitamin deficiencies complicating the severe forms of protein calorie malnutrition with special reference to vitamin A. In McCance, R. A. and Widdowson, E. M. (eds.). *Calorie deficiencies and protein deficiencies* (London: Churchill)

55. Pereira, S. M. and Begum, A. (1969). Prevention of vitamin A deficiency. *Am. J. Clin. Nutr.*, **22**, 858

56. Srikantia, S. G. and Reddy, V. (1970). Effect of single massive dose of vitamin A on serum and liver levels of the vitamin. *Am. J. Clin. Nutr.*, **23**, 114

57. Swaminathan, M. C., Susheela, T. P. and Thimmayamma, B. V. S. (1970). Field prophylactic trial with a single annual oral massive dose of vitamin A. *Am. J. Clin. Nutr.*, **23**, 119

58. Mujibur Rahman, M., Rahman, M., Guda, B., Khazir, S. M. K. and Alam, M. A. (1975). Vitamin A deficiency: Preventive programmes in Bangla Desh. p. 212. *Proc. X. Inter. Cong. Nutr.* Kyoto, Japan

59. Santoso, Tarwotjo, S. and Karyadi, D. (1975). Protecting children from vitamin A deficiency in Indonesia with special reference to crash preventive programmes. *Proc. X. Inter. Cong. Nutr.*, p. 210. Kyoto, Japan

60. Arroyave, G. and Brenes, E. B. (1973). Control of vitamin A deficiency in Guatemala: Fortification of sugar with retinol palmitate. *Nutr. Abstr. Reviews.*, **43**, 741

61. Arroyave, G. (1977). Evaluation of sugar fortification with vitamin A at the national level. *Xerophthalmia Club. Bull.*, **12**, 1

62. Arroyave, G., Mejia, L. A. and Aguilar, J. R. (1981). The effect of vitamin A fortification of sugar on the serum vitamin A levels of preschool Guatemalan children: a longitudinal evaluation. *Am. J. Clin. Nutr.*, **34**, 41

63. Arroyave, G., Aguilar, J. R., Flores, M. and Guzmán, M. A. (1979). Evaluation of sugar fortification with vitamin A at the national level. Scientific publication 384, pp. 1–66. Pan American Health Organization, 525 23rd Sreet N.W., Washington D.C. 20037

64. Vijayaraghavan, K., Naidu, A. N., Rao, N. P. and Strikantia, S. G. (1975). A simple method to evaluate the massive dose vitamin prophylaxis programme in pre-school children. *Am. J. Clin. Nutr.*, **28**, 1189

7
Protein energy malnutrition (PEM) in children

S. G. SRIKANTIA

INTRODUCTION

Deficiency diseases due to nutritional inadequate diets constitute public health problems in several developing countries. Among these, protein energy malnutrition (PEM) is the most widespread. It is a disease predominantly of young children living under unsatisfactory socioeconomic conditions. The severe forms carry a high mortality rate unless they receive prompt attention. The less severe forms impose handicaps not only during childhood but also in later life. A very large volume of data is available on PEM, but only the very salient features are presented here with emphasis on the public health aspects. No attempt has been made to be exhaustive.

PREVALENCE

The prevalence of PEM is high in developing parts of the world. It varies between countries and within a country, from one area to another. PEM covers a wide spectrum of clinical stages, the extreme forms being kwashiorkor and marasmus while the mild and moderate forms express themselves as varying grades of growth retardation. Results of community surveys involving large numbers of children have shown that among children below the age of 5 years, about 2–3 % suffer from the severe forms – kwashiorkor and marasmus, while almost 20 % suffer from the moderate forms. In some countries the mild forms are seen in as high as 50 % of the child population[1]. The relative frequencies of kwashiorkor and marasmus show considerable geographic variations, the reasons for which are not as yet fully clear, although urbanization with consequent changes in breast feeding practices is known to be an important cause.

SEVERE FORMS OF PROTEIN ENERGY MALNUTRITION
Clinical manifestations

There are several excellent detailed descriptions of the clinical features of kwashiorkor and marasmus[2-4]. The characteristic features of kwashiorkor are growth retardation, oedema and obvious mental changes which include apathy and irritability. Some degree of muscle wasting is almost always present. These, in addition to low levels of serum albumin, constitute the minimum diagnostic criteria. Other features which are variable, include changes in the hair and skin, hepatosplenomegaly, anaemia, diarrhoea and signs of associated vitamin deficiency, particularly of vitamin A and B complex vitamins. Hair changes include sparseness, dyspigmentation and easy pluckability. Changes often seen in the skin are dryness, scaliness and the more severe flaky dermatosis and crazy pavement dermatosis.

The cardinal features of marasmus are severe growth retardation, marked loss of subcutaneous tissue, muscle wasting and an absence of oedema. Levels of serum albumin are normal or only marginally reduced. Skin and hair changes are infrequent. Associated vitamin deficiencies are, however, seen. In addition to these differences in clinical manifestations, the biochemical profile in marasmus has been shown to be different from that in kwashiorkor[5, 6, 8]. Another major difference between the two conditions is the extensive fatty infiltration which is invariably seen in kwashiorkor, and characteristically absent in marasmus.

Evolution

It has long been held that these two clinical syndromes are separate entities arising as a result of differences in the protein–calorie ratio of the habitual diet. It has been believed that kwashiorkor arises from consuming diets which are predominantly deficient in protein with normal or near normal calorie content, and that marasmus is due to the consumption of diets which provide adequate protein but which are low in calories. It is possible to produce syndromes somewhat similar to these in experimental animals, by the dietary manipulation of protein and calorie in the diet. There is no evidence that these dietary situations, in fact, are responsible for the development of these clinical features in man.

An observation of considerable importance which has been made during the last decade is that the primary limiting nutrient in the diets of children among whom PEM is widespread, is not protein as was hitherto believed, but energy. This is particularly so in situations where cereals form the staple food and some legumes enter the diets[7]. In situations where roots and tubers and bananas constitute the staple food, primary insufficiency of protein in the diet can exist. The central feature in large parts of the developing world, where PEM is a problem, is thus an inadequate intake of food whose protein content is satisfactory but with a consequent deficit in energy intake. As a result of these findings, the earlier theory of two separate dietary aetiologies for kwashiorkor and marasmus has been questioned. It is now proposed that both groups of children suffer from primary calorie inadequacy and secondary protein deficiency, and that the ability to successfully adapt to the nutritional stress determines the clinical outcome and manifestations[8,9].

Hormones have an important role to play in the process of adaptation, with the adrenal hormones having a central role. It was postulated that in response to the stress of inadequate protein and calories, the adrenal cortex would secrete increased amounts of cortisol and that as a consequence, muscle protein would break down releasing amino acids. These amino acids would then be taken up and utilized preferentially by organs with a high rate of protein turnover such as the liver, pancreas and the intestines. Thus, visceral integrity would be maintained at the expense of muscle – a situation characteristic of marasmus. Failure of adequate breakdown of muscle due to sub-optimal response of the adrenal cortex could lead to a breakdown of the adaptation mechanism leading to kwashiorkor.

Determination of the hormonal profile has indeed lent strong support to this hypothesis. Levels of plasma cortisol are elevated both in kwashiorkor and marasmus, but to a much greater extent in marasmus[10,11]. The response of the adrenal cortex to corticotropin has been found to be exaggerated in marasmus and not in kwashiorkor[11]. Levels of plasma growth hormone are raised in kwashiorkor[12,13] and not in marasmus[13], and following a stimulus, levels further increase in kwashiorkor while no changes are seen in marasmus[13]. The action of growth hormone on cartilage is known to be mediated through somatomedins which are generated in the liver. Levels of circulating somatomedins are depressed in kwashiorkor, but normal in marasmus[14] – an observation in line with the observation made earlier with respect to several other proteins of hepatic origin. Most of the biochemical differences between kwashiorkor and marasmus can be explained on the basis of differences in their hormonal profile.

However, the nature of factors which contribute to the breakdown of the adaptation needs to be further explored. An abrupt and drastic reduction in the quantity of food consumed, which is already low, may be a factor. Repeated attacks of infection in quick succession may be another.

MILD AND MODERATE FORMS OF
PROTEIN ENERGY MALNUTRITION
Growth retardation

As indicated earlier, the severe forms of the disease are seen in 1–3 % of the child population, but the mild–moderate forms are seen in a much higher proportion. Growth status as judged by anthropometry has been widely used to assess nutritional status of children. Among measurements most frequently used are height, weight, arm circumference and skin fold thickness at selected sites of the body. Using these measurements and also indices derived from them, a variety of classifications have been developed to grade and quantitate malnutrition[15–17]. The method most widely used is the Gomez classification which makes use of the extent of deficit in weight for age[18]. Other more elaborate methods employed are those wherein weight for height, the extent of wasting, presence or absence of oedema are also considered[19].

Growth standards

Two widely used reference values for height and weight are the Boston standards for American children[20] and the Tanner figures for the UK[21]. The validity of the use of either set of figures for children in developing countries has often been raised. Data now available from some of the developing countries, where PEM is widespread, on the pattern of physical growth of children belonging to the privileged groups where there are no nutritional and environmental constraints, show that they are essentially similar to those of the Boston and Tanner standards[22-26]. Although growth status is extensively used to measure nutritional status, the validity of this concept may be questioned, particularly in the case of mild–moderate PEM. There are several studies in severely malnourished children which show that several biochemical and functional parameters are altered. Similar data on children suffering from the mild–moderate forms are scanty. The results of a few recent studies have shown that in mild–moderate PEM, intestinal absorption of xylose, fat and vitamin B_{12} is normal[27]. Antibody responses to several bacterial antigens were found unaltered[28]. Phagocytosis by leukocytes and the cell-mediated immune response were normal in the mild forms and impaired only in a small proportion of the moderate forms[28]. This was also true of the secretory immunoglobulins in several body fluids. These observations suggest that the functional status in mild–moderate PEM may not be seriously impaired. This is obviously an area where more information must be obtained, and there is need to investigate on a global basis the relationship that exists between growth retardation and vital body functions including mental function. It is also important to determine the functional status of different types of growth retardation, particularly of nutritional dwarfs who seem to constitute a high proportion of malnourished children.

AETIOLOGY OF PROTEIN ENERGY MALNUTRITION

Protein energy malnutrition is an outcome of the interaction of several factors, predominant among which are a dietary insufficiency of proteins and calories and repeated infective episodes. Economic factors leading to poor family purchasing capacity is of prime importance. There has been, in the past, a tendency to overemphasize the role of protein inadequacy in the development of the disease. It has now been recognized that in parts of the world where cereals, millets and legumes are included in habitual diets, the primary inadequacy is energy and not protein, despite dietary protein being of vegetable origin. Analyses of such diets have shown that if consumed in amounts sufficient to meet energy needs, protein requirements would be more than met. This, however, is not to say that there is no protein inadequacy in children. Almost a fourth to a third of children in communities, where PEM is seen, consume quantities of diet which are low enough to lead to a situation where both protein and calorie intakes are inadequate.

Apart from inadequate food intake, repeated infections, particularly of the gastrointestinal and respiratory systems constitute a major cause for the development of PEM. The precipitating effects of infectious diseases such as measles, whooping cough, chicken pox, tuberculosis and diarrhoeas in the development of kwashiorkor have been well documented. In addition to the metabolic effects of such infections which tend to raise nutrient requirements, reduced food intake during and after the infection due to loss of appetite, and also to culturally determined feeding practices during sickness, considerably influence ultimate nutritional status. In addition, the lack of minimal and timely medical care are important additional contributory factors.

. Delayed introduction of food supplements to infants and young children, faulty feeding practices including inadequate amounts being given because of lack of knowledge, large family size with short inter-pregnancy intervals are also among the important aetiological factors.

ASSOCIATED DEFICIENCIES

Severe forms of PEM usually show signs of vitamin deficiencies, which vary depending upon the dietary pattern. Signs of vitamin A deficiency – particularly the serious forms involving the cornea – leading to irreversible blindness is the most widespread. Iron deficiency anaemia of moderate severity is a common associated feature. Signs of B-complex vitamin deficiencies such as glossitis, cheilosis and angular stomatitis are not uncommon.

BIOCHEMICAL CHANGES

A number of biochemical changes in the blood, endocrine glands and tissues have been described in PEM, and there are several excellent reviews dealing with these changes[29, 30]. All of them, however, concern changes seen in the severe forms. Important among the changes is the marked reduction in circulating levels of total proteins and albumin. As a rule, albumin levels are below 2.5 g/dl in kwashiorkor. Measurement of albumin levels is one of the most useful biochemical indicators, since it is easily performed and a reduction is a clear indication of protein energy inadequacy except in marasmus, where levels may be only marginally lowered. Together with changes in body weight, serum albumin level is a useful indicator of PEM.

Over the last two decades, there have been innumerable efforts made to identify simple, sensitive and reliable biochemical parameters which would help identify early stages of PEM. Among indices looked for have been alterations in the ratio of essential to non-essential amino acids in plasma, hydroxyproline index – the ratio of hydroxyproline to creatinine per kg body weight excreted in urine, 3-methyl histidine in urine, transferrin, ceruloplasmin, prealbumin and a host of circulating enzymes. None of these has been found to satisfy the criteria of being both reliable and sensitive.

TREATMENT

The treatment of mild PEM calls for the administration of an adequate diet and control of infection, which can be done at home. The severe forms need hospitalization, particularly if there are complications such as dehydration, electrolyte imbalance and severe infection.

Diets containing skimmed milk as the source of protein have been extensively used in the past with success in the dietary management of kwashiorkor and marasmus. It is now accepted that diets based exclusively on vegetable protein sources are almost as effective as those containing skimmed milk[31, 32]. Legumes and oilseeds, particularly Bengal gram (*Cicer aeritinum*) and peanut (*Arachis hypogea*) have been extensively used. Also, a mixture of three parts of vegetable protein and one part of milk protein brings about clinical and biochemical responses identical with those seen with milk protein alone. Optimal responses are usually achieved with diets[33, 34] which provide 150–200 calories and 3–4 g protein (kg body weight)$^{-1}$. To provide such high levels of calories, without unduly increasing the bulk, it is necessary to include fairly large amounts of fat in the diet. Contrary to earlier held beliefs, it is now known that even severely malnourished children tolerate dietary fat well. As much as 30–40 % of total calories have been fed as fats. With the institution of dietary therapy and control of infection, the response is quite rapid. Most children shed their oedema within 8–10 days, serum albumin levels show a clear increase by this time and the acute manifestations are usually reversed by the 3rd or 4th week; although at this time, they are still far from being normal. Failure to control infections is often associated with a delay in the clinical and biochemical responses.

Kwashiorkor can be treated successfully with oral feeding alone. The use of plasma, whole blood, amino acid mixtures and protein hydrolysates are not only not associated with improvement either in the rate of recovery or survival, but carry an element of risk due to adverse side-effects. Their use is now severely restricted to children who are in a moribund state and who are in a state of dehydration and shock.

Mortality during treatment varies considerably depending upon age, duration of illness, severity of the disease and presence of complications. With adequate hospitalized care, mortality rates can be kept to around 15 %.

SEQUELAE OF PROTEIN ENERGY MALNUTRITION

With the increase in the number of children who survive even the severe forms of PEM, there has been a growing concern about the longterm effects of early childhood malnutrition. A number of studies in experimental animals have shown that even moderate malnutrition during critical phases of growth and development in early life, if persistent, can lead to permanent and irreversible physical and functional deficits in later life. Among the late effects are those related to physical size, physical work capacity and work output and mental development. However, there have been limited studies on the subsequent growth of children who had recovered from kwashiorkor. Increments in height and weight of such children, appeared not to be different from those seen in matched children who had not suffered the acute, severe episode of malnutrition[35, 36]. Although it has been suggested that long continued marginal malnutrition is responsible for the permanent stunting of growth seen in developing countries[37], there have been very few studies of a longitudinal nature where young children from communities whiċh have a high rate of PEM, have been followed into adult life. The results of a recent follow-up study of large numbers of children whose nutritional experience during childhood was known, have shown that the height at 5 years of age significantly influences adult height, and children who had experienced malnutrition in early life had short statures in later life[38]. In this study there were no interventions to correct the nutritional situation. The important question as to whether there would have been catch-up growth, had there been the necessary inputs, cannot, therefore, be answered.

Some recent studies on maximum work capacity as well as work output in actual life situations have shown that both are related to body weight, lighter subjects performing less well than do heavier subjects. However, expressed in terms of unit body weight differences tended to disappear[39–42]. These findings suggest that malnutrition during childhood may affect work capacity in adult life through its influence on body size and not through qualitative changes.

Of equal or even greater concern has been the suggestion that malnourished children may lack the ability to fully express their intellectual potential. This aspect of childhood malnutrition has been intensively investigated during the last decade and much of the information available in man has recently been comprehensively reviewed[43, 44]. Among parameters used in these studies have been head circumference, brain weight, special techniques to study intracranial contents, biochemical analysis of brain to determine cell number and cell size, lipid content and lipid profile, intellectual performance and neurointegrative competence. It has been demonstrated that severe PEM during early childhood is associated with biochemical changes in the brain and more importantly with function. Disturbances in neurological and psychological functions have been documented both during the acute state and during the recovery period. Children who have completely recovered from kwashiorkor when examined several years later have shown impaired cognitive development and neurointegrative competence, when compared with their siblings or with children of similar socioeconomic status who had not had the severe acute episode. The association between altered mental capacity and the less severe forms of PEM is controversial and far from clear. Although this association between malnutrition and impaired mental function is believed to be causal, there is as yet no conclusive evidence that it is in fact so and even if they are causally related, the extent to which malnutrition contributes to poor intellectual performance is not known with any degree of certainty. This is because malnutrition invariably occurs in the context of poor physical and intellectual environment, and dietary inadequacy forms only a part of the potentially detrimental environment to cognitive development. Non-nutritional factors are now believed to contribute to an unknown but significant extent to the poor intellectual function of malnourished children. These include the loss of learning time, interference with learning during critical periods, family environment with particular reference to mother–child interactions and the extent of stimulation which the child receives. There are several well designed prospective studies currently in progress in several parts of the world and their results may be expected to provide important information on the interrelationship between childhood malnutrition and mental function.

Whether the impaired mental function seen in malnourished children is permanent or can be reversed, has also been a subject of considerable controversy. Longterm follow-up studies on children who had completely recovered from acute severe PEM have shown conflicting results – some studies showing an improvement and some not. In most situations, the severely malnourished children have gone back to the unsatisfactory environment which predisposes to both malnutrition and poor mental development. It has very recently been suggested that if children with severe PEM receive adequate intellectual stimulation during and after recovery, their mental performance shows considerable improvement.

The extensive fatty changes which are characteristic of kwashiorkor at the height of the disease, and the high incidence of liver cirrhosis in adults in areas where PEM is a major public health problem, had, in the past led to the speculation that adult cirrhosis may be a sequel of severe childhood malnutrition. Longterm follow-up studies of children in different parts of the world who had recovered from kwashiorkor have conclusively shown that this is not so[45-47].

CONTROL AND PREVENTION

PEM has a multifaceted aetiology with several factors acting in a synergistic manner. It should not be viewed as a mere nutritional deficiency disorder, which can be corrected simply by providing more food, although this is a prerequisite. Most causes of PEM are in some way or other related to underdevelopment, such as poor living conditions, unsatisfactory environmental sanitation and personal hygiene, lack of primary health care and ignorance. Programmes aimed at the control and prevention of PEM must take into account all these factors.

Among dietary practices which have an important bearing on the widespread prevalence of PEM in late infancy and early childhood, is the delayed introduction of supplementary foods, because of the wrong belief among many mothers that as long as the child is receiving some breast milk its nutritional needs are met. It is essential to encourage breast feeding for as long as possible; at the same time communities must be encouraged to introduce additional foods around the 6th month of life. In many parts of the developing world, foods suitable for infant feeding have now been developed using exclusively indigenous foods, which can be processed at the home level. There are usually mixtures of cereals and legumes with or without milk which are nutritionally balanced and not expensive. Bulk is often cited as a problem in the feeding of the young child mainly because their diets have a low calorie density, and enough food is not consumed to meet the protein and calorie needs. This can be overcome by increasing the fat content of the diet which would raise the calorie density. In several countries where PEM is widespread, dietary fat is an expensive article of food and beyond the reach of the poor. By increasing the frequency of feeding of the young child, it is possible to satisfy his nutrient needs without altering the calorie density. Creating awareness of these factors among rural mothers may be expected to reduce, at least partly, the extent of the problem.

Control of infection is an important aspect in the control and prevention of PEM. Immunization programmes are effective against a limited number of childhood diseases, but unfortunately, there is no immunization against diarrhoeal disease, which is perhaps the most important single infection in influencing PEM. They have to be prevented by improving the sanitary conditions, making available adequate water supplies and treating the attacks as early as possible.

In addition to other measures, surveillance of children at risk is important in the control and prevention of PEM.

References

1. DeMaeyer, E. M. (1976). Protein energy malnutrition. In Beaton, G. H. and Bengoa, J. M. (eds.). *Nutrition in Preventive Medicine.* pp. 23–54 (World Health Organization, Geneva)
2. Trowell, H. C., Davies, J. N. P. and Dean, R. F. A. (1954). *Kwashiorkor* (London: Edward Arnold)
3. Gopalan, C. and Ramalingaswami, V. (1955). Kwashiorkor in India. *Ind. J. Med. Res.,* **43,** 751
4. Waterlow, J. C., Craviato, J. and Stephen, J. M. L. (1960). Protein malnutrition in man. In Anfinsen, C. B., Anson, M. L., Baily, K. and Edsall, J. T. (eds.). *Advances in Protein Chemistry.* **15,** 131 (London: Academic Press)
5. Srikantia, S. G., Jacob, C. M. and Reddy, V. (1964). Serum enzyme levels in protein calorie malnutrition. *Am. J. Dis. Child.,* **107,** 256
6. Whitehead, R. G. (1968). Biochemical changes in kwashiorkor and marasmus. In McCance, R. A. and Widdowson, E. M. (eds.). *Calorie Deficiencies and Protein Deficiencies.* p. 109 (London: Churchill)
7. Gopalan, C. and Narasinga Rao, B. S. (1971). Nutritional constraints on growth and development in current Indian dietaries. *Proc. Nutr. Soc. India,* **10,** 111
8. Gopalan, C. (1968). Kwashiorkor and marasmus: Evolution and distinguishing features. In McCance, R. A. and Widdowson, E. M. (eds.) *Calorie Deficiencies and Protein Deficiencies,* p. 49 (London: Churchill)
9. Jaya Rao, K. S. (1974). Evolution of kwashiorkor and marasmus. *Lancet,* **1,** 709
10. Alleyene, G. A. O. and Young, V. H. (1966). Adrenal function in malnutrition. *Lancet,* **1,** 911
11. Jaya Rao, K. S., Srikantia, S. G. and Gopalan, C. (1968). Plasma cortisol levels in protein calorie malnutrition. *Arch. Dis. Child.,* **43,** 365
12. Pimstone, B. L., Wittmann, W., Hansen, J. D. L. and Murray, P. (1966). Growth hormone and kwashiorkor: Role of protein in growth hormone homeostasis. *Lancet,* **2,** 779
13. Raghuramulu, N. and Jaya Rao, K. S. (1974). Growth hormone secretion in protein calorie malnutrition. *J. Endocrinol. Metab.,* **38,** 176
14. Mohan, P. S. and Jaya Rao, K. S. (1979). Plasma somatomedin activity in protein energy malnutrition. *Arch. Dis. Child.* (In press)
15. Jelliffe, D. B. (1966). The assessment of the nutritional status of a community. *WHO Monograph Series* **53,** Geneva
16. Classification of infantile malnutrition (1970). *Lancet,* **2,** 302
17. Seoane, N. and Latham, M. C. (1971). Nutritional anthropometry in the identification of malnutrition in children. *J. Trop. Pediatr. Environ. Hlth.,* **17,** 98

18. Gomez, F., Galvan, R. R., Frenk, S., Munoz, J. C., Chavez, R. and Vazquez, J. (1956). Mortality in second and third degree malnutrition. *J. Trop. Pediatr.*, **2,** 77
19. Waterlow, J. C. (1976). Classification and definition of protein energy malnutrition. In Beaton, G. H. and Bengoa, J. M. (eds.). *Nutrition in Preventive Medicine.* (Geneva: WHO)
20. Stuart, H. C. and Stevenson, S. S. (1959). In Nelson, W. E. (ed.) *Textbook of Pediatrics.* (Philadelphia: Saunders)
21. Tanner, J. M., Whitehouse, R. H. and Takaishi (1966). Standards from birth to maturity for height, weight, height velocity and weight velocity. *Arch. Dis. Child.*, **41,** 613
22. Asheroft, M. T. and Lovell, H. G. (1974). The heights and weights of Jamaican children of various racial origins. *Trop. Geogr. Med.*, **16,** 346
23. Vijayaraghavan, K., Darshan Singh and Swaminathan, M. C. (1971). Heights and weights of wellnourished Indian children. *Ind. J. Med. Res.*, **59,** 648
24. Villarejos, V. M., Osborne, J. A., Payne, F. P. and Arguedas, V. J. A. (1971). Heights and weights of children in urban and rural Costa Rica. *J. Trop. Pediatr. Environ. Chld. Hlth.*, **17,** 31
25. Amirhakimi, G. H. (1974). Growth from birth to two years of rich urban and poor rural Iranian children compared with Western norms. *Ann. Hum. Biol.*, **1,** 427
26. Habicht, J. P., Martorell, R., Yarbrough, C., Malina, R. M. and Klein, R. E. (1974). Height and weight standards for preschool children: How relevant are ethnic differences in growth potential? *Lancet*, **1,** 611
27. Reddy, V. and Mammi, M. V. I. (1976). Intestinal function in malnourished children. *J. Trop. Pediat. Environ. Child Hlth.*, **22,** 3
28. Reddy, V., Jagadeesan, V., Raghuramulu, N., Bhaskaram, C. and Srikantia, S. G. (1976). Functional significance of growth retardation in malnutrition. *Am. J. Clin. Nutr.*, **29,** 3
29. Waterlow, J. C. and Alleyene, G. A. O. (1971). Protein malnutrition in children: Advances in knowledge in the last ten years. In Anfinsen, C. B., Edsall, J. T. and Richards, F. M. (eds.). *Advances in Protein Chemistry*, **25,** 117 (London: Academic Press)
30. Whitehead, R. G. and Alleyene, G. A. O. (1971). Pathophysiological factors of importance in protein calorie malnutrition. *Br. Med. Bull.*, **28,** 72
31. Dean, R. F. A. (1953). Plant proteins in child feeding. *Med. Res. Coun. Spl. Rep. Ser.*, **279** (London: HM Stationery Office)
32. Srikantia, S. G. (1969). Protein malnutrition in Indian children. *Ind. J. Med. Res.*, **57** (Suppl.), 36
33. Waterlow, J. C. (1961). The rate of recovery of malnourished infants in relation to the protein and calorie levels of the diet. *J. Trop. Pediatr.*, **7,** 16
34. Srikantia, S. G., Venkatachalam, P. S., Reddy, V. and Gopalan, C. (1964). Protein and calorie needs in kwashiorkor. *Ind. J. Med. Res.*, **52,** 1104
35. Briers, P. J., Hoorweg, J. and Stanfield, J. P. (1975). The long-term effects of protein energy malnutrition in early childhood on bone age, bone cortical thickness and height. *Acta Paed. Scand.*, **64,** 853
36. Srikantia, S. G. (1979). Repercussions of early malnutrition in later intellectual development. In Brozek, J. (ed.) *Behavioural Effect of Energy and Protein Deficits.* Proceedings of an International Conference (In press)
37. Alleyne, G. A. O., Hay, R. W., Picou, D. I., Stanfield, J. and Whitehead, R. G. (1977). The long-term effects of protein energy malnutrition on growth and development. In *Protein Energy Malnutrition.* p. 122 (London: Edward Arnold)
38. Satyanarayana, K., Naidu, A. N. and Narasinga Rao, B. S. (1979). Nutritional deprivation in childhood and the body size, activity and physical work capacity of young boys. *Am. J. Clin. Nutr.* (In press)
39. Areskog, N. H., Selinus, R. and Vahlquist, B. (1969). Physical work capacity and nutritional status in Ethiopean male children and young adults. *Am. J. Clin. Nutr.*, **22,** 471
40. Davies, C. T. M. (1973). Physiological response to exercise in East African children. II. The effects of schistosomiasis, anaemia and malnutrition. *Environ. Child Hlth.*, **19,** 115
41. Satyanarayana, K., Naidu, A. N., Chatterjee, B. and Narasinga Rao, B. S. (1977). Body size and work output. *Am. J. Clin. Nutr.*, **30,** 322
42. Satyanarayana, K., Naidu, A. N. and Narasinga Rao, B. S. (1978). Nutrition, physical work capacity and work output. *Indian J. Med. Res.*, **68** (Suppl.) 88
43. Dodge, R. P., Prensky, A. L. and Feign, R. D. (1975). Influence of protein calorie malnutrition of the human nervous system. In *Nutrition and the Developing Nervous System.* p. 205 (St Louis: C. V. Mosby)

44. Pollit, E. and Thomson, C. (1977). Protein calorie malnutrition and behaviour: A view from psychology. In Wurtman, R. J. and Wurtman, J. J. (eds.). *Nutrition and the Brain*, 2, 261 (New York: Raven Press)
45. Higginson, J., Grobbelaar, M. B. and Walker, A. R. P. (1957). Hepatic fibrosis and cirrhosis in man in relation to malnutrition. *Am. J. Pathol.*, 33, 29
46. Suckling, P. V. and Campbell, J. A. H. (1957). A five year follow up of coloured children with kwashiorkor in Cape Town. *J. Trop. Pediatr.*, 2, 173
47. Srikantia, S. G., Sriramachari, S. and Gopalan, C. (1958). A follow up study of fifteen cases of kwashiorkor. *Indian J. Med. Res.*, 46, 121

8
Endemic pellagra

S. G. SRIKANTIA

INTRODUCTION

Pellagra is a nutritional disorder associated with nicotinic acid deficiency. Since the essential amino acid tryptophan can be converted by man into nicotinic acid, the dietary intakes of both nicotinic acid and tryptophan assume importance in the development of pellagra. More recently, it has been suggested that the disease may be due to an amino acid imbalance leading to conditioned niacin deficiency. All cases of pellagra, however, can be cured by the administration of nicotinic acid, clearly showing that it is a disease of nicotinic acid inadequacy.

EPIDEMIOLOGY

As a clinical disease, pellagra was first reported in Spain by Casal in the middle of the 18th century. The disease occurred in epidemic form in parts of southern Europe, North Africa, Latin American countries, the southern United States, Egypt and India. Because of its widespread occurrence in epidemic proportions, pellagra was considered to be an infectious disease. During the early part of this century, the dietary aetiology of the disease was established when Goldberger[1] showed that it occurs only among the poor and malnourished segments of the population, whose staple diet is maize, and that it could be cured by the inclusion of flesh foods or by yeast in the diet. Pellagra was also at one time believed to be a protein deficiency disease, until it was shown that protein free liver extracts containing what was termed as 'pellagra preventing factor' (PP) could cure pellagra. The PP was subsequently identified as nicotinic acid[2]. It was later that the ability of mammalian tissues to convert dietary tryptophan to nicotinic acid was discovered – an observation which could explain the curative and preventive effect of large amounts of protein. Pellagra has been experimentally produced in man on diets low in niacin and tryptophan[3].

The global incidence of the disease is on the decline and it has almost completely disappeared from Europe and USA, although it is still reported

209

from several countries in the Middle East and from some Asian countries. Even in these areas, it no longer occurs in epidemic form, but in endemic foci, particularly in rural areas where it constitutes a public health problem. It occurs predominantly among agricultural labourers, whose diets are generally unsatisfactory. It is a disease of adults and is rarely seen in infants and children below the age of 12 years, for reasons as yet unknown. The disease is more frequently seen in men than in women.

Pellagra has a strong seasonal incidence, it being considerably higher during the cool winter months than during the rest of the year, although in some countries, it is reported to occur during summer. Seasonal variations in the pattern of food availability and consumption have been held responsible, but these alone do not explain fully the clear-cut seasonal trend.

AETIOLOGY

Pellagra has traditionally been associated with diets wherein maize is the staple food. In the past, epidemics of pellagra have spread following the cultivation of maize and have disappeared when maize in the diet was replaced with wheat. During the last two decades, endemic pellagra has been reported to occur in India among populations whose staple food is sorghum (a similar grain to maize) and whose diets do not contain any maize[4]. Such a situation has also been found in Egypt[5]. Pellagra among maize eaters has been ascribed to two major factors. Although maize contains a good amount of niacin, it exists in a bound form and thus is not biologically available; but it can be made available by hydrolysis with either sodium hydroxide or lime water[6]. Maize is a poor source of tryptophan and this along with niacin being in a bound form, therefore, leads to a niacin deficiency. In experimental pellagra, the disease has been found to develop more rapidly and is more severe with corn diets than with wheat diets, which contain similar levels of niacin and tryptophan[7]. Also, the disease develops more readily with whole corn than with degerminated corn[8]. Development of pellagra on sorghum diets is difficult to explain, since it contains niacin in an available form and its tryptophan content is not low[9]. Therefore, factors responsible for the development of pellagra on maize diets do not operate in the case of sorghum. A feature common to both sorghum and maize grain is the high concentration of the essential amino acid leucine; it constitutes over 12% of the protein in both, as compared to a level of below 8% in other staple foods[4]. A series of biochemical and experimental studies have shown that excess dietary leucine is related to the development of the disease. These studies have been reviewed in recent publications[10,11]. The administration of leucine to normal human volunteers has been found to alter the pattern of excretion of tryptophan–niacin metabolites in urine, inhibit the synthesis of nicotinamide nucleotides[12,13] which are the functional forms of nicotinic acid, and to modify the metabolism of serotonin[7] (5-hydroxytryptamine).

Changes in the pattern of urinary excretion of niacin metabolites have not been found by other workers[14,15]. This may be due to differences in experimental procedures including the nature of the diet, natural versus amino acid mixtures, the tryptophan content and the protein content of the experimental diets. Also, using baby chicks and weanling rats the addition of supplementary leucine did not exacerbate the development of niacin deficiency when they were fed diets containing low levels of niacin and tryptophan[16]. Essentially similar findings were made when these studies were extended to dogs[16a]. The reasons as to why other workers have not been able to confirm that excess intake of dietary leucine may influence nicotinic acid deficiency are not clear. It is possible, and has been suggested, that this relates to a special set of conditions rather than to be a generally reproducible phenomenon[16a].

Black tongue has been produced in pups maintained on sorghum based diets[17] and by feeding casein based diets to which leucine was added[18]. Casein based diets by themselves are not pellagragenic. It has been suggested that even in pellagra seen amongst maize eaters, excess dietary leucine may have a role, since pups fed the opaque-2 maize, whose protein has a leucine content of around $8 g\%$, did not develop black tongue in contrast to those fed the conventional varieties of maize whose protein contained over 12% leucine. The mere addition of leucine to opaque-2 maize made it pellagragenic[19].

Although maize is the staple food in Mexico and Central America, pellagra is less common in these areas. Maize is consumed here mainly as tortillas, after the millet has been subjected to treatment with lime water. This procedure is known to release some of the niacin which is present in the bound form, and it also causes some lowering of the leucine content. Apart from this, the consumption of coffee, which is a rich source of nicotinic acid, may also be responsible for the lower prevalence of the disease. A cup of coffee can contain between 1 and 3 mg of niacin, depending upon the darkness of the roast, the amount of coffee used and the method of preparation[20]. Niacin from coffee has been shown to be biologically available[21].

More recently, it has been reported that it is the leucine–isoleucine balance that may be more important in the pathogenesis of pellagra. Many of the biochemical changes seen with leucine supplements can be counteracted by the simultaneous administration of isoleucine[22,23], and even the clinical manifestations could be controlled[24].

Results of studies undertaken to determine the site at which excess dietary leucine acts, leading to nicotinic acid deficiency and the subsequent development of pellagra, have shown that it depresses the activity of the enzyme – quinolinate phosphoribosyl transferase (QPRT) – a key enzyme in the synthesis of nicotinamide nucleotides from tryptophan[25]. The precise mechanism by which leucine inhibits QPRT is not known. However, this cannot be the whole explanation, since only a part of the nucleotides formed in the body are obtained through the tryptophan–niacin pathway.

Pellagra is not seen to the same extent in all areas where sorghum is the staple food, suggesting that factors other than the leucine–isoleucine balance may be involved in the pathogenesis of the disease. The pyridoxine status of the individual appears to be important in this respect. Leucine induced changes have been found to be largely prevented by the administration of vitamin B_6[26]. Pellagrin sufferers show biochemical evidence of vitamin B_6 deficiency, and their ability to clear leucine from plasma after a leucine load which is impaired is corrected by treatment with vitamin B_6[27].

Thus, the aetiology of pellagra appears to be more complex than was hitherto believed. Not only can it arise from a dietary inadequacy of niacin or its precursors, it can also be the result of an amino acid imbalance. Three essential amino acids – tryptophan, leucine and isoleucine – and two vitamins – niacin and vitamin B_6 – appear to be involved. Endemic pellagra may be the outcome of the interaction of these nutrients, and it is possible that future studies may reveal the participation of additional nutrients.

Apart from these nutrients, the regular consumption of alcohol is clearly related to the development of pellagra. In the Middle East, pellagra is associated with parastic disease, particularly schistosomiasis and intestinal helminthic infestations. Pellagra has been reported to be cured just by treating the infestation, without changing the diet[5].

CLINICAL FEATURES

Early symptoms of pellagra include weakness, easy fatiguability and several other non-specific complaints. Dermatitis, diarrhoea and dementia have in the past been considered as characteristic features. It is now recognised that of these manifestations, dermatitis is the diagnostic feature, since diarrhoea and dementia are variable clinical manifestations.

The skin lesions are typical of the disease. They are bilateral, symmetrical and occur on the exposed parts of the body, specially on the dorsal surfaces of the forearms, legs and feet. The head may or may not be affected. The neck and the exposed part of the chest are often involved (Casal's necklace). The lesion starts as an erythema, soon followed by scaling and exfoliation with the affected part showing areas of pigmentation and depigmentation. It is typical of the dermatitis that the demarcation between the normal and the affected skin is very clear cut. In chronic lesions, there is considerable hyperkeratosis of the affected area. In some cases, atypical areas of the skin do show pellagrous dermatitis.

Diarrhoea occurs in only a proportion of pellagrins, and in some constipation has been reported. Other gastro-intestinal manifestations include glossitis, cheilosis and angular stomatitis, which are usually due to associated deficiencies of other B-complex vitamins.

Symptoms relating to the central nervous system are variable and protean. A great majority have mental changes of a mild nature, which are often missed unless specifically looked for. Insomnia and apprehension are present in almost all and the insomnia is unrelated to the physical discomfort. Severe mental changes are seen in $1-2\%$ of hospital admitted cases, and include confusion, disorientation, hallucination, loss of memory and loss of orientation to space and time. Depression and severe paranoid symptoms can also occur. Pellagrins, who have mild skin lesions, but have severe mental changes, have sometimes been admitted to mental hospitals. Other changes related to the nervous system include paresthesias and peripheral neuritis.

BIOCHEMICAL BASIS OF THE CLINICAL MANIFESTATIONS

Skin changes

Although skin changes are diagnostic of pellagra, the biochemical basis of the dermatitis has not been adequately investigated. The results of limited studies have revealed that the skins of pellagrins show alterations of the collagen nitrogen content in the dermis, although there are no changes in the total nitrogen content[28]. This leads to a grossly reduced collagen to non-collagen ratio. Additionally, the amino acid profile of dermal protein has been found to be different from that seen in normal individuals, there being a reduction in the concentrations of hydroxyproline and arginine and an increase in aspartic acid, threonine, serine, methionine, leucine, isoleucine and phenylalanine[28]. The urocanic acid content of skin in pellagra sufferers is lower than that found in normal controls, due to a reduction both in the concentration of the precursor amino acid, histidine, and the activity of the enzyme – histidase[29]. Since urocanic acid acts as a trap for ultraviolet light, this reduction may have an aetiological role in the photosensitive rash.

Mental changes

As in the case of dermatitis, the biochemical basis of the altered mental status is not well understood. A study of the electroencephalographic (EEG) changes in pellagrins has shown that irrespective of whether or not obvious mental changes were present, EEG changes were present. Normal α-rhythm was absent in a great majority of pellagrins. Excess θ-activity and high voltage δ-activity were the other abnormalities[30]. Serotonin (5-hydroxytryptamine) is present in the brain in appreciable amounts, and there is enough evidence to show that it is one of the biogenic amines which modulates behaviour[31]. Pellagrins excrete low amounts of 5-hydroxyindole acetic acid (5-HIAA) – a metabolite of serotonin – in urine[11]. The serotonin content of platelets in pellagrins is low[32] as are the 5-HIAA levels in the cerebrospinal fluid[33], suggesting that serotonin metabolism is altered in pellagra. Brains of rats fed a sorghum diet had concentrations of serotonin well below those fed a casein diet[34]. Similarly, rats fed a diet containing an excess of leucine had lower levels of brain serotonin[34, 35]. These findings suggest that the mental changes in pellagra may, at least in part, be due to alterations in serotonin metabolism. This is an area where obviously more information is needed.

TREATMENT

The administration of nicotinic acid produces dramatic improvement. It is usually administered in doses of 300 mg daily (100 mg thrice a day) orally. Mental symptoms disappear quite rapidly — sometimes within hours, while the dermatitis takes a few days to show improvement. Intramuscular or intravenous administration is rarely needed, except in rare instances where severe mental changes warrant its use. A proportion of subjects show unpleasant side-effects such as flushing, nausea, vomiting, a burning sensation of skin and sometimes hypotension. Nicotinamide is equally effective and has fewer side-effects.

Since most pellagrins have associated B-complex vitamin deficiencies, it is desirable to administer these vitamins as well.

PREVENTION AND CONTROL

As long as maize and sorghum continue to be staple foods, and as long as the habitual diets do not contain sufficient amounts of protective foods, such as milk, meat, eggs and legumes, endemic pellagra will continue to be a public health problem. In the USA and Europe, pellagra has been controlled primarily for two reasons. Diets were diversified so that maize ceased to be the staple component, and in addition maize flour meals and grits and other items of foods were enriched with niacin. Both these approaches have limitations in developing countries where pellagra is endemic. The poorest segments of the population who are at risk, consume either maize or sorghum because it is the cheapest food. Often, agricultural labourers who are victims of the disease receive their wages not in cash but in kind – usually in the form of the cheapest food grain which is either maize or sorghum. Fortification or enrichment of foods with niacin is not a practical suggestion, since in rural areas food is eaten off the land and families mill their grains at home. It will be, therefore, difficult to replace sorghum and maize as the staple item in the diet; it will also be difficult in the near future to improve these diets because of economic and socio-cultural considerations. While these efforts to improve the quality of the diet as a whole have to continue, other avenues need to be explored. Since there is adequate evidence that in both sorghum and maize, high levels of leucine are aetiologically related to the development of the disease, efforts may be directed towards identifying and breeding varieties of these food grains with the necessary leucine–isoleucine balance. The existence of marked varietal differences in the chemical composition of food grains is well known and the opaque-2 maize has relevance in this context. Selective propagation of such varieties of sorghum and maize may, therefore, be one of the methods of controlling the problem. The advantage of this approach is that it does not call for either nutritional education or a change in dietary habits. In view of the fact that the genetic expression is considerably influenced by agricultural practices and location, it needs to be ascertained that the low leucine trait in maize is stable.

Pellagra can be prevented and cured by nicotinic acid even when the diet is otherwise pellagragenic. Most varieties of sorghum contain around 4 mg of nicotinic acid/100 g grain. Two Ethiopian varieties of sorghum have been reported to contain over 10 mg of the vitamin/100 g[36]. Both these varieties, however, are low yielders and have a shrivelled appearance with poor consumer acceptability. If the high nicotinic acid trait of these varieties can be transferred to varieties now most widely cultivated, some impact can be made on preventing endemic pellagra. Thus, a combination of nutritional education, improvement in socioeconomic status leading to diversification in the habitual diet, and improvement in the nutritional quality of maize and sorghum with special reference to their amino acid make up and nicotinic acid contents would effectively control endemic pellagra.

References

1. Goldberger, J. and Wheeler, G. A. (1920). Experimental production of pellagra in human subjects by means of diet. *Hyg. Lab. Bull.*, **120**, 7
2. Elvehjem, C. A., Madden, R. J., Strong, F. M. and Woolley, D. W. (1937). Relation of nicotinic acid amide to canine black tongue. *J. Am. Chem. Soc.*, **59**, 1767
3. Goldsmith, G. A., Sarett, H. P., Register, U. D. and Gibbens, J. (1952). Studies on niacin requirement in man: 1. Experimental pellagra in subjects on corn diets low in niacin and tryptophan. *J. Clin. Invest.*, **31**, 533
4. Gopalan, C. and Srikantia, S. G. (1960). Leucine and pellagra. *Lancet*, **1**, 954
5. Barakat, M. R. (1947). Some of the problems of nutrition in Egypt. *J. Trop. Med. Hyg.*, **50**, 95
6. Kodicek, E. (1960). The availability of bound nicotinic acid to the rat. ii: The effect of treating maize and other materials with sodium hydroxide. *Br. J. Nutr.*, **14**, 13
7. Goldsmith, G. A., Rosenthal, H. L., Gibbens, J. and Unglaub, W. G. (1955). Studies of niacin requirement in man, ii: requirement of wheat and corn diets low in tryptophan. *J. Nutr.*, **56**, 371
8. Goldsmith, G. A., Gibbens, J., Unglaub, W. G. and Miller, O. N. (1956). Studies of niacin requirement in man, iii: Comparative effects of diets containing lime-treated and untreated corn in the production of experimental pellagra. *Am. J. Clin. Nutr.*, **4**, 151
9. Belavady, B. and Gopalan, C. (1966). Availability of nicotinic acid in jowar (*Sorghum vulgare*). *Ind. J. Biochem.*, **3**, 44
10. Gopalan, C. and Jaya Rao, K. S. (1975). Pellagra and amino acid imbalance. *Vitamins Horm.* (NY), **33**, 505
11. Srikantia, S. G. (1978). Endemic pellagra among jowar eaters. *Ind. J. Med. Res.*, **68** (Suppl), 38
12. Belavady, B., Srikantia, S. G. and Gopalan, C. (1963). The effect of oral administration of leucine on the metabolism of tryptophan. *Biochem. J.*, **87**, 652
13. Srikantia, S. G., Narasinga Rao, B. S., Raghuramulu, N. and Gopalan, C. (1968). Pattern of nicotinamide nucleotides in the erythrocytes of pellagrins. *Am. J. Clin. Nutr.*, **21**, 1306
14. Nakagawa, I., Ohguri, S., Sasaki, A., Kajimoto, M., Sasaki, M. and Takahashi, T. (1975). Effects of excess intake of leucine and valine deficiency on tryptophan and niacin metabolites in humans. *J. Nutr.*, **105**, 1241
15. Truswell, A. S., Goldsmith, G. A. and Pearson, W. N. (1963). Leucine and pellagra. *Lancet*, **1**, 778
16. Manson, J. A. and Carpenter, K. J. (1978). The effect of a high level of dietary leucine on the niacin status of chicks and rats. *J. Nutr.*, **108**, 1883
16a. Manson, J. A. and Carpenter, K. J. (1978). The effect of a high level of dietary leucine on the niacin status of dogs. *J. Nutr.*, **108**, 1889
17. Belavady, B. and Gopalan, C. (1965). Production of black tongue in dogs by feeding diets containing jowar (*Sorghum vulgare*). *Lancet*, **2**, 1220
18. Belavady, B., Madhavan, T. V. and Gopalan, C. (1967). Production of black tongue in pups fed diets supplemented with leucine. *Gastroenterology*, **5**, 749
19. Belavady, B. and Gopalan, C. (1969). The role of leucine in the pathogenesis of canine black tongue and pellagra. *Lancet*, **2**, 956
20. Goldsmith, G. A., Miller, O. N., Unglaub, W. G. and Kercheval, K. (1959). Human studies of biological activity of niacin in coffee. *Proc. Soc. Exp. Biol. Med.*, **102**, 579
21. Teply, L. J., Krehl, W. A. and Elvehjem, C. A. (1945). Studies on nicotinic acid content of coffee. *Arch. Biochem.*, **6**, 139
22. Kamala Krishnaswamy and Raghuram, T. C. (1972). Effect of leucine and isoleucine on brain serotonin in rats. *Life Sci.*, **11**, 1191
23. Belavady, B., Udayasekhara Rao, P. and Lateefa Khan (1973). Effect of leucine and isoleucine on nicotinamide nucleotides in erythrocytes. *Int. J. Vit. Nutr. Res.*, **43**, 442

24.   Kamala Krishnaswamy and Gopalan, C. (1971). Effect of isoleucine on skin and electroencephalogram in pellagra. *Lancet*, **2,** 1167

25.   Ghafoorunissa and Narasinga Rao, B. S. (1973). Effect of leucine on enzymes of the tryptophan–niacin metabolic pathway in rat liver and kidney. *Biochem. J.*, **134,** 425

26.   Kamala Krishnaswamy, Bapurao, S., Raghuram, T. C. and Srikantia, S. G. (1976). Effect of vitamin B_6 on leucine induced changes in human subjects. *Am. J. Clin. Nutr.*, **29,** 177

27.   Bapurao, S. and Kamala Krishnaswamy (1978). Vitamin B_6 nutritional status of pellagrins and their leucine tolerance. *Am. J. Clin. Nutr.*, **31,** 819

28.   Vasantha, L. (1970). Collagen content and dermal amino acid pattern in pellagra. *Clin. Chim. Acta*, **27,** 543

29.   Vasantha, L. (1970). Histidine, urocanic acid and histidine α-deaminase in the stratum corneum in pellagrins. *Ind. J. Med. Res.*, **58,** 1079

30.   Srikantia, S. G., Veeraraghava Reddy, M. and Kamala Krishnaswamy (1968). Electroencephalographic changes in pellagra. *Electroencephal. Clin. Neurophysiol.*, **25,** 386

31.   Woolley, D. W. and Shaw, E. N. (1957). Evidence for the participation of serotonin in mental processes. *Ann. N.Y. Acad. Sci.*, **66,** 649

32.   Kamala Krishnaswamy and Ramanamurthy, P. S. V. (1970). Mental changes and platelet serotonin in pellagrins. *Clin. Chem. Acta*, **27,** 301

33.   Raghuram, T. C. and Kamala Krishnaswamy (1975). Serotonin metabolism in pellagra. *Arch. Neurol.*, **32,** 708

34.   Ramanamurthy, P. S. V. and Srikantia, S. G. (1970). Effect of leucine on brain serotonin. *J. Neurochem.*, **17,** 27

35.   Yuwiler, A. and Geller, E. (1965). Serotonin depletion by dietary leucine. *Nature (London)*, **208,** 83

36.   Pant, K. C. (1975). High nicotinic acid content of two Ethiopian sorghum lines. *J. Agric. Food. Chem.*, **23,** 608

9
Nutritional eccentricities

J. H. YOUNG

Some years ago an imaginative promoter in the southern part of Illinois, USA, calling himself Silent George of Shawneetown, had a good thing going. Removing the labels from small cans of condensed milk, Silent George sprayed the cans with gold paint, then affixed new labels bearing the name Swamp Rabbit Milk[1]. The labels described the cans' contents as 'a balanced product for unbalanced people, rich in Vitamins J, U, M and P', indeed much richer in the last of these vitamins than beer or watermelon. Like many labels, these bore a warning, aimed at women, slyly suggesting the product's indications for use: Do not imbibe the potent fluid 'in (the) absence of your husband, sparring partner, boy friend, or running mate, as the action is fast and it is two jumps from a cabbage or lettuce picnic to a cruise down the Nile with your dream version of Mark Anthony.'

Southern Illinois is known as Little Egypt, so reference to the Nile may not have been inappropriate. Nonetheless, Silent George's audacity makes his Swamp Rabbit Milk seem a travesty on the traditional nostrum. Not so. The Shawneetown promoter intended his 'vitamins' to lure real customers, and at a dollar a can he was doing a land office business until agents of the State Department of Agriculture terminated his scheme. Silent George's gaudy if short-lived venture points toward three key propositions that may be borne in mind profitably when considering nutritional eccentricities.

First, from time immemorial what has been taken in through the mouth has far transcended nutriment. The milk of the swamp rabbit became the joy of sex. Food, like the air we breathe, but in a more complex and varied way, is an indispensable ingredient of life. Because of this, food inevitably mingles with other important ingredients in life's vast pot. Food has served as taboo, as poison, as potent marvel, as status symbol and as a handmaiden to beauty[2, 3]. Food has penetrated to the mysterious inner recesses of religion, has adorned patriotic banners, has fuelled speculation about proper personal behaviour and about the ideal society. 'For all people,' three psychiatrists have written, '... what goes into their mouths ... is very strongly associated with good and evil'[4]. Such diverse and powerful symbolic roles for food have been vulnerable to manipulation, sometimes earnest but misguided, at other times calculating and mischievous.

Second, folklore of ancient coinage may retain currency for centuries, even millennia. Cleopatra's Nile flowed fertilely in the Little Egypt of twentieth century Illinois, just as garlic, renowned in old Egypt for healing potency, has maintained its powers in popular thought from those remote pharaonic times into our own, helping enrich contemporary promoters[5-7]. Nor could Silent George's rabbit reference have been accidental in his marketing of a mating medicine. Eons of history remain firmly embedded in current quackery.

Third, if the very old teaches profitable lessons to the unorthodox, so does the very new. Although pseudoscience and science play by different rules, and pseudoscience constantly berates true science, nonetheless, the specious continually does the genuine the signal honour of apeing it. To promote his lactational fraud, Silent George flaunted the word 'vitamin'. Granted that proclaiming vitamin P an aphrodisiac is easier to establish than vitamin B_1 as a cure for beriberi, nonetheless, the glamour of 'vitamin' may embrace both P and B among a certain audience, to a quack's profit. Countless promoters, like Silent George, have, in fabricating images for their wares, fused with traditional folk beliefs those elements stolen from respected science.

Important constituents in the structure of popular ideas sustaining recent American nutritional eccentricities were laid down more than a century ago. Part of the vast reform movement associated in politics with Jacksonian democracy focused upon food. American eating habits of the time (late 18th–early 19th century) warranted criticism, but the thrust of attack and the purpose of remedial action went much further. Disturbed by changes in society being wrought by the first wave of industrialism and growing urbanization, hygiene reformers, reworking ancient ideas, saw in food a major means of salvation from the sins of too much civilization[8,9]. The more man had removed himself from a pure state of nature and had adopted an artificial mode of life, wrote Sylvester Graham, leading theorist of the movement, the more had disease afflicted him[10,11]. Reviving a diet resembling that consumed in the Garden of Eden would lead to health, vigour and the supposed longevity of Old Testament patriarchs[12]. Such a diet also promised enhanced intelligence, improved morals, and a less violent, more benevolent society. 'There is a far more intimate relation', Graham wrote, 'between the quality of bread and the moral character of a family than is generally supposed.'

What Graham meant by 'the food of the first family and the first generations of mankind' he summed up as 'Fruits, nuts, farinaceous seeds, and roots, with perhaps some milk, and it may be honey'[12]. No 'artificial preparation' had been required beyond shelling the nuts. Graham and like-minded reformers condemned meat, alcohols, tea, coffee, salt and spices. They criticized overeating, castigated hotel and steamboat cuisine, put great stress on extensive mastication and daily bowel movements, and bemoaned the cruelty of slaughtering animals for flesh food. They deemed grain a more efficient utilization of land than livestock, and worried about grain grown on exhausted soil which had been 'debauched' by fertilizer[9,11-13]. The use of '[f]louring mills and bolting-cloths, and ... innumerable culinary and other utensils' Graham condemned as inimical to man's digestion which God had created for a state of nature[12]. Bakery bread, even when not adulterated, served man poorly. Bread should be baked in the home, not by servants, but by loving mothers and wives. The best flour for the purpose, milled from wheat and unbolted, still bears Graham's name.

Graham and his 19th century allies and successors saw no conflict between Christian morality and emerging physiological science in relation to diet. As James C. Whorton recently has shown, the Grahamites turned that science into 'grist for an ideological mill', perusing it for items, sometimes torn from context, which seemed to substantiate their doctrines, and for items that required refutation or skewing so as to make them accord with Grahamite principles[13]. For example, Graham, to discredit meat, reinterpreted William Beaumont's data so as to turn Beaumont's conclusions completely around. While criticizing case studies offered by their opponents, Grahamites relied on enthusiastic vegetarian testimonials as experimental evidence. And they found reasons to excuse failures by Grahamites to live the promised hundred years – a necessity upon the death of Graham himself, who had reached 56 years of age. Graham and his peers, Whorton grants, grappled bravely with the 'great modern dilemma, the question of how to use science to improve the human condition without alienating man from nature in the process'. Yet, however laudable their goals, Grahamites did incalculable 'violence ... to logic and to science'.

These ideas lay close beneath the surface of the soil ready to crop up again and again as new worries developed about the state of an increasingly industrializing and urbanizing society, especially its ever more commercially processed food supply. Graham's doctrines influenced the dietary practices of new religious sects, such as the Seventh Day Adventists[14], and were borrowed to cloak commercial ventures. A hydrotherapist created the first cold breakfast cereal out of Graham flour, and that form of corn flakes later known as Post Toasties, invented in Battle Creek, centre of Adventist strength, first bore the name Elijah's Manna[11,15].

A major heir of Grahamite doctrines early in the 20th century, Bernarr Macfadden, preached about how to get back to nature in the city[16,17]. Although he had gone to grade school only briefly, Macfadden launched a magazine called *Physical Culture* and compiled an encyclopaedia to promote his version of nature's way to health. On the streets of New York City he exhibited his own muscled body as his most potent advertisement. Like Graham, Macfadden favoured exercise, regarded clothing with some suspicion, condemned 'the baneful habit of over-eating', and thought ill of meat and well of raw vegetables. The carrot became Macfadden's symbol.

Macfadden propagated his simple regimen during the same years that nutrition matured into a truly sophisticated field[18]. 'In 1900', Elmer McCollum has said, 'we were (still) almost blind to the relation of food to health.' Casimir Funk coined the word 'vitamine' in 1911, and by 1940, as a result of burgeoning research throughout the world, more than 40 vitamins and other nutrients had been proved necessary for an adequate diet in man, and a number had been synthesized. This 'newer knowledge of nutrition', as McCollum called it[19], did not remain secret from the popular press, in either article or advertising pages. Advertising techniques by the 1920s had just reached the stage to make the most of such a glorious opportunity[20]. 'Health' became a major marketing constituent of many traditional foods, a theme so distorted and exaggerated that Food and Drug Administration officials warned both industry and the public. Label claims, charged Commissioner Walter G. Campbell in 1929, led the consumer 'to believe that our ordinary diet is sorely deficient in such vital substances as vitamins and minerals, and that these so-called *health foods* are absolutely necessary to conserve life and health'[21]. The next year Campbell's deputy, Paul Dunbar, frankly told canners and wholesale grocers that '(t)he magic words *health giving* are today the most overworked and loosely applied in the advertising lexicon', and scolded those who marketed 'Jones' carrot bread or Smith's turnip breakfast food' with the claim that they contained 'all known vitamins'[22].

The word 'vitamin' had acquired a golden glamour. Yeast and chocolate bars – as well as turnip breakfast food – vaunted their vitamin content[23]. Cod liver oil, long a staple in the proprietary drug field, enjoyed a new vogue with the discovery that it was a source of vitamin D. So-called extracts of this oil were promoted, with false claims of vitamin value devoid of fishy taste. The vitamin pill came on the market, like Mastin's Vitamon Tablets, promising to 'Give You That Firm Flesh Pep'. The 'Zestful New Health Tonic' Vita-Pep guaranteed to 'Restore ... Youthful Vitality' with a mixture of vitamin B and sherry wine[24].

That time-tested promotional ploy which wedded ancient folk beliefs with modern scientific discoveries adapted itself to vitamins. Royal Lee, a non-practising dentist in Milwaukee, destined throughout a long career to meet the Food and Drug Administration a number of times in court, marketed Catalyn[25, 26]. Made of wheat bran, milk sugar, and epinephrine (adrenaline), Catalyn bore a label boasting potency in all vitamins from A through G, and claiming to cure high and low blood pressure, Bright's disease, dropsy, and goitre. When convicted for making false and fraudulent claims under the 1906 law, Lee modified his formula and moved his claims. The new formula contained wheat flour, wheat bran, milk sugar, powdered rice bran, powdered carrots, and glandular material[27, 28]. The claims – in no way abated – departed from the package and entered into circulars and pamphlets, which Lee shipped to dealers separately from the Catalyn with instructions to place such literature with the product at the point of sale. This ruse, the Circuit Court of Appeals for the Seventh District decided, violated the new Food, Drug, and Cosmetic Act passed by the US Congress in 1938. The joining of product and promotion at the end of their separate interstate journeys, the judges ruled, meant that labelling had accompanied product in the eyes of the law.

This stronger New Deal food and drug measure provided regulators with various weapons to combat nutritional deception. Yet the new law itself may be viewed as one of the host of factors responsible for an upsurge in the misleading promotion of vitamins and nutritional supplements that began about 1940, a boom, it seems fair to assert, that, despite constant criticism by responsible nutritionists and periods of intense regulatory attack, has accelerated ever since. The 1938 law aided nutritional quackery by making it seem a greener field for exploitation than were the more traditional forms of quackery[23]. As the FDA began to use its new powers to curtail long standing patent medicine abuses, besieged promoters escaped into what they deemed to be a less risky form of promotion.

Less risk stemmed in part from greater complexity. Too many essential food factors had been discovered for the layman to keep track of, and new ones turned up every now and then. The mathematics of adequate daily dosages beggared comprehension. The twisting and distorting of these circumstances by shrewd promoters proved easy to do. The basic premise of the newer nutrition could also be phrased so as to provoke alarm. Even while eating enough of what you usually ate, you might get sick. Your health lay hostage to food factors you could neither see nor taste. Without them, you could wither away or succumb to horrendous symptoms. To stay healthy, mysterious extras were required.

Worry about the adequacy of American food had been intensified by diet surveys of depression America – cited for years in the promotional pamphlets of health food vendors – and by food shortages[23] during World War 2. These concerns made people vulnerable to specious assurances from quacks. The unscrupulous could also traffic on the publicity associated with legitimate remedial ventures, like the war-spurred enrichment programme of bread and other grain products and the first 'Recommended Daily Allowances for Specific Nutrients,' issued in 1941 by the Food and Nutrition Board of the National Academy of Sciences/National Research Council.

Besides exploiting the newer nutrition, the growing breed of food supplement salesmen tapped the great mythical storehouse of ancient ideas about food, including elements of Grahamism which had retained currency in the folk mind. Refashioned to take account of 20th century circumstances, reiterated in uncountable repetitions in print and speech, a major nutritional myth came to underwrite commerce in the health food area[23, 29]. This mighty myth held that almost all disease resulted from improper diet, mainly because of poor eating habits and the abominable state of the standard food supply. Food bought at the grocery store lacked important elements having been grown on worn-out soil and over-processed by industry, and moreover, such food contained dangerous poisons stemming from chemical fertilizers and pesticides used in the cultivation, and from additives used in the processing. Even though a person did not have cancer or heart disease, indeed, though he might display no severe symptoms at all, food had nonetheless made him sick: he suffered from subclinical deficiencies. Weariness, tension, gloominess – a host of life's day-to-day difficulties and moods – were harbingers of catastrophic decline. Prevention and cure required remedial action – the consumption only of 'natural' foods grown by 'organic' farming[30, 31] – a special reliance on alfalfa, garlic, yoghurt, wheat germ, blackstrap molasses, or vinegar and honey, sometimes alone, sometimes in combinations – dosage with vitamins, mammoth quantities of those recognized by nutritional science as needed at lesser levels, and purported new ones, like Silent George's J, U, M and P. In the wake of Catalyn, many promoters entwined elements of the older folklore and the newer nutrition into single entities, sometimes containing dozens of ingredients[32].

Millions of Americans came to regard the new nutrition myth as truth. A social science survey of the health opinions and self-treatment practices of

American adults, sponsored by seven federal agencies and published in 1972, demonstrated the effectiveness with which the health food industry had got its message across[33]. In most facets of self-treatment, the study revealed, no coherent body of theory, true or false, dictated behaviour. Americans acted impulsively, practising a sort of 'rampant empiricism'. However, with respect to food faddism, different circumstances prevailed. Buyers of health foods did bolster their action with theory, and this apologia turned out to be essentially the same myth that promoters of nutritional wares had been trumpeting for years. Three out of four adult Americans were persuaded that no matter how nutritionally adequate their diet, using extra vitamins would imbue them with extra pep.

Little of the tremendous propaganda blitz that conditioned the public to the nutritional myth appeared in product labelling. The 1938 law made this legally hazardous. Even more devious approaches, as Royal Lee had discovered with Catalyn, might prove troublesome. One major effort to avoid difficulty relied on oral communication[23, 31]. This approach reduced risk of detection and put huckster face to face with potential customers. Two score or more lecturers took to the circuit, making speeches, sometimes holding classes, promoting books, kitchen gadgetry and a variety of packaged products. A much larger enterprise involved door-to-door salesmanship. Pioneered by the promoters of a vitamin, mineral, alfalfa, parsley and watercress mix called Nutrilite, who built up a force of 20 000 doorbell-ringing salesmen, this method of selling was later imitated in several major waves[23]. Nutri-Bio at its height enlisted a sales force of 75 000, outnumbering all employees of the Food and Drug Administration by 40 to 1. Nonetheless, the FDA won many cases in court, presenting evidence of outrageously false claims which had been tape recorded unbeknown to spieler or house-to-house salesman. In time such taping came to be considered an unwarranted invasion of privacy. Even in their heyday, recorders had caught only a few of the millions of fleeting words by which the nutritional myth became established.

During the 1960s the site of face-to-face encounters shifted. Sales in the home by itinerant agents declined as sales in health food stores accelerated. Such stores, a rarity in earlier decades, proliferated. Scarcely a shopping mall escaped without one. The boom was made possible by would be customers taking the initiative, and travelling to the place where what they wanted was kept in stock. To be sure, conversations with store employees might broaden the customer's horizons and expand his purchases. 'Health food stores', observed a food and drug official in California, 'are hotbeds of over-the-counter prescribing'[34]. But the customer's zeal had been provoked, or at least his curiosity aroused, before he entered the emporium's portal.

A vast flood of words proclaiming the nutritional myth poured over the American consumer, arousing his anxiety and urging him to modify his dietary ways. Talk shows featuring food-oriented gurus on radio and television became very popular[35]. If false and misleading claims went forth over the airways about a brand name product – a transgression Carlton Frederick was once guilty of[36] – regulatory officials could take action. But in most appearances no brand of vitamins or supplements was sold; counsel was merely given. To be sure, the publicity received from television booking could be counted upon to help fill in a lecturer's itinerary and to sell an author's books. In the wake of a major television appearance by one author it was claimed that 65 000 copies were sold of his book offering a nutritional approach to relieve arthritis[37]. It was the printed word that played the major role, not only in miseducating the broad public to the tenets of the myth, but also in misinforming which ancient botanicals or supposed new vitamins might be purchased for salvation[38]. Again, if the mention of specific brand names and certain trade practices converted books into labelling – as happened with a best-seller called *Calories Don't Count* – law officials might take the offenders to court. Otherwise the First Amendment's protection of free speech legitimately safeguarded expression of even the wildest pseudoscientific doctrines, and the boldest promises of life, health, and the pursuit of happiness to be derived from common foods and from uncommon vitamins. 'I have yet to know', Adelle Davis wrote in *Let's Get Well*, 'of a single adult to develop cancer who has habitually drunk a quart of milk daily'[39]. ' ... (I)n our view', John A. Richardson wrote in *Laetrile Case Histories*, 'cancer ... is a disease caused by a deficiency of vitamin B_{17}, pancreatic enzymes, or both'[40].

Dozens of books filled with distorted doctrine made their appearance. 'Diet books take up about 20 feet of shelf space', remarked a librarian in Seattle's main public library. 'They're among the most popular books we have[41],' A number of the diet books are issued by respectable publishers. Harcourt Brace Jovanovich published five books by Adelle Davis, all best-sellers, books sharply criticized by nutritional specialists for their inaccuracies, distortions, misuse of sources, and sometimes dangerous counsel[39, 42, 43]. Davis had been trained as a nutritionist herself. McGraw-Hill in 1975 issued a *Nutrition Almanac* which is on sale in many health food stores, naturally enough, because it contains references to and cites exaggerated claims without serious critique, for such vitamins, not credited by scientific nutrition, as B_{13}, B_{15}, T, U and P – this last one not Silent George's contribution but bioflavonoids[44]. Besides books, magazines have played a role in conveying the nutritional myth, special magazines like *Prevention* wholly focused upon food, and the sensationalist press particularly. Even magazines deemed most respectable occasionally include an article marred by nutritional distortions. When challenged, editors sometimes reply that they strive to present a 'balance' in the debate 'between the scientific establishment and the popular nutritionists'[45]. The unwary lay reader, however, may well presume that all nutrition news found in such familiar pages is fit to print. 'In effect', as Stephen Barrett has put it, 'the media have become the label'[46]. This kind of label engraved in the mind of the consumer absolves the promoter from the need to affix a label to his product, and reduces his risks of meeting food and drug regulators in court.

Moreover, vulnerability to nutritional quackery vastly increased during the third quarter of the 20th century as a result of a series of deep interacting currents that have perplexed, frightened, and angered the populace. Their world felt increasingly out of joint, and prospects for setting it right seemed dim. Such a period of rapid social change and uncertain prospects, as in Sylvester Graham's day, cast its shadow over food. Indeed, some worrisome aspects of the total scene related explicitly to food.

During the decade of the 1950s, sharp doubts arose about the food supply. Magazine articles put such queries in their titles as 'Poison in Every Pot?'[47], 'How Much Poison Are We Eating?'[48], and 'Is It Safe Enough to Eat?'[49]. The Congress held extensive hearings, and in due course enacted laws providing for premarket testing to assure safe levels of pesticide residues and to determine the safety of food and colour additives[50]. These events, raising sober questions about the science and ethics of food processing, occurred within a broader climate of suspicion: physicians, scientists, 'egg-heads' generally, surveys revealed, were regarded by a significant minority with antagonism[4].

Events beginning in the following decade, from the Vietnam War on through Watergate, broadened and deepened mistrust of established leadership. Health scientists continued suspect. As articulate anti-establishment organizations became rooted and as inflation worsened, attacks on bureaucrats intensified, creating what *Newsweek* has called 'the nation's new anti-regulatory religion'[51]. Both bureaucrats and businessmen shared in the critique from awakened environmentalism, following the publication in 1962 of Rachel Carson's *Silent Spring*. Renewed worries about the food supply, often much exaggerated, accompanied this significant movement. On the international scene, the rising power of the Third World stimulated knowledge and quickened conscience about the malnourished majority of the planet's population.

These and other trends precipitated such major changes in attitudes and actions about food that they may fairly be called – as Sam Keen does call them in *Psychology Today* – 'a nutritional revolution'[52,53]. As in Graham's day, the dominant theme is 'back to nature'. Such a primitivistic response characterizes periods of widespread frustration, when the troubles of complex society seem too overwhelming to be borne. Even in elegant cuisine, chefs have sought simplicity in lighter, more natural creations, composed of the least chemically treated raw products available[54]. Many middle class homemakers, reading about the 'spongy, squooshy, ghastly white, dehumanized, denutritized, flavorized, propionated, artificialized, shot-up, brought-down item more closely related to a styrofoam cup than the staff of life' which allegedly they had been buying, sought literally to revive the whole wheat loaf on which Sylvester Graham's vision had centred[55].

Other seekers, especially among the young, went much further in a search for salvation through nutrition. In the contest between a myth stressing consumption as the nation's proper goal and the myth imbuing conservation with the highest values, Keen suggests, 'food seems to have replaced sex as a source of guilt'. One owner of a health food store told Keen that 'people come to him as they once went to Lourdes seeking a nutritional priest'[52]. Vegetarianism, 'not a mere way of eating' but 'a form of sensibility, ... a philosophy of life', gained many recruits, its proponents repeating arguments current a century ago[56]. More radical alternatives, like the macrobiotic diet, overlaid with loose Buddhist symbolism, lured to their deaths several deeply dedicated converts who sought to subsist on brown rice alone[53,57].

The dilemma concerning the roles of science and nature in man's welfare has become even more acute and anguishing than it was in Graham's day. Yet one need not resolve all factual disputes in a congeries of major debates in order to sense how such a mixture of fear and faith, passion and persuasion, as has just been sweepingly suggested, offers enormous opportunities for the misguided and the unscrupulous. Not only have they found a constantly increasing supply of eager customers. Many of those customers have been so imbued with the zeal of converts as to sign petitions, write letters, picket offices, attend hearings, and, in other ways, prompted by cues from the leaders of unorthodoxy, to demonstrate fervent opposition to any restraints upon free and unlimited access to any and all vitamins and food supplements whatever. In the nation's bicentennial year this crusade for irrational nutrition won a significant victory.

Although finding the 'small army of food quacks'[58] a slippery foe to grapple with, the Food and Drug Administration fought them vigorously[59]. In 1954, a year in which the nation's nutritional quackery toll was estimated at half a US billion dollars, the FDA sought for a more effective means of control than that of assuming the burden of proving each case which made misleading therapeutic claims in court[60]. Might not rational standards of identity be devised to govern ingredients and formulas for vitamin–mineral preparations and food supplements to which manufacturers would have to conform or be automatically in violation of the law? FDA requested the Food and Nutrition Board to provide scientific support on which the government might base such regulations. The Board replied by saying the situation was still too complex to permit the supplying of evidence on which dosage and labelling standards could be founded[61]. The FDA was left with its product-by-product enforcement effort.

When, 8 years later, the FDA again sought to achieve new regulations which might introduce scientific rationality into the realm of nutritional wares, the agency found itself pitted against a powerful foe. In 1955 a group of promoters, mainly of nutritional products – Royal Lee among them, but also of health devices and cancer cures, established the National Health Federation[25, 62]. Some founding members had already been convicted of violating food and drug laws, and others later would so transgress. The NHF emblazoned on its banner the slogan 'freedom of choice' with regard to health affairs. And they fought regulatory pressure however they could. Within 2 years a high FDA official spoke of a 'bitter attack from an apparently well-organized and vocal association of pseudonutritionists'[63]. Communications were particularly aimed at Congressmen by the Federation's generals and by its increasing body of enthusiastic troops. FDA officials also received such mail. In response to the 1962 proposed regulations, some 54 000 letters and cards poured in, 40 000 of them generated by the NHF[64].

A new version of the regulations, issued in 1966, underwent marathon hearings which generated 32 000 pages of testimony, used to formulate a final revised version of regulations announced in 1973[2]. Hoping to thwart the threat such regulations would pose to sales, the health food industry, led by the NHF, turned its attention to the Congress. The industry deluged Congressmen with over 2 million letters – the issue was said to have spurred more mail than Watergate – protesting the FDA regulations and demanding a law to stay the agency's hand. During 1973 a number of bills to that end were introduced, one of which received Senate approval by a vote of 81 to 10. This vote showed the way political winds were blowing. A wide spectrum of groups opposed the food supplement measure, including the American Institute of Nutrition, the American Society of Clinical Nutrition, the American Dietetic Association, the American Medical Association, the Society of Food Technologists, the Committee on Nutrition of the American Academy of Pediatrics, Consumers Union, Ralph Nader's associates, and the American Association of Retired Persons. The Congress acted as if they had not heard a word of comment unfavourable to the bill. The trend of events struck a trade newsletter as 'one of the "legislative miracles" in a lifetime'[65]. Without serious opposition, in 1976, the amendment became law[66], the first retrogressive step in federal legislation respecting self-treatment wares since enactment of the initial Pure Food and Drugs Act in 1906.

The law not only wiped out more than a decade of effort by the Food and Drug Administration to secure tougher regulations over nutritional products. It repealed statutory authority given to FDA by the Congress in the 1938 law. The agency summed up what the amendment forbade it henceforth to do: 'Limiting the potency of vitamins and minerals in dietary supplements to nutritionally useful levels; classifying a vitamin or mineral preparation as a "drug" because it exceeds a nutritionally rational or useful potency: requiring the presence in dietary supplements of nutritionally essential vitamins and minerals; (and) prohibiting the inclusion in dietary supplements of useless ingredients with no nutritional value'[67].

Court action further diminished the FDA's policing of vitamins. Because of toxicity hazards from huge doses of vitamins A and D, the agency required by regulation in 1973 that capsules and tablets containing more than a given level deemed safe for self-dosage would require prescriptions. The National Nutritional Foods Association and the Solgar Company challenged FDA's authority and won a 1977 decision in the Court of Appeals for the Second Circuit. If the agency desired to restrict the potency of vitamins offered as dietary supplements, the judges ruled, it must employ the adulterated food provisions, not the prescription drug provisions, of the law. The Department of Justice decided not to appeal the ruling[68-70].

During the course of the legislative venture leading to the Vitamin Amendments of 1976, the then FDA Commissioner Alexander M. Schmidt had spoken of the pending bill as 'a charlatan's dream'[71]. After the court defeat of efforts to restrict popular dosage forms of vitamins A and D. Commissioner Donald Kennedy remarked: 'I think some regulation of vitamins is necessary, but we are not allowed to do anything. The health food industry ... beat us eight ways to Sunday'[72].

Nutritional eccentricity, in such a climate, bids fair to become the dominant doctrine rather than an odd wayward pathway. In Sam Keen's explication in *Psychology Today* of food's role in current American consciousness, the space given to extreme dietary practices, the tolerance shown to unscientific spokesmen, the meagreness of critique cited from scientific nutritionists, the mildness of the author's occasional questioning, and his obvious sympathy for the basic forces leading to 'the nutritional revolution' all seem conducive to establishing a sympathy in the reader's mind for some far-out and even hazardous approaches to food[52, 53]

In the pages of other magazines, short-cuts to weight reduction march in an endless parade of deceptive promises[73,74], and the money spent for questionable reducing aids, according to a market research firm, totals 10 (US) billion dollars a year[75]. One recent example is a pair of plastic earrings offered as a 'behavioral stimulating device for dietary weight control' through 'acupressure'[76]. Sometimes the promises can be dangerous indeed. In this category must be included the boom in low calorie predigested liquid proteins touched off by the publication in 1976 of *The Last Chance Diet* by Robert Linn, operator of obesity clinics in Philadelphia and Washington[77-79]. The book sold more than 2 million copies. Some 50 brands of such proteins came on the market, with powdered protein formulas following. A dramatic drop in poundage was promised to users who substituted such a product for food at every meal, with lesser but still substantial weight loss when the protein product was used to replace only one or two daily meals. Disastrous consequences began to appear among a few of the customers who undertook such a spartan regimen without medical supervision. Reports of illnesses with many distressing symptoms and even of deaths led to investigations by the Food and Drug Administration and the Centers for Disease Control. The agencies confirmed at least 16 deaths in which protein diets were a contributing factor. Most of the diets, upon analysis, turned out to be nutritionally incomplete, especially lacking essential amino acids and potassium. Animal tests suggested that perhaps heart attacks could be precipitated by reliance on the regimen of liquid protein 'modified fasting'. The FDA moved from requests for voluntary labelling warnings, to requirements for mandatory warnings that such an approach to dieting should not be undertaken without supervision by a physician.

Laetrile, the much ballyhooed cancer treatment, furnishes the most striking example of recent widespread trooping into the protective tent of nutritional unorthodoxy[80]. This brand name for amygdalin, extracted from apricot kernels, appeared on the market about 1951 under the guise of an investigational chemotherapeutic drug which could release its cyanide component to kill a high proportion of cancers[81]. In the mid-1960s, coinciding with an increase in regulatory pressure by both California officials and the Federal Food and Drug Administration, a change occurred in Laetrile's stance. The chemotherapeutic drug became transmogrified into vitamin B_{17}, and in the process cancer became redefined as a deficiency disease[82,83]. Everyone was 'severely deficient' in this protective anti-cancer vitamin, asserted its sponsors, a circumstance which explained cancer's epidemic proportions.

To those interested in the commercial side of Laetrile, the new vitamin posture offered advantages. One anticipation might be greater immunity from regulatory pressure, because the food provisions, under which vitamins were classified, tended to be more lenient than the drug provisions of the law. Further, conjoining the most feared word in the disease catalogue, 'cancer', with one of the most buoyantly hopeful words in the popular lexicon, 'vitamin', promised to attract the attention of that increasing segment of the population aggressive about do-it-yourself health. The suggestion that vitamin B_{17}, besides controlling cancer when the disease had appeared, could also prevent its

227

occurrence, certainly expanded the potential for its sale. If every American took Laetrile regularly, a physician who prescribed it told a subcommittee of the United States Senate, 'in 20 years cancer would be relegated to the dusty pages of history'[84].

Numerous nutritionists with the most respected credentials refuted the absurdity of Laetrile's claimed vitamin status[85-87]. And the Food and Drug Administration found effective ways to challenge such new over-the-counter products containing amygdalin as Bee-Seventeen and Aprikern[88]. Yet the Laetrile boom continued, until this false vitamin achieved notorious distinction as the unorthodox brand name health promotion which had generated the greatest public furore in all the nation's history. Rooted in the deep fear of cancer, Laetrile's commercial success depended on extremely shrewd promotion, particularly on the part of leaders, many of them members of the John Birch Society, of a new organization established to fight Laetrile's battles[89-91]. Although some of the leaders might make a great deal of money from the underground distribution of Laetrile smuggled in from Mexico, they nonetheless believed zealously in a highly circumscribed role for government. Control of medications did not properly fall within the powers granted by the Constitution. The very name of the organization, the Committee for Freedom of Choice in Cancer Therapy, incorporated the same gospel which the National Health Federation kept preaching. Much mutual support linked these two groups. Committee leaders borrowed from the NHF techniques for marshalling the fervour of loyal followers to build up political pressure, which had proved so successful in achieving the Vitamin Amendments of 1976, and applied these approaches to state legislatures, in quest of laws giving Laetrile some type of state-level legality[92]. The NHF helped out by making this campaign its own Number 1 priority[93]. In the 2 years following September 1976, 17 states had placed pro-Laetrile laws upon their statute books.

The goal, for which the noble word 'freedom' served in this effort, aimed at bypassing Laetrile around rules the national Congress had set up to govern the admission of new drugs to the marketplace, rules requiring sponsors first to prove the drugs safe and effective for their proposed therapeutic uses. Such proof Laetrile's sponsors had not provided. Congress had decided, as Commissioner Kennedy pointed out in an agency analysis of Laetrile, issued in 1977, 'that the absolute freedom to choose an ineffective drug was properly surrendered in exchange for the freedom from danger to each person's health and well-being from the sale and use of worthless drugs'[94]. In any case, the Commissioner asserted, the choice on the part of a cancer sufferer to use Laetrile, made in an atmosphere of double stress created by dread of the disease and by the high pressure promotion of Laetrile advocates, with 'seldom any rational laying out of competing arguments', could seldom properly be described as free.

In court actions, too, Laetrile users who could secure from physicians affidavits that their cancer cases were terminal, won the right to import Laetrile made by foreign producers[95]. The expanding use of an unproven drug – some 75000 Americans had resorted to Laetrile[96] – and its enlarged public acceptance as indicated in polls and in the rash of state laws, caused some cancer specialists and newspaper editors to make an extreme suggestion[97,98]. Granted that Laetrile's sponsors would not follow the established rules about drug testing, perhaps the public good, in view of all the clamour, required the testing of Laetrile, even if that step did breach the rules. A properly controlled test under the most respectable auspices, it was argued, should it establish Laetrile's lack of value in cancer therapy, could be counted upon to persuade public opinion and end the Laetrile nightmare. In 1978 the National Cancer Institute determined to move forward toward such a test[99].

That such a trial would satisfy everybody seemed unrealistic optimism. Laetrile's proponents had not accepted several series of animal tests suggesting the drug's lack of effectiveness in cancer, indeed, as had Graham with Beaumont's experiments, they had sought to reinterpret several of them to turn the results around[100]. And, with respect to human trials, the Laetrile leaders made it abundantly clear, they would trust no results that came from experiments they did not control. A pro-Laetrile physician told a Senate subcommittee: unless the National Cancer Institute study should be conducted 'in the way that the proponents of Laetrile ... are urging that it be done', then 'it will be an absolute sham'[101]. Many followers could be expected to concur in judgments of the clinical trials on Laetrile which their leaders would see fit to form, continuing the sense of confusion in broad public opinion.

A further factor must yet be introduced, one even more chilling to any expectation of universal persuasiveness to be achieved from carefully conducted trials. The Laetrile odyssey had not stopped with its journey from chemotherapeutic drug to vitamin. The next stage blurred Laetrile's sharpness of identity by mingling it with other elements in a 'total metabolic therapy'. In a 1977 book entitled *Now That You Have Cancer*, written by the head of the Committee for Freedom of Choice in Cancer Therapy, the metabolic programme was likened to a crown containing nine jewels, with Laetrile 'the crown jewel within that diadem'[102]. Vitamin B_{17} retained an indispensable place in the regimen aimed at controlling cancer, but it must be supported by a complex programme involving such other variables as diet, exercise, rest, detoxification, a positive mental attitude, minerals, enzymes, vitamins A, C and E, and that other major promotion of Laetrile's inventor, so-called vitamin B_{15} or pangamic acid. Moreover, only metabolic physicians with faith in their theories could successfully practise these therapeutic regimens embracing Laetrile. Those inside and outside the movement dwelt 'in ... different universe(s)'[103]. Those sympathetic to the expanding metabolic universe will not trust discouraging results from experiments conducted in the universe of scientific orthodoxy, especially by an agency of government. So complex is the new metabolic regimen, and so enshrouded within it is Laetrile, that devising protocols to test the present professed approach of Laetrile's proponents seems impossible. Even to make the effort breaches the efficacy provisions of federal drug law and thus establishes a precedent portending mischief for the future.

The multiproduct approach of metabolic therapy exceeds in complexity, although it resembles in psychology, the Swamp Rabbit Milk of Silent George of Shawneetown. The new wave will prove to be a much thornier nettle for regulators to grasp. Clinics dispensing such treatment based on vitamins, enzymes, orotates, and other ingredients are having no great difficulty attracting enthusiastic customers, and it may be considered a growth industry. Public acceptance of unorthodox health practices has become 'so well established, and [is] so little challenged', in the sad but seasoned judgment of Thomas H. Jukes, 'that its impact will produce a decline of scientific medicine, and its replacement by quackery'[104].

References

1. Anon. (1961). *Food Drug. Rev.*, **45**, 218
2. Young, J. H. (1978). The agile role of food. In Hathcock, J. N. and Coon, J. (eds.). *Nutrition and Drug Interrelations*. pp. 1–18. (New York: Academic Press)
3. Pyke, M. (1968). *Food and Society*. (London: John Murray)
4. Marmor, J., Bernard, V. W. and Ottenberg, P. (1960). Psychodynamics of group opposition to health programs. *Am. J. Orthopsychiatry*, **30**, 330
5. Raspadori, D. (1966). Un medicamento sempre usato: l'aglio. *Med. Nei Secoli*, **3**, 8
6. Anon. (1947). *Food Drug Rev.*, **31**, 219
7. Young, J. H. (1967). *The Medical Messiahs*. p. 352. (Princeton, NJ: Princeton University Press)
8. Walker, W. B. (1955). The Health Reform Movement in the United States. (*Ph.D. dissertation*, Johns Hopkins University)
9. Whorton, J. C. (1975). "Christian physiology": William Alcott's prescription for the millennium. *Bull. Hist. Med.*, **49**, 466
10. Shryock, R. H. (1966). Sylvester Graham and the popular health movement. In Shryock, R. H., *Medicine in America*. pp. 111–125. (Baltimore: Johns Hopkins)
11. Cole, E. W. (1975). Sylvester Graham, Lecturer on the Science of Human Life. (*Ph.D. dissertation*, Indiana University)
12. Graham, S. (1883). *Lectures on the Science of Human Life*. (New York: Fowler and Wells; 1st ed., 1839)
13. Whorton, J. C. (1977). "Tempest in a flesh-pot": the formulation of a physiological rationale for vegetarianism. *J. Hist. Med.*, **32**, 115
14. Numbers, R. L. (1976). *Prophetess of Health: A Study of Ellen G. White*. (New York: Harper and Row)
15. Carson, G. (1957). *Cornflake Crusade*. p. 183. (New York: Rinehart)
16. Macfadden, B. and Gauvreau, E. (1953). *Dumbbells and Carrot Strips*. (New York: Holt)
17. Young, J. H. (1977). Macfadden, Bernarr. In Garraty, J. A. (ed.), *Dictionary of American Biography, Suppl. 5*, pp. 452–454. (New York: Scribner's)
18. McCollum, E. V. (1957). *A History of Nutrition*. (Boston: Houghton Mifflin)
19. McCollum, E. V. (1918). *The Newer Knowledge of Nutrition*. (New York: Macmillan)
20. Pease, O. (1958). *The Responsibilities of American Advertising* (New Haven: Yale)
21. Food and Drug Administration (1929). Press release, May 22
22. Anon. (1930). *Food and Drug Rev.*, **14**, 41
23. Young, J. H. (1967). *The Medical Messiahs*. pp. 333–359, 401–405
24. Cramp, A. J. (1936). *Nostrums and Quackery and Pseudo-Medicine*. pp. 213–214. (Chicago: American Medical Association)
25. Food and Drug Administration. (1963). Report on the National Health Federation, Oct. 21
26. *U.S. v. Lee*. (1939). 107 F.2d 522
27. Food and Drug Administration. (1943). *Drugs and Devices*. Notice of Judgment No. 821
28. *U.S. v. Lee*. (1942). 131 F.2d 464
29. Bell. J. R. (1958). Let 'em eat hay. *Today's Hlth*, **36**, 22
30. Jukes, T. H. and Barrett, S. (1976). The genuine fake. In Barrett, S. and Knight, G. (eds.). *The Health Robbers*. pp. 125–137. (Philadelphia: George F. Stickley)
31. Deutsch, R. M. (1977). *The New Nuts Among the Berries*. pp. 305–314. (Palo Alto: Bull)
32. Food and Drug Administration. (1963). *FDA's Campaign Against Nutritional Quackery*, Progress Report

33. National Analysts, Inc. (1972). *A Study of Health Practices and Opinions.* (Springfield, VA: National Information Service)
34. Deutsch, R. M. (1961). *The Nuts Among the Berries,* p. 215. (New York: Ballantine)
35. Gunther, M. (1976). Quackery and the Media. In Barrett, S. and Knight, G. (eds.), *The Health Robbers.* pp. 285–300. (Philadelphia: George F. Stickley)
36. Deutsch, R. M. (1977). *The New Nuts Among the Berries.* pp. 225–227. (Palo Alto: Bull)
37. Ibid., p. 266
38. Ladimer, I. (1967). Literature and advertising. In *Proceedings, Third National Congress on Medical Quackery.... 1966,* pp. 69–82. (Chicago: American Medical Association)
39. Rynearson, E. H. (1973). Adelle Davis' books on nutrition. *Med. Insight,* **13,** 32 (July–Aug.)
40. Richardson, J. A. and Griffin, P. (1977). *Laetrile Case Histories,* p. 6. (New York: Bantam)
41. Evans, V. (1976). Watching your weight. *Mainliner, United Airlines and Western International Hotels Mag.,* p. 40 (Aug.)
42. Anon. (1971). Adelle Davis celebrates 25 years with Harcourt. *Publishers' Weekly,* **199,** 56 (June 21)
43. Nutrition information and food faddism. (1974). *Nutr. Rev.,* **32,** Suppl. 1
44. Nutrition Search, Inc. (1975). *Nutrition Almanac.* (New York: McGraw-Hill)
45. Deutsch, R. M. (1977). *The New Nuts Among the Berries.* pp. 265–279 (Palo Alto: Bull)
46. Barrett, S. (1976). Health frauds and quackery. *FDA Consumer,* **11,** 12 (Nov.)
47. Rorty, J. (1952). Poison in every pot? *Am. Mercury,* **75,** 73 (Nov.)
48. Martin, R. G. (1955). How much poison are we eating? *Harper's,* **210,** 63 (Apr.)
49. Anon. (1960). Is it safe enough to eat? *Newsweek.* p. 99 (Mar. 21)
50. Janssen, W. F. (1964). FDA since 1938. The major trends and developments. *J. Publ. Law,* **13,** 205
51. Pauly, D. and Walcott, J. (1978). The FTC under fire. *Newsweek.* p. 94 (Dec. 4)
52. Keen, S. (1978). Eating our way to enlightenment. *Psychol. Today,* **12,** 62 (Oct.)
53. Keen, S. (1978). The pure, the impure, and the paranoid. *Psychol. Today,* **12,** 67 (Oct.)
54. Francke, L. B., Sullivan, S. and Goldschlager, S. (1975). Food: the new wave. *Newsweek.* p. 50 (Aug. 11)
55. Hess, J. L. (1973). A trend toward "oldtime" bread. *Atlanta Constitution* (Oct. 6). Quotation cited from J. Beard, *Beard on Bread*
56. Carson, G. (1968). Vegetables for breakfast ... and lunch ... and supper. *Natural Hist.,* **77,** 18 (Dec.)
57. Stare, F. J. (1968). Nutritional quackery. Presented at the *Fourth National Congress on Health Quackery,* October 2–3, Chicago
58. Anon. (1951). *Food Drug Rev.,* **35,** 141
59. Food and Drug Administration Annual Reports chronicle this regulatory effort through the years.
60. Anon. (1954). *FDC Reports,* **15,** 4 (Feb. 20)
61. Anon. (1954). *FDC Reports,* **16,** 2 (Nov. 27)
62. Barrett, S. (1976). The unhealthy alliance. In Barrett, S. and Knight, G. (eds.), *The Health Robbers.* pp. 189–201 (Philadelphia: George F. Stickley)
63. Harvey, J. L. (1957). Progress and problems. *Food, Drug, Cosmetic Law J.,* **12,** 430
64. Public Health and Environment Subcommittee. (1973). *Vitamin, Mineral, and Diet Supplements* (Committee Print No. 11). Committee on Interstate and Foreign Commerce, U.S. House of Representatives. 93d Congress, 1st Session
65. Anon. (1975). *FDC Reports,* **37,** 5 (Sep. 1)
66. Health Resources and Health Services Amendments. (1975). 90 Stat. 401
67. Food and Drug Administration. (1976). *FDA Talk Paper,* Apr. 27
68. Anon. (1977). Restrictions voided on vitamins A and D. *FDA Consumer,* **11,** 3 (Oct.)
69. Anon. (1978). Rule limiting vitamin dosage revoked. *FDA Consumer,* **12,** 24 (July–Aug.)
70. The National Nutritional Foods Association and Solgar Co. v. Mathews. (1977). 557 F.2d 325
71. Food and Drug Administration. (1974). *FDA Talk Paper,* Aug. 14
72. Food and Drug Administration. (1978). *Highlights of the Ad Hoc Professional Meeting Held in Atlanta, Georgia,* Apr. 21
73. Mayer, J. (1976). Weight control and 'diets': facts and fads. In Barrett, S. and Knight, G. (eds.), *The Health Robbers.* pp. 47–59. (Philadelphia: George F. Stickley)

74. Anon. (1973). Dietmania. *Newsweek*, p. 74 (Sep. 10)
75. Anon. (1977). $10 billion a year to fight fat. *Atlanta Constitution*, Dec. 7
76. Anon. (1978). Manufacturer recalls diet control earrings. *Atlanta Constitution*, Nov. 16
77. Conn, R. (1977). Protein: big diet boom, but ... *Charlotte Observer*, Oct. 30
78. Anon. (1978). Protein diets. *Charlotte Observer*, Apr. 30
79. Glick, N. (1978). Low calorie protein diets. *FDA Consumer*, **12**, 7 (Mar.)
80. Young, J. H. (1980). Laetrile in historical perspective. In Markle, G. E. and Petersen, J. C. (eds.), *Politics, Science and Cancer: the Laetrile Phenomenon*, pp. 11–60. (Boulder: Westview)
81. White, R. C. and Taylor, D. L. (1952). Report to San Francisco District, Dec. 15. *Food and Drug Administration File on Labeling and Composition of Laetrile*, FDA Records (Rockville)
82. Krebs, E. T., Sr. (1963). Letter to FDA, Apr. 18. San Francisco District File CF: 10 183, *John Beard Memorial Foundation*, **6**, FDA Records (San Francisco)
83. Krebs, E. T., Jr. (1970). The nitrilosides (vitamin B-17). Their nature, occurrence, and metabolic significance. *J. Appl. Nutr.*, **22**, 75
84. Richardson, J. A. (1977). Testimony, p. 247. *Banning of the Drug Laetrile from Interstate Commerce by FDA*. Hearing before the Subcommittee on Health and Scientific Research, Committee on Human Resources, U.S. Senate. 95th Congress, 1st Session
85. Greenberg, D. M. (1975). The vitamin fraud in cancer quackery. *West. J. Med.*, **122**, 345
86. National Nutrition Consortium, Inc. (1976). *Statement on Laetrile-Vitamin B_{17}*, Dec. 21
87. Jukes, T. H. (1977). Is Laetrile a vitamin? *Nutr. Today*, **12**, 12 (Sept.–Oct.)
88. Food and Drug Administration. (1975 and 1978). *Notices of Judgment* 29 (Oct. 1975), 31 (Nov. 1975), and 32 (Apr. 1978)
89. Bradford, R. W. (1973). Form letter from The Committee for Freedom of Choice in Cancer Therapy. In *File AF 26-731*, **22**, FDA Records (Rockville)
90. Petit, C. (1976). The Laetrile connection–disputed cancer drug. *San Francisco Chronicle*, Aug. 11
91. Lyons, R. D. (1977). Credentials on Laetrile figures found exaggerated. *New York Times*, June 26
92. Nightingale, S. L. and Arnold, F. D. (1978). How Laetrile laws affect MDs. *Legal Aspects of Med.*, **6**, 31
93. National Health Federation. (1977). Form letter promoting "Fund to stop government ban on Laetrile". *Decimal file 439.ILX*, **33**, FDA Records (Rockville)
94. Food and Drug Administration. (1977). Laetrile: Commissioner's decision on status, *Fed. Reg.*, **42**, 39768
95. Rutherford v. U.S. (1975, 1976, 1977, 1978). 399 F. Supp. 1208. 542 F.2d 1137. 438 F. Supp. 1287. 582 F.2d 1234
96. Newell, G. R. (1978). Statement (Jan. 26) ... on retrospective evaluation of Laetrile anticancer activity in man. *NCI Information Kit*
97. Moertel, C. G. (1978). A trial of Laetrile now. *N. Engl. J. Med.*, **298**, 218
98. Anon. editorial. (1977). The cancer drug dilemma. *New York Times*, Feb. 11
99. Ellison, N. M., Byar, D. P. and Newell, G. R. (1978). Special report on Laetrile: the NCI Laetrile review. *N. Engl. J. Med.*, **299**, 499. The NCI-sponsored trials of Laetrile were authorized; early results showed no evidence of its effectiveness against human cancer
100. Burk, D. (1977). Letter to Edward Kennedy, Nov. 16, with exhibits, pp. 384–419. *Banning of the Drug Laetrile from Interstate Commerce by FDA*. Hearing before the Subcommittee on Health and Scientific Research, Committee on Human Resources, U.S. Senate. 95th Congress, 1st Session
101. Halstead, B. (1977). *Testimony*, p. 261. Ibid.
102. Bradford, R. W. (1977). *Now That You Have Cancer*. (Los Altos: Choice Publications)
103. Krebs, E. T., Jr. (1977). FDA Administrative Record, Laetrile. Docket No. 77N-0048, vol. 0-1
104. Jukes, T. H. (1978). Letter to author, Aug. 11

10
Laetrile, the bogus 'vitamin B₁₇'

T. H. JUKES

The name 'laetrile' was coined by Ernst Krebs, Jr. as a condensation of *lae*vorotatory aminoni*trile* β-glucuronic acid[1]. The term laetrile as presently used refers to any one of a group of compounds that include amygdalin, prunasin, linamarin, and dhurrin. These compounds are correctly called 'cyanogenic glycosides.' The laetrile that is being used illicitly to treat cancer is amygdalin, a β-glucoside containing gentiobiose and the cyanhydrin, mandelonitrite, formed by condensation of benzaldehyde and hydrocyanic acid (HCN)[2]. Its structural formula is shown in Figure 1 from Conn[3]. Liebig and Wohler in 1837, described the hydrolysis of amygdalin by an enzyme they called 'emulsin' (actually, a mixture of enzymes) present in almonds to yield benzaldehyde, glucose and HCN (cyanide). These products are shown in Figure 1. The other cyanogenic glycosides all contain HCN, condensed with a ketone or aldehyde, and a carbohydrate in β-linkage. A list of some of these is shown in Table 1 taken from Conn[2].

The cyanogenic glycosides are a group of compounds that are included among 'toxicants occurring naturally in foods'. Since they are often poisonous to animals that eat the plants containing them, it is concluded that the evolutionary development of the cyanogenic glycosides helped plants to protect themselves against animals. In the Darwinian sense, plants containing these compounds would tend to survive because their enemies were killed. This interpretation receives interesting support from the fact that plants containing the compounds also contain enzymes that hydrolyse them with the liberation of cyanide. Furthermore, the enzyme specifically hydrolysing a cyanogenic glycoside occurs in the plant in which the glycoside originates[3]. Animals do not produce these enzymes. The enzyme in the plant is sequestered so that it does not reach the glycoside until the plant tissue is crushed or macerated. This accounts for the liberation of cyanide from the crushed fresh leaves of the European laurel, and these are used by insect collectors to kill a butterfly that is placed in a jar containing the crushed leaves. The same reaction is fatal to farm livestock that eat the leaves of certain plants, such as choke cherries and immature sorghum[2].

However, the amount of cyanide ingested may be insufficient to cause death, and, if this lower dosage is given day after day, chronic subacute cyanide poisoning may result. Two forms of this have been described. The first of these,

Table 1 Some cyanogenetic glycosides

Glycoside	Plant source	Hydrolysis products
Amygdalin	Members of the Rosaceae, including almond, apple, apricot, cherry, peach, pear, plum, quince	Gentiobiose + HCN + benzaldehyde
Prunasin	Members of the Rosaceae, including cherry laurel; *Eucalyptus cladocalyx*, *Linaria striata* Dc.	D-Glucose + HCN + benzaldehyde
Sambunigrin	*Sambucus nigra* L. (elderberry), *Acacia* sp. (Australian acacias)	D-Glucose + HCN + benzaldehyde
Vicianin	*Vicia* sp. (common vetch)	Vicianose + HCN + benzaldehyde
Dhurrin	*Sorghum* sp. (sorghums, Kaffir corns)	D-Glucose + HCN + p-hydroxybenzaldehyde
Taxiphyllin	*Taxus* sp.	D-Glucose + HCN + p-hydroxybenzaldehyde
Linamarin	*Phaseolus lunatus* L. (lima bean, many varieties); *Linum usitatissimum* L. (linen flax); *Manihot* sp. (cassava or manioc); *Trifolium repens* L. (white clover), *Lotus* sp. (trefoils); *Dimorphotheca* sp.	D-Glucose + HCN + acetone
Lotaustralin	Occurs with linamarin	D-Glucose + HCN + 2-butanone
Acacipetalin	*Acacia* sp. (South African acacias)	D-Glucose + dimethylketene cyanohydrin
Triglochinin[5]	*Triglochin maritimum* L. (arrow grass)	D-Glucose + HCN + triglochinic acid

(From Conn[2])

is the more acute form, called tropical ataxic neuropathy. This is characterized by blindness, nerve degeneration and loss of hearing[2]. The milder form of chronic cyanide poisoning is caused by the transformation of cyanide to thiocyanate by the enzyme rhodanese. Thiocyanate is one of the most important and prominent members of a group of compounds called thyroid inhibitors or 'goitrogens', which are widely distributed in foods, especially in members of the cabbage family. The action of a goitrogen is to inhibit iodine uptake by the thyroid gland. This sets in motion a 'feedback mechanism' in which the pituitary gland produces increased amounts of the thyroid stimulating hormone, thyrotropin. The stimulation causes the thyroid gland to become enlarged, hypertrophic, and eventually after prolonged stimulation, carcinomatous changes take place. The 'laetriles', therefore, are potential

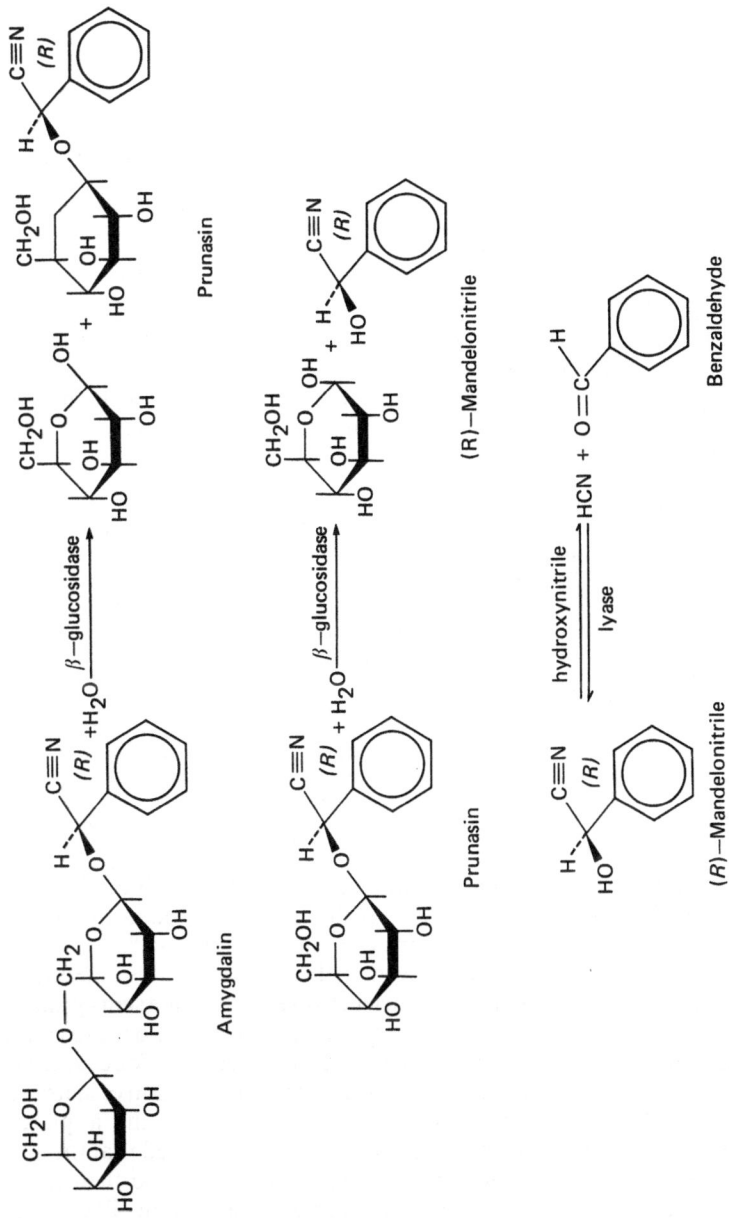

Figure 1 Enzymatic steps in hydrolysis of amygdalin (From Conn, 3)

carcinogens. Chronic effects of cyanide poisoning are common in tropical countries, where cassava is a major article of diet. Cassava contains linamarin (Table 1). The products of hydrolysis of linamarin are traditionally removed by pounding and washing cassava. However, enough cyanide remains to cause health problems. For example, according to Dorozynski[4]

'... a team of Belgian researchers, headed by Dr. Andre-Marie Ermans of the Department of Radioisotopes at the Saint-Pierre Hospital, University of Brussels, ... a study of the population of Idjwi Island on Lake Kivu, Zaire, ... have shown that a steady diet of cassava inhibits iodine uptake by the thyroid gland. When iodine supply is marginal, this can cause endemic goiter, cretinism, and mental retardation.

... In the past ten years or so, epidemiological studies in Africa, South America and Asia have revealed that more than 200 million people may be affected by goiter. How much cassava as a staple food, may contribute to this is yet to be determined.

... Cassava contains cyanogenic glucosides; when ingested, these glucosides are detoxified, yielding thiocyanate as a by-product which inhibits iodine uptake by the thyroid.'

The superimposition of iodine deficiency upon the goitrogenic action of thiocyanate serves to increase the hazard of goiter in cassava eating countries.

A theory without experimental support, for treating cancer with amygdalin was proposed some years ago by Krebs. This theory and its absence of validity, have been cogently discussed by Greenberg[5]:

'The cyanide is presumed to kill cancer cells, but not normal tissue, because in the latter there is postulated to be present large amounts of the enzyme thiosulphate transferase (rhodanese) which converts the cyanide to the less toxic thiocyanate. Cancer tissue is presumed to be rich in beta-glucosidase.

There are several flaws in this hypothesis:

. The available information shows the presence of only traces of beta-glucosidase in animal tissues and even less in amount in experimental tumors than in such organs as liver and kidney.

. The beta-glucosidase values reported for tumor tissue give a false picture, since the substrate commonly employed to test for this enzyme was p-nitrophenyl-β-D-glucoside. This compound has been observed in the laboratory of Dr. E. Conn at the University of California, Davis, to be an order of magnitude more active as a substrate than amygdalin or prunasin when all are subjected to the action of glucosidase from liver.

. There is no evidence that there is any pronounced differential between the rhodanese content of comparable normal and cancerous tissue.'

Nevertheless, the advocates of laetrile continue to promote it on the basis of this spurious theory. No experimental results have appeared in the scientific literature, either with human beings or experimental animals[1,6], that show an anti-cancer effect for laetrile. Going even further, the advocates of laetrile tell their victims that cancer is a dietary deficiency disease, just like scurvy and, just as vitamin C prevents or cures scurvy, so will laetrile prevent or cure cancer[7]. The origin of this nonsense dates back to 1969 when the Food and Drug Administration turned down an application for the introduction of laetrile as a new drug[1,6]. Before denying this request, the FDA had the application reviewed by an outside panel of cancer experts, who concluded that the claims made for laetrile had no validity[1,6]. The sponsors of laetrile then had the ingenious idea of concocting a story that laetrile was a vitamin. They called it 'Vitamin B_{17}'. Of course, laetrile, and the cyanogenic glycosides, in general have no resemblance to vitamins. The name was just a 'sales gimmick'. Vitamins are substances that are needed in a diet in small amounts, and in their absence, a specific nutritional deficiency disease develops that is prevented or cured by the vitamin. Vitamins are not minerals. The essential amino acids found in proteins are also not vitamins. Laetrile is not a vitamin for several reasons, one of which is that laboratory animals can grow and reproduce normally on diets that do not contain laetrile. The Committee on Nomenclature of the American Institute of Nutrition has stated that it

'finds no scientifific evidence for the existence of a nutrient' identified as vitamin B_{17}. 'This terminology is neither recognized nor used by qualified nutritionists.' 'The Committee ... finds no scientific evidence that Laetrile has nutrient properties or is in any way of nutritional value for either animals or humans.'

Furthermore, cancer is not a nutritional deficiency disease; indeed, it has been shown repeatedly that cancers grow more slowly in experimental animals when they are undernourished. The testimonials and anecdotes of patients who say that they have been helped by laetrile often reveal that either they have had some form of additional treatment, such as X-rays, surgery, or standard anti-cancer drugs. Some patients have had temporary spontaneous remission after which the cancer later returns. In very rare cases, cancer spontaneously disappears without treatment, perhaps due to the immunity processes of the body. Some of the patients were not diagnosed as having cancer. The National Cancer Institute (NCI) mailed 455 000 letters to physicians and health professionals asking for information on patients who have received benefit from laetrile, and received only 93 reports that could be evaluated. Of these, 26 cases were not scientifically diagnosed as cancer, 11 of the remaining cases had insufficient data, 35 others were patients who had received other forms of anti-cancer treatments, leaving 22 patients to be judged. Seven of the 22 were cases of progressive cancer, nine had been stabilized, leaving 6 cases of possible remission in the 93 case histories, all that were obtained, as I said, from 455 000 inquiries. One would expect at least this many spontaneous remissions from such a survey without use of any treatment.

Deaths have been attributed to dosage with laetrile. One of these was a child who swallowed her father's laetrile tablets, and another was a young woman who drank a solution of laetrile[3]. There have also recently been several cases of non-fatal poisoning with laetrile. Some of these were in people who consumed 'apricot seed milkshakes' and allegedly made according to a recipe in a 'health food' magazine[6]. Another incident of poisoning took place when children made a drink by crushing choke cherries.

The fact that the advocates of laetrile refer to it by the spurious name 'vitamin B_{17}' is of considerable significance. One falsification leads to another. The fraud is augmented by the fact that the dispensers of laetrile offer this material as part of a 'quackery package' that includes laetrile tablets and injections, pancreatic enzyme tablets, 'vitamin B_{15}', vitamin C, amino acid tablets, chelated minerals, 'Supergran', vitamin E and 'liquid protein'. All animal protein, including dairy products, is excluded. Dr. Victor Herbert has commented adversely on this regime[8]. In the components of the above list, 'vitamin B_{15}' is a non-vitamin. It is a trade name that was invented by Mr. Krebs for so-called Pangamic acid, which has never been defined. Various mixtures of nutritionally worthless ingredients are sold as 'vitamin B_{15}

(pangamic acid)'. These substances include calcium gluconate, dimethylglycine, di-isopropylammonium dichloracetate and, sometimes, glycine. Enzyme tablets are nutritionally and therapeutically worthless; they are destroyed by pepsin in the gastric juice. The other components of the regime have no value in the treatment of cancer, and are ingredients of what has been termed 'acute remunerative therapy'.

Through the years, there has been a long series of spurious remedies for cancer, including krebiozen, 'Hoxsey's remedy', 'Glyoxylide' and others listed by Fishbein in 'History of Cancer Quackery'[12], but none of these have reached the level of notoriety attained by laetrile. This state of affairs is due in part to vigorous advocacy, and in part to the media, which have given extensive coverage to pro-laetrile anecdotes, and to appearances by laetrile pushers. None of these efforts has been substantiated scientifically. One of the most prominent pro-laetrile organizations is called 'Committee for Freedom of Choice in Cancer Therapy'. It is headed by Robert Bradford, who has described himself as a 'nuclear engineer'. Richard Lyons, in the *New York Times* (6-26-77) has commented as follows on Bradford

> Mr. Bradford, 46 years old, a poised spokesman for the group, has at various times described himself as a scientist, an engineer who attended Georgia Tech, and an electronics specialist who helped develop guidance systems for missiles. Each point is open to question.
> Asked in an interview last week if he had attended Georgia Tech, Mr. Bradford answers: 'Yes, for two years.'
> Yet employees of the Georgia Institute of Technology in Atlanta said a search of their registration and alumni records failed to turn up the name Robert W. Bradford.
> Records on file with the United States Attorney's office in San Diego, where Mr. Bradford was convicted earlier this year of conspiracy to smuggle laetrile into the country and was fined $40,000, indicate that in 1950 he attended San Jose Community College for one semester, studying police administration.
> John McLain, a spokesman for what is now San Jose State University, confirmed that Mr. Bradford had attended the institution. He added that the records indicated that 'he wasn't a very good student.'
> After leaving the college, Mr. Bradford enlisted in the Air Force. David Rorvik, a freelance journalist, has said that Mr. Bradford described himself as having 'helped develop the guidance system for the first United States tactical guided missile' in his service at Cape Kennedy and as having directed 'the Air Force electronics and guidance systems program.'
> Yet the records indicate that Mr. Bradford's highest rank was that of staff sergeant, which would hardly have qualified him for such important positions.
> After leaving the Air Force, Mr. Bradford was employed by several defense contractors in the San Francisco Bay area and in the early 1960's was hired by Stanford University, which was then developing one of the world's largest linear accelerators for research into subatomic physics.
> Mr. Bradford described himself as an engineer and was listed on the Stanford employment records as such. Yet his supervisor there, Carl Olsen, said Mr. Bradford's duties would be more accurately described as those of an 'expert technician.'
> Federal and state investigators have testified that Mr. Bradford had taken part in laetrile sales transactions involving hundreds of thousands and even millions of dollars; he said, however, that he had only a modest income. He would not be specific.
> Grant Leake, an agent of the California Food and Drug Bureau, estimated that Mr. Bradford, who has openly conceded that he was a distributor of laetrile, takes in $150,000 to $200,000 a month on laetrile sales.
>
> Herbert Hoffman, the Assistant United States Attorney in San Diego who prosecuted Dr. Richardson and Mr. Bradford, testified that hundreds of thousands of dollars had been made by the men in smuggling operations between Mexico and the United States.

Mr. Hoffman said that according to Mr. Bradford's own records, he had made a profit of $675,000 on $1.4 million in sales of laetrile over two and a half years. He testified further that letters that Mr. Bradford had sent to his Mexican suppliers, letters seized by Federal agents, had complained that the substance was being shipped to other American distributors and demanded that that be stopped.

The National Health Federation (NHF) strongly advocates laetrile. This organization is described in *The Health Robbers* by Stephen Barrett. A number of its founders and leading figures have records of 6 convictions for fraud. Barrett says in part

Many of them write or publish books and other materials which support unscientific health theories and practices. Many sell questionable 'health' products and some have even been convicted of crimes while engaged in this kind of activity.

. Fred J. Hart was NHF's founder. ... In 1954, Hart and the Electronic Medical Foundation were ordered by a U.S. District Court to stop distributing electrical devices with false claims that they could diagnose and treat hundreds of diseases and conditions. In 1962, Hart was fined by the court for violating this order. Hart died in 1975.

. Royal S. Lee, ... helped Hart found NHF and served on its board of governors. In 1962, he and the vitamin company which he owned were convicted of misbranding 115 special dietary products by making false label claims for the treatment of more than 500 diseases and conditions. Lee received a one-year suspended prison term and his company was fined $7,000.

. Andrew G. Rosenberger, ... has been listed as NHF 'nutrition chairman'. ... In 1962, he and his brother Henry were fined $5,000 each and were given six-month suspended prison sentences for misbranding dietary products.

. Kurt W. Donsbach, chairman of NHF's board of governors, is a chiropractor and naturopath by background. In 1970, while Donsbach operated a 'health food' store, agents of the Fraud Division of the California Bureau of Food and Drug observed him represent that vitamins, minerals and herbal tea would control cancer, cure emphysema and the like. Charged with nine counts of such illegal activity, Donsbach pleaded guilty to practicing medicine without a licence and agreed to cease 'nutritional consultation'.

. V. Earl Irons, vice-chairman of NHF's board of governors, received a one-year prison sentence in 1957 for misbranding 'Vit-Ra-Tox,' a vitamin mixture sold door-to-door.

. Roy F. Paxton, while serving as an NHF governor in 1963, was sentenced to three years in prison for misbranding 'Millrue' as effective in treating cancer, arthritis and other serious diseases.

. Clinton Miller, vice-president and Washington lobbyist, had a quantity of 'dried Swiss whey' seized from his Utah wheat shop in 1962. The FDA charged that the product was misbranded as effective in treating intestinal disorders.

. Bob Hoffman, another NHF governor, owns a publishing firm and sells 'health' products through his company, York Barbell Co. In 1960, the company was charged with misbranding its 'Energol Germ Oil Concentrate' because literature which accompanied the oil claimed falsely that it could prevent or treat more than 120 diseases and conditions, including epilepsy, gallstones and arthritis.

. Emory Thurston, another NHF governor, has been an active promoter of 'Laetrile.' When approached by an agent of the California Bureau of Food and Drug, who told him she had cancer of the uterus, Thurston said he could supply her with Laetrile. Thurston sold Laetrile to the agent – and advised her not to have surgery! After additional evidence against Thurston was gathered, he was convicted, fined $500 and placed on probation for two years.

One of the most publicized physicians involved in administration of laetrile is Dr. John A. Richardson of Albany, California. His licence to practise medicine was suspended in 1976 for

Aiding or abetting unlicensed practice, prescribing dangerous drugs without good faith prior medical examination. Violation of California Health and Safety Code involving possession of misbranded and adulterated drug, receipt or delivery of adulterated drug, or commerce. Laetriles for treatment of cancer, unlawful sale of drugs for alleviation of cancer. Gross negligence and incompetence. Revoked. November 29, 1976.

A Grand Jury indictment recently revealed that Dr. Richardson had banked 2.6 million dollars between 1973 and 1975. Dr. Richardson is the co-author of a paperback book *Laetrile Case Histories*. This book has been exhaustively criticized in the voluminous FDA publication[1] which has pointed out that,

> 'It is absolutely incredible that anyone would expect to show the effectiveness of a drug by describing 62 out of over 4000 patients with a selection process of the type Richardson describes. The Commissioner has no means of knowing what happened to the other 3938 or more patients. No details are given to show how the 500 patients representing a 'cross-section' of the 4000 were chosen. The failure 'to establish contact and a working relationship' with half of the patients that were chosen illustrates a serious lack of follow up. Logic suggests that those patients who were not benefited by Laetrile would be less likely to be willing to develop a 'working relationship' with Dr. Richardson's office. Clearly patients who had died would not be available for such a relationship. The discarding of weak medical histories has never been an accepted practice in the study of any drug. What constitutes the weakness of a medical history is not explained.'

The National Cancer Institute proposes to conduct clinical experiments with laetrile. This proposal is open to criticism on the following grounds. There is no evidence that laetrile is effective against cancer, and there is no indication that laetrile is safe. The enzyme β-glucosidase that liberates cyanide from laetrile is present in common foods, and cyanide may be liberated in the stomach before this enzyme becomes inactivated by the gastric juices, so that laetrile poisoning may take place. Advocates of laetrile specify that it be used as a component of a treatment including various worthless or deleterious ingredients, without which it may be anticipated that the advocates will declare any negative result to be unacceptable[9]. The ethics of the proposal are open to serious question. It is proposed to use human beings as experimental subjects in a procedure which *Time* magazine has characterized as being undertaken for 'political purposes'. Consent by the patients involved does not exempt the perpetrators of the experiment from liability. Finally, there is the question of precedent. The proponents of various other spurious cancer remedies may demand equal consideration at public expense. The fundamental premises of scientific medicine are being violated by the excursion of the National Cancer Institute into the realm of quackery.

Collaboration by the FDA has been furnished for the NCI clinical experiment. This collaboration represents an abrupt turnabout from the following statement made by FDA in 1977[1]

> One submission objected to the possible use of Laetrile by terminal patients on the grounds that approval of such use constitutes sanction of an inhumane fraud upon the patients involved, one which wastes the financial resources of the patients and their families uselessly (R 190 at ¶17). Two other arguments were expressed by a number of submitters: (1) there is no such thing as a 'terminal' patient and (2) allowing use by a subgroup of cancer patients would lead to increased use by patients who could be helped by legitimate therapy.
>
> The Commissioner concludes that approval of Laetrile restricted to 'terminal' patients would lead to needless deaths and suffering among (1) patients characterized as 'terminal' who could actually be helped by legitimate therapy and (2) patients clearly susceptible to the benefits of legitimate therapy who would be misled as to Laetrile's utility by the limited approval program or who would be able to obtain the drug through the inevitable leakage in any system set up to administer such a program.

If, in the NCI experiment terminal cancer patients receive a mixture of remedies in addition to laetrile, it will be impossible to deduce which component of the mixture had an effect.

The history of laetrile has been carefully documented and chronicled by Young[10], and the current activities of laetrile promoters have been-exhaustively documented by Herbert[11].

References

1. *Federal Register*, **42**, No. 151, pp. 39768–39806. No. 151
2. Conn, E. E., Cyanogenetic glycosides, 1973. In *Toxicants Occurring Naturally in Foods*, 2 eds, pp. 299–308. Washington, DC: National Academy of Sciences
3. Conn, E. E., Cyanogenic glycosides. In *Biochemistry of Nutrition* (in press)
4. Dorozynski, A., 1978. *Nature*, **272**, 121
5. Greenberg, D. M. 1975. *Western J. Med.*, **122**, 345
6. Jukes, T. H. 1976. *J. Am. Med. Assoc.*, **13**, 1284
7. Court record, The People of the State of California, Plaintiff and Ernst Krebs Jr and Malvina Cassese, Defendants, trial ending Feb 15, 1977, Municipal Court, San Francisco, Calif.
8. Herbert, V. 1978. *J. Am. Med. Assoc.*, **240**, 1139
9. A spokesman for NHF, in C & EN, Nov. 20, 1978, p. 5 proposed that "Laetrile-enzyme-nutritional therapy" be used in the NCI, and stated "The present protocol proposal by NCI is unacceptable".
10. Young, J. H. 1980. Laetrile in Historical Perspective. In Markle, G. E. and Petersen, J. C. (eds.) *Politics, Science and Cancer, The Laetrile Phenomenon*, pp. 11–60. (Colorado: Westview Press). See also Young, J. H., this volume, pp. 227–29
11. Herbert, V. 1980. Laetrile, the Cult of Cyanides. In *Nutrition Cultism* pp. 1–73 (Philadelphia: George F. Stickley)
12. Fishbein, M. (1965). History of Cancer Quackery. *Perspect. Bio. Med.*, **8**, 140

Index